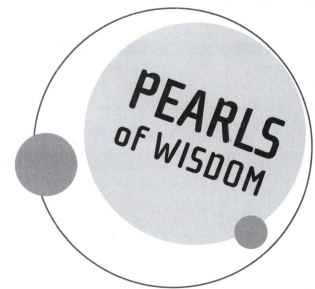

PEARLS OF WISDOM

Physician Assistant
EXAMINATION REVIEW
Fourth Edition

Editor-in-Chief

Daniel Thibodeau, MPH, PA-C

Associate Editor

Scott Plantz, MD

D0139127

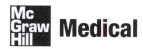 **Medical**

New York Chicago San Francisco Lisbon London Madrid Mexico City Milan
New Delhi San Juan Seoul Singapore Sydney Toronto

Physician Assistant Examination Review, Fourth Edition

Copyright © 2010, 2006 by The McGraw-Hill Companies, Inc. All rights reserved. Printed in the United States of America. Except as permitted under the United States Copyright Act of 1976, no part of this publication may be reproduced or distributed in any form or by any means, or stored in a database or retrieval system, without the prior written permission of the publisher. Previous editions © Boston Medical Publishing Corporation.

1 2 3 4 5 6 7 8 9 0   WDQ/WDQ   14 13 12 11 10

ISBN 978-0-07-162771-9
MHID 0-07-162771-5

Notice

Medicine is an ever-changing science. As new research and clinical experience broaden our knowledge, changes in treatment and drug therapy are required. The authors and the publisher of this work have checked with sources believed to be reliable in their efforts to provide information that is complete and generally in accord with the standards accepted at the time of publication. However, in view of the possibility of human error or changes in medical sciences, neither the authors nor the publisher nor any other party who has been involved in the preparation or publication of this work warrants that the information contained herein is in every respect accurate or complete, and they disclaim all responsibility for any errors or omissions or for the results obtained from use of the information contained in this work. Readers are encouraged to confirm the information contained herein with other sources. For example and in particular, readers are advised to check the product information sheet included in the package of each drug they plan to administer to be certain that the information contained in this work is accurate and that changes have not been made in the recommended dose or in the contraindications for administration. This recommendation is of particular importance in connection with new or infrequently used drugs.

The book was set in Adobe Garamond by Aptara®, Inc.
The editor was Kirsten Funk.
The production supervisor was Sherri Souffrance.
Project management was provided by Deepa Krishnan, Aptara®, Inc.
The cover designer was Ty Nowicki.
Worldcolor Dubuque was the printer and binder.

The book is printed on acid-free paper.

Library of Congress Cataloging-in-Publication Data

Physician assistant examination review. – 4th ed. / [edited by] Daniel Thibodeau.
    p. ; cm. – (Pearls of wisdom)
  Includes bibliographical references.
  ISBN 978-0-07-162771-9 (pbk. : alk. paper)   1. Physicians' assistants–Examinations, questions, etc.
I. Thibodeau, Daniel. II. Series: Pearls of wisdom.
  [DNLM: 1. Physician Assistants–Examination Questions. W 18.2 P5784 2010]
  R697.P45P483 2010
  610.76–dc22   2009033162

McGraw-Hill books are available at special quantity discounts to use as premiums and sales promotions, or for use in corporate training programs. To contact a representative, please e-mail us at bulksales@mcgraw-hill.com.

DEDICATION

I dedicate this work to my two sons Alex and Mason,
my parents, brothers and sisters, and my close friends who keep me grounded.

DT

CONTENTS

Contributors vii

Foreword ix

Preface xi

Acknowledgments xiii

1. Examination Preparation and Test-Taking Strategies 1

2. Cardiovascular 9

3. Pulmonary 49

4. Endocrine 97

5. Eyes, Ears, Nose, Throat (EENT) 119

6. Gastrointestinal/Nutritional 135

7. Genitourinary 157

8. Reproductive 183

9. Musculoskeletal 225

10. Neurology 257

11. Psychiatry/Behavioral Science 283

12. Dermatology 305

13. Hematology 319

14. Infectious Disease 339

15. Pediatrics/Geriatrics 375

16. Surgery 391

17. Trauma 421

18. Pharmacology/Toxicology 439

19. Health Policy 487

CONTRIBUTORS

Anthony Brenneman, MPAS, PA-C
Director of Clinical Education and Clinical
   Assistant Professor
Physician Assistant Program
University of Iowa
Iowa City, Iowa
Hematology

Michael G. Clark, PhD, PA-C
Vice-Chair, Clinical Education in PA Program
Associate PA Program Director
Associate Professor, Department of Physician
   Assistant Studies and Department of Internal
   Medicine/Division of Cardiovascular Medicine
University of North Texas Health Science Center
Cardiovascular

Kimberly K. Dempsey, MPA, PA-C
Associate Director of Academic Education
Assistant Professor
Physician Assistant Program
Eastern Virginia Medical School
Norfolk, Virginia
Dermatology

Michael Dryer, DrPH, PA-C
Chair and Program Director
Physician Assistant Program
Arcadia University
Glenside, Pennsylvania
Health Policy

Travis Kirby, MPAS, PA-C
Private Practice
Yorktown, Virginia
Gastrointestinal/Nutritional

David J. Klocko, MPAS, PA-C
Assistant Professor and Clinical Coordinator
Department of Physician Assistant Studies
UT Southwestern Medical Center
Dallas, Texas
Eyes, Ears, Nose, Throat (EENT)

John Oliphant, MHP, MS Ed, PA-C, ATC
Clinical Coordinator
Rochester Institute of Technology
Rochester, New York
Musculoskeletal

Jacqueline Jordan Spiegel, MS, PA-C
Assistant Professor and Clinical Coordinator
Physician Assistant Program
Midwestern University College of Health
   Sciences
Glendale, Arizona
Endocrine
Reproductive

Michel Statler, MLA, PA-C
Associate Director and Associate Professor
Department of Physician Assistant Studies
UT Southwestern Medical Center
Dallas, Texas
Neurology

Daniel Thibodeau, MHP, PA-C
Assistant Professor
Physician Assistant Program
Eastern Virginia Medical School
Norfolk, Virginia
Examination Preparation and Test-Taking Strategies
Pulmonary
Genitourinary
Psychiatry/Behavioral Science
Infectious Diseases
Pediatrics/Geriatrics
Pharmacology/Toxicology

Jeffrey G. Yates, MPA, PA-C
Assistant Professor
Physician Assistant Program
Eastern Virginia Medical School
Norfolk, Virginia
Surgery
Trauma

FOREWORD

"Learning is fun, exciting and personal. The fun varies from person to person. It's a chance to sample what possibilities are in the world, but first one must sit at the table before beginning the feast. It begins first by starting with the problem and then in finding its solution."

Dr. Eugene Stead

Learning is fun and it is lifelong experience for physician assistants. *Pearls of Wisdom: Physician Assistant Examination Review, Fourth Edition* is a fun and engaging way for PAs to prepare for the National Commission on Certification of Physician Assistants (NCCPA) PANCE/PANRE or to just reinforce their knowledge base.

A book *for* PAs, written totally *by* PAs, *Pearls of Wisdom* is not intended as a primary text, rather it is a concise yet comprehensive review book. Using a self-study/quiz format for questions and short case scenarios, *Pearls of Wisdom* provides the problem and its solution. Chapters are organized by organ system with the question format following the NCCPA's "blueprint". Content areas include history, physical examination, etiology, signs and symptoms, laboratory diagnostics, treatment and health maintenance. In addition, there is an entire chapter devoted to examination preparation and test taking strategies.

It was Socrates who told us the best way to teach is to question. As physician assistants we are confronted with questions in all aspects of our work. Knowing the right question and its answer is one of the core principles in the practice of medicine. Users of this review book are provided with a wide variety of commonly encountered questions spanning all areas of medicine. With the question and answer format the PA can review essential information efficiently. Answers can be covered while reading the question and revealed immediately to reinforce the material. Answers are short and succinct to allow the PA to digest large volumes of material in a short period of time.

Medical knowledge is one of the six core competencies for the physician assistant profession. As PAs we spend our lives building and enhancing our knowledge base. Our knowledge is reinforced through clinical work and practical application. However, our knowledge is also reinforced through didactic applications such as the question-answer format found in *Pearls of Wisdom*. So whether you are preparing for your initial PA certification examination or your final recertification examination, *Pearls of Wisdom* is a great place to begin - it starts with the problem and then finds its solution.

Cynthia Booth Lord, MHS, PA-C
Clinical Associate Professor and PA Program Director
Quinnipiac University
Hamden, CT

Immediate Past President and Chair of the Board
American Academy of Physician Assistants

PREFACE

Welcome to the fourth edition of the *Pearls of Wisdom Physician Assistant Examination Review*. The authors are delighted that you have chosen this book as a study guide in your quest to pass the national certification examination. We believe that we have prepared this fourth edition with several people in mind. First, for the student who is graduating and getting ready to prepare for taking the Physician Assistant National Certification Examination (PANCE), and second for the graduate who will be taking the Physician Assistant National Recertification Examination (PANRE). Lastly, we believe that not only does this book prepare you well for the national examination but there is also value for the PA student on clinical rotations. Each section is dedicated to a system-based approach that will guide you in a recall of the essential elements that make up the examination. In addition, this format of a bulleted question with a single answer allows you to focus on the necessary information without having to weed through other answers that are incorrect. The rapid-fire method of learning works well for those who need instant feedback into their own study habits.

For the fourth edition, we have totally restructured this book and have added several hundred new questions. First, we wanted to be sure that we were addressing the necessary content that you will see on the national examination. Next, we have organized the chapters as they would appear for the content on the examination. There are a couple of exceptions. In this book, we have taken the time to provide you with a detailed chapter in pharmacology, which should enhance the value of all the other chapters as pharmacology encompasses material into every subject matter. In addition, we have added a short chapter on test preparation as well as test taking strategies. Many of you are confident with the material that you have faced every day in clinical practice or in school. However, to sit and take a test to assess your knowledge of this material can be difficult for some. The test taking strategies chapter will try to allow you to see ways of helping choose the best answer on the examination. It will also assist you into helpful tips in preparing for sitting for the examination.

Many of you who are reading this book are coming right out of school and preparing for the PANCE. While you want to feel as prepared as possible for the examination, you will never feel 100% about going in to take a test such as this. Because you have just finished or are about to finish PA school, my advice is to take the examination as soon as you are able. At our institution we have seen people wait to take the examination for a period longer than three months, feeling that they are going to prepare during the time off. We have also seen the opposite where students graduate and take the examination within weeks of graduation. While this observation has no scientific basis, we have noticed that individuals taking the examination earlier when they graduate perform better than those that wait. It is thought that this may be due to the student being fresh off of clinical rotations and test taking as a regular routine in their academic life.

For graduates who need to prepare to take the PANRE, this is a different story. Because of work restraints and your regular life schedule, it is wise to prepare in a manner that allows you sufficient time to study. Having said that, I would still recommend taking the examination during the first year of eligibility so that by the off chance you do not pass the recertification, you will have enough time to study again and take the test. Vast majorities of PAs (>95%) who take the recertification test pass on the first time.

I want to wish you well in your studies for this examination. The time you spend preparing for the big test will be well worth the time and effort. We certainly hope that the *Pearls of Wisdom* book will be a big reason for you passing the test.

All the best,

Dan Thibodeau MHP, PA-C

ACKNOWLEDGMENTS

I love my profession. The years that I have spent being able to care for people in my community, as well as teach future physician assistants has been incredibly rewarding. This book is one facet to the body of work I have tried to accomplish. I have many more challenges ahead.

One hundred percent of my royalties will go to the Physician Assistant Foundation. The philanthropic arm of the American Academy of Physician Assistants strives to generate funds and allocate resources that empower the physician assistant profession to impact the health and wellness of the communities they serve. I hope that you will be supportive of this wonderful organization. http://www.aapa.org/pa-foundation

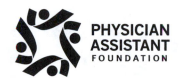

Daniel Thibodeau, MPH, PA-C
Norfolk, Virginia
2010

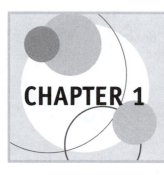

CHAPTER 1

Examination Preparation and Test-Taking Strategies

Daniel Thibodeau, MHP, PA-C

• • • INTRODUCTION • • •

After you have finished a long and distinguished journey from your physician assistant program, you are now faced with the reality of taking and passing the Physician Assistant National Certification Examination (PANCE). Those who have graduated in the past, i.e., practicing PAs, are required to take the Physician Assistant National Recertification Examination (PANRE) every 6 years to remain certified. The certifying examination is not just another test; it is a comprehensive assessment of the knowledge you have accumulated through courses and clinical experiences. Because we do not take examinations like this on a regular basis, you should have a careful plan of action in preparing to take such an important test. This chapter will help prepare you to sit for this examination—whether it's your first time or you are recertifying for the third time.

• • • ABOUT THE EXAMINATION • • •

The PANCE and PANRE are single-day examinations covering multiple aspects of clinical medicine. The PANCE comprises 360 multiple-choice questions that are broken into six blocks of 60 questions. Each block is 60 minutes long, so you have approximately 1 minute per question. The PANRE comprises 300 questions that are divided into five 60-minute blocks.

The framework of content on the examination is built around a "blueprint." The blueprint focuses on two large areas that the questions will cover—task areas and questions related to organ system. The National Commission on the Certification of Physician Assistants (NCCPA) determines the percentage of the content of questions on the examination. Their most recent blueprint is shown here:[1]

Task Area	Examination Content
History taking and performing physical examinations	16%
Using laboratory and diagnostic studies	14%
Formulating most likely diagnosis	18%
Health maintenance	10%
Clinical intervention	14%
Pharmaceutical therapeutics	18%
Applying basic science concepts	10%
Total	**100%**

Organ System	Examination Content
Cardiovascular	16%
Pulmonary	12%
Endocrine	6%
EENT	9%
Gastrointestinal/nutritional	10%
Genitourinary	6%
Musculoskeletal	10%
Reproductive	8%
Neurological	6%
Psychiatric/behavioral	6%
Dermatologic	5%
Hematologic	3%
Infectious disease	3%
Total	**100%**

[1] *NCCPA Connect.* Retrieved May 1, 2009, from National Commission on Certification of Physician Assistants (www.nccpa.net).

The organization of this book is based on the content of the blueprint and covers the majority of topics found in the test. However, the test is random and does not group the type of questions being asked from one section to the next. You must be prepared to answer any question from any category at any time.

You may answer the questions within a given block in any order, and you may review and change responses within a block during the time allotted for that section. As you navigate through the examination, you may encounter a question that is more difficult for you to answer. Try to remember that you must use good time management skills in taking the test. If the question requires more time than normal to think about, skip the question and move on. You can always come back to it later.

As you finish each section you will be given a summary of that section and if all the questions have been answered. If you have not answered all of the questions for that section, go back and answer every question in the block. A blank answer counts as an error, so it is in your best interest to take an educated guess on every question. Keep in mind that once you exit a block of questions or the time expires for that block, you cannot review or change your answers.

• • • PREPARING FOR YOUR EXAMINATION • • •

We all have different ways of learning. Each of us has different experiences of how we are able to retain knowledge and remember certain items. For new graduates, you have the recent experience of completing a vigorous program in which you have been tested numerous times throughout that the last couple of years. The PANCE will be an examination similar to your tests at school but much longer and with a lot more at stake. For practicing PAs taking the PANRE, getting back in to the habit of studying may be a bit of a challenge. Because you have been out of school for years, compounded with schedule restrictions such as full-time employment, the thought of preparing for and taking a large test can be intimidating. Here are some suggestions when preparing to study for the examination:

- **Commitment:** You need to pledge to yourself that you will do everything needed to properly prepare for the examination. Your certification/recertification depends upon it.
- **Confidence:** If you have just graduated from PA school, build confidence from the fact that you were able to successfully handle a lot of complex material. This test is an assessment of the knowledge that you have already obtained while in school. For recertification as a practicing PA, you have gained knowledge in your everyday practice over the past 5–6 years (or more) and so apply this experience toward the content of the examination. If you keep a positive attitude about preparing for the examination, you will feel better about going into the examination on a positive note.
- **Time management:** Whether you are a new graduate or a professional recertifying, make the most of your time studying. Consider the amount of material that you will need to prepare for and try to estimate the amount of preparation you will need for those areas. Look at a calendar and plan backward from your examination date to ensure you allow yourself enough time to review. Set up a schedule that you can follow and a routine that you can commit to. If you can keep up with this strategy, you will not feel rushed at the end to cram a lot of material into the last minute.
- **Comfortable environment:** Choose a study area that has the fewest distractions so that you can focus. The content of a test like this is complicated at times. Having a comfortable environment can be helpful to your concentration. Whatever the place, make sure that you can study in this area with your undivided attention.
- **Nutrition and exercise:** Make sure that as you prepare you not only take care of studying but you take care of yourself as well. Proper nutrition and exercise can be very helpful in preparing for a test.

Another facet of preparation for the examination is to familiarize yourself with the testing software. The NCCPA offers a practice self-assessment module for a nominal fee.

• • • EXAMINATION DAY TIPS • • •

The day of the examination will usually start early for you. Here are some important reminders for you to consider:

- When registering for the test, make your time in accordance with your own biological clock. If you are an early riser, think about registering for a morning time slot. If getting up in the morning is tough for you, consider starting at a later time.

- Leave plenty of time getting to the testing facility. Showing up late not only causes unneeded stress on the day, but you could jeopardize being able to take the test if you are late.
- Make sure that you have a good meal before you go into the testing center so you don't tire while taking the examination.
- Take breaks during the examination to refresh yourself mentally and physically.

You will be taking the test in an independent testing facility called a Prometric Test Center. It is important that you be prepared for the examination before you enter the facility. Make sure that you have the following materials with you when entering the testing center:

- Your testing certificate that states you are registered for the examination.
- Two valid forms of photo identification card (driving license, passport).
- Comfortable clothing (dress in layers in case you get warm/cold).

Once you enter the facility and sign in, you will have to verify who you are each time you step into the testing area. Leave any nonessential items in your car because you cannot take anything into the examination room except your identification. You can use a locker to store other personals that you have, but try to bring in as little as possible. You will be asked to empty out your pockets so that you enter the testing area only with the clothes you have on. You will then be asked to give your fingerprint prior to entering the testing room, and then would be escorted to the computer where you will take the test. From the moment you enter the examination room, you will be videotaped as well as recorded for sound. Once seated, you will be offered some earplugs to drown out noise. I would recommend accepting a pair and holding on to them in case you need them. The testing assistant will help you log onto the computer and you are on your way!

• • • TEST-TAKING STRATEGY • • •

Believe it or not, taking a test like this involves a bit of strategy on your part. You just have to know how to think about answering a question so that you can narrow down your choices.

Questions are usually written in a format that follows a consistent formula. For example, you might have a question that focuses on a particular clinical problem. You will be given four to five choices, all of which will either be a physical examination finding, a diagnosis, a laboratory test to order, or treatment plan. The hard part for you is to figure out which of these similar answers is correct. This is where test-taking strategy can help. First, let's focus on types of questions, then discuss answer types, and conclude on making the best choice.

Most questions asked on the examination can be placed into certain categories. In general, questions will be based on either a major medical problem or a situation that requires you to think about the next step in a clinical scenario. Before we describe type of questions that will be on the examination, here are some question types that you **will not see** on the examination:

- True/False questions
- Matching
- Questions of negation (i.e., . . . all of the following EXCEPT. . .)
- "Type K" questions (i.e., choices that have more than one answer, e.g., A and B)

Almost all of the questions will come in the form of clinical vignettes. These types of questions are used because they can assess an individual's knowledge in many different ways. The questions are generally straightforward and most good questions will test an individual to the general knowledge of a subject. With that in mind, you need to take your time in reading the question carefully to determine what it is asking. The first part of the question that you will read is called the stem. The stem is the precursor to the actual question that will be asked. Take this question for example:

A 22-year-old male patient has a 4-day history of periumbilical pain that has migrated to the right lower quadrant over the last 24 hours. He complains of fever, nausea, and a sharp pain to the right lower quadrant on movement. On examination, he has a temperature of 100.7°F, P: 92, R: 16, BP 133/88; head and neck examination is normal and cardiac examination has a regular rate and rhythm. Abdominal examination reveals a flat abdomen without scars, normal active bowel sounds are present, and pain on palpation to the right lower quadrant with rebound tenderness at McBurneys point. Laboratory results

reveal a WBC count of 12,000/mm³ with a left shift, urinalysis is negative, and acute abdominal series X-ray has nonspecific bowel gas patterns. Which of the following is the most appropriate diagnosis?

You will notice that the first part of the question is the clinical vignette—this is the stem. By reading the vignette, you should be able to determine that the case is pointing to an acute appendicitis as the most likely diagnosis. The next part of the question, usually the last sentence, is what will determine how you need to answer. Based on the last sentence, this same scenario could change and ask you to determine the next step in treatment, or whether or not to give a certain medication, or if evaluation by a surgeon is warranted. Regardless of any question being asked in the last sentence, you should be able to read the vignette (stem), think about the entire clinical situation (symptoms, examination findings, predictable laboratory results, diagnostic tests, and treatment plans), and be able to answer questions that relate to that clinical scenario.

If you notice the question above, you will see that there is a pattern to how the question is written. Most of the questions that are written in clinical vignette format have a basic flow to the stem.

Here are some basics to most clinical scenario questions:

- Patient demographics (age, gender, ethnicity)
- Presenting problem or chief complaint
- Past history including:
  - Medical history
  - Surgical history
  - Medications
  - Family/social history may also be listed
- Details of the physical examination
- Laboratory data and any testing (CT, MRI, X-rays, etc.)

Why is this important to know? If you can learn how questions are written, then you can start to try to understand how to think about what may be asked. A good test taker has the ability to infer all of the necessary information about a clinical scenario from the stem that will be needed to answer any question that comes from the information supplied. In the case of the acute appendicitis question above, while reading the question one should be already thinking about appendicitis and the details associated with the condition: presenting signs and symptoms, typical physical examination findings, differential diagnosis, laboratory and testing findings, and lastly treatment plans. By using this technique, you can make a reasonable guess to what possible questions could be asked, and by the time you get to the actual question you have already assessed possible paths that may need to be taken to get to the correct answer. By the time you get to the answer options to the question, you can already have a good idea on the correct choice without having even looked at them yet. This can help minimize making an incorrect choice. As you look to the choices, try to think in terms of the *most* common issue or most commonly treated condition. Try to avoid thinking in terms of what is done sometimes in practice. This may not always be the treatment of choice or standard of care.

Some questions will require you to answer about treatment plans. These questions are trying to test you on the gold standard for a condition or treatment of a disease. Remember, these questions are not here to trick you. In this type of examination, you should not see questions that would be considered too detailed or too specific in nature. The "zebras" that can be seen in medicine are usually not the type of questions that are asked in an examination such as the PANCE or PANRE. The questions are written to assess your basic knowledge of medicine and are written in a way to make sure that you understand the basic concepts of the material that is listed within the blueprint of the examination. They are also written in a way to assess your ability to take a question, think about the question from a standpoint of clinical practicality, and be able to choose the best answer based on the information provided. A majority of the questions that are asked should be formatted in a way where you will be able to have an idea on what the answer is even before looking at the choices given.

Now that we have looked at how questions are presented, let's think about choosing an answer. There will be questions that may have more than one *correct* answer that you can choose. You need to determine not only what you think is correct, but what is the **best** choice available. In many of the questions your objective should be to seek out the answer that is the "most common," "most likely," or "next best step" in regards to the clinical scenario provided. This means that you have to know the general knowledge of a disease or pathology as well as how to prioritize these choices into a list from most correct to least. Let's give some examples of how this works:

The pathogen that is most responsible for community-acquired pneumonia in an outpatient setting is:

A. *Haemophilus influenza*
B. *Streptococcus pneumoniae*
C. *Moraxella catarrhalis*
D. *Staphylococcus aureus*
E. *Mycoplasma pneumoniae*

From this question, you can see that there are several correct answers to this question. While it is true that *H. influenza*, *S. aureus*, and *M. pneumoniae* can all cause community-acquired pneumonia, the **best** choice for this question is **B** (or *Streptococcus pneumoniae*). To dig a little deeper into the question, you could also consider *M. catarrhalis* as a choice. However, this pathogen is seen more in patients with comorbidity like COPD. You have to consider what the *most likely* pathogen would be. Let's give another example:

What test is the standard test for confirmation of a pulmonary embolus?

A. **Chest X-ray**
B. **Ventilation to perfusion scan**
C. **CT scan**
D. **Pulmonary angiography**
E. **MRI**

There are a few correct answers that could be used clinically to find a pulmonary embolus. However, when considering the **best** choice and what is considered the gold standard, the answer for this question is **D** (or Pulmonary angiography). This is one of the aspects to this test that you must remember—many of the questions will be looking for the gold standard of care. While you may remember that there are other choices that can be used in everyday medicine to either diagnose or treat a disease, the test question is looking for the *best* choice, not just *any* correct choice. Having clinical experience is very helpful when testing. However, be careful to remember the standards of care as some clinical practices are more advanced than what a question will ask.

For some questions, you may read the entire scenario but still fall short on knowing what the correct answer is. In this situation, try to think about the most common findings that are associated with this clinical question and then look at the choices. In some cases, you may be able to deduce what the best possible guess may be. A goal in the completion of taking the test is to answer every question that is given to you. Not answering a question can mean points against you, thus lowering your overall performance on the examination.

● ● ● OTHER CONSIDERATIONS ● ● ●

There are aspects to many questions where you will be given an image to evaluate in order to answer the question or test results. Some things you will see on the examination are:

- ECG
- An X-ray, CT scan, or MRI
- Laboratory values (blood, urine, other tests)
- Photographs, usually of a physical examination finding

A question will usually refer to the information provided by these visual aides. It is worth spending a little time discussing what you need to think about when confronted with these types of questions.

Most of the electrocardiograms that will be given to you will have some basic pathology on the ECG. The tracing will either be in a rhythm strip, and in some cases a 12-lead ECG. You should consider a simple approach to determine what the basic problem may be. Think of each ECG in this easy to remember rhyme: "Narrow or wide, fast or slow, kill my patient, yes or no." If you can approach the ECG and ask yourself what could be the most life-threatening thing that you may see on the ECG, you should be able to figure out what the question is trying to ask. Try to think about the most common types of ECG rhythms/problems that you will encounter in medicine and have a good general knowledge of their etiology, different presentations, and lastly treatment for the problem.

Several questions may be present that will give you one or two views from an X-ray, a CT scan, or an MRI. With regard to X-rays, try to keep a methodical approach in looking at the films. First understand what you are viewing with regard to anatomy and the type of film that was performed. Next, make sure you can identify anatomic reference points on the film that will help you assess the entire film. For example, let's consider a chest X-ray. For starters, think about your **ABCs** as an easy approach.

- **A** (Airway): Look at the airway, alignment, and the lung tissue and note in your mind any abnormalities. Infiltrates, nodules, masses, atelectasis, and loss of lung tissue as in a pneumothorax and any fluid that may be present are some things to consider.
- **B** (Bone): Look at the boney structures for any abnormalities. Look at the contour of the ribs and at spine from the AP view and try to determine if there are any abnormalities that stick out on the film.
- **C** (Cardiac): Look at the cardiac silhouette. Is it large or normal appearance in size? Is there any evidence that there is obstruction of the silhouette by another structure such as a widened mediastinum, mass, or fluid?
- **D** (Diaphragm): Does the diaphragm appear to be normal? Is there an effusion present that obscures your view of the diaphragm, and do the borders anatomically appear to be in the correct position?
- **E** (Everything else): Look at the soft tissue for any abnormalities (free air, foreign body, etc.).

This is one way to try to stay organized while taking the test. That way, as you look at the picture or X-ray on the screen, you can determine what the abnormality is, which can give you a better idea on how to answer the question before you see the choices.

In several of the questions you will be given a series of laboratory results, blood, urine, and other tests. Remember, the testing material that you are given will provide you with a list of all laboratory tests and their normal values. These are usually available to you at all times on the test in a separate page on the computer that is easy to pull up at any time. Just remember that if you cannot recall what a normal value is, reference it by utilizing the laboratory value page that is provided. That way, if you get stuck on a question where you may not recall the significance of a laboratory test, you can try to work through the problem by understanding how the laboratory value is abnormal (either elevated, low, positive when a normal value is negative, and so forth).

In some cases, you will encounter a photo that will be provided with a question. In most instances the photo will be directly related to the condition that you are being questioned. This will be in the form of a physical examination finding, a blood smear, a gram stain photo, or some other type of photo that will aid in the question. Remember to use a methodical approach in trying to answer in your mind what you are looking at before you make a decision on the choices that will be given.

••• CONCLUSION •••

Not everyone is a great test taker. But the good news is, you don't have to be. If you can take a methodical approach to your study time and preparation, along with reminding yourself of some basic test-taking strategies, you can better your chances of improving your test score. Good luck!

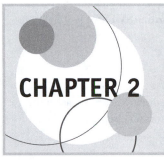

CHAPTER 2 Cardiovascular

Michael G. Clark, PhD, PA-C

● ● ● **CARDIOMYOPATHIES** ● ● ●

○ **Which is the most common type of cardiomyopathy?**

Dilated cardiomyopathy (dilation of all four chambers). This condition is often idiopathic but can be induced by progression of ischemia, myocarditis, alcohol consumption, Adriamycin, diabetes, pheochromocytoma, thiamine deficiency, thyroid disease, and valve replacement. The other type of cardiomyopathies are hypertrophic and restrictive.

○ **What is the abnormality seen in the 2-D echocardiogram shown in Figure 2-1?**

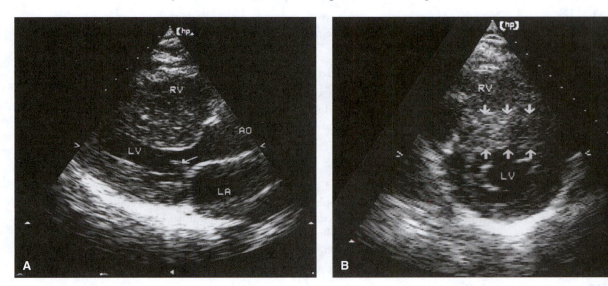

Figure 2-1 (Reproduced, with permission, from Fuster V et al. *Hurst's The Heart.* 12th ed. New York, NY: McGraw-Hill: 2008, Fig. 16-106.)

Hypertrophic cardiomyopathy. Note the very thickened septum.

○ **What drugs have been shown to regress LV hypertrophy and reduce LV mass?**

Beta-blockers, alpha-methyldopa (Aldomet), ACE inhibitors, and thiazide diuretics.

○ **What is the most common mechanism responsible for supraventricular tachycardia (SVT)?**

AV node reentry.

○ **What are the common causes of SVT?**

Myocardial ischemia, myocardial infarction, congestive heart failure, pericarditis, rheumatic heart disease, mitral valve prolapse, preexcitation syndromes, COPD, ethanol intoxication, hypoxia, pneumonia, sepsis, and digoxin toxicity.

○ **What are the physiologic characteristics of dilated cardiomyopathies?**

Reduced ventricular ejection fraction, high end-diastolic filling volumes and pressures, reduced cardiac output, and high pulmonary capillary wedge pressures.

○ **What are the common clinical presentations that can occur with a dilated cardiomyopathy?**

Fatigue, exertional dyspnea, and orthopnea. They commonly have an S_3 and a LV/RV heave. Other presentations that could occur include mitral and/or tricuspid regurgitation, jugular venous distention, rales and edema, low voltage on EKG, and signs of cardiomegaly by CXR.

○ **What are the physiological aspects of restricted cardiomyopathy?**

Normal systolic contractility, reduction in diastolic relaxation and filling capacity, high LV end-diastolic filling pressures, and high pulmonary wedge pressures especially with exercise.

○ **What are the common causes of restrictive cardiomyopathy?**

Most are idiopathic but other causes include infiltrative diseases, e.g., sarcoid and amyloid, and storage diseases, e.g., hemochromatosis. Other potential causes include radiation exposure and cancer.

○ **What are the common clinical presentations associated with restrictive cardiomyopathy?**

Symptoms are very similar to dilated cardiomyopathy with fatigue, exertional dyspnea, and orthopnea but could present with syncope/near syncope and palpitations. Restrictive cardiomyopathy is more likely to have an S_4 as opposed to S_3. The symptoms often present with a resting tachycardia and typically will not show signs of cardiomegaly on CXR.

○ **What is hypertrophic cardiomyopathy?**

It is a genetic disorder resulting in abnormal hypertrophy of the ventricular walls. It often results in asymmetric hypertrophic changes, which can create outlet obstruction. Typically, there is normal LV systolic contractility but increased diastolic stiffness resulting in reduced LV filling volumes. Patients often present with high pulmonary capillary wedge pressures and pulmonary hypertension.

○ **What are the common clinical presentations of hypertrophic cardiomyopathy?**

In young patients, clinical signs and symptoms may be difficult to ascertain. Commonly, they may present with complaints of palpitations, chest pain, dyspnea, syncope, or dizziness. Sudden death is not an uncommon presentation for this disorder. Resting tachycardia is common.

○ **What are the key management options for patients with hypertrophic cardiomyopathy?**

Patients may be advised to avoid vigorous physical activity. Avoid preload and afterload reducing agents and positive inotropes such as digoxin. Beta-blockers and calcium channel blockers may be used to slow the heart rate. Myomectomy and septal ablation by catheter or chemical means may be needed to decrease outflow tract obstruction. ICDs are often considered because of the increased risk for ventricular dysrhythmias in these patients. Also, the immediate family should be screened for undiagnosed individuals at risk.

● ● ● CONDUCTION DISORDERS ● ● ●

○ **What are the common causes of multifocal atrial tachycardia?**

COPD, CHF, sepsis, valvular heart disease, and methylxanthine toxicity. Treat the arrhythmia with magnesium, verapamil, or beta-blocking agents.

○ **How is atrial flutter treated?**

Initiate AV nodal blockade with beta-blockers, calcium channel blockers, or digoxin. If necessary, treat a stable patient with chemical cardioversion by using a class IA agent, such as procainamide or quinidine, after digitalization. If this treatment fails or if the patient is unstable, electrocardiovert at 25 to 50 J.

○ **What are some causes of atrial fibrillation?**

Hypertension, rheumatic heart disease, pneumonia, thyrotoxicosis, ischemic heart, pericarditis, ethanol intoxication, PE, CHF, valvular heart disease, and COPD.

○ **How is atrial fibrillation treated?**

Control rate with beta-blocker or calcium channel blocker (such as verapamil or diltiazem), and then convert with procainamide, quinidine, or verapamil. Digoxin may be considered, although its effect will be delayed. Synchronized cardioversion at 100 to 200 J should be performed on an unstable patient. In a stable patient with a-fib of unclear duration, anticoagulation should be considered for 3 weeks prior to chemical or electrical cardioversion. *A transesophageal echocardiogram is commonly used to determine the timing of cardioversions.* Watch for hypotension with the administration of negative inotropes.

○ **What is the treatment of SVT caused by digitalis toxicity?**

Stop the digitalis, treat hypokalemia, and administer magnesium or phenytoin. Provide digoxin-specific antibodies to the unstable patient. Avoid cardioversion.

○ **What is the treatment for stable SVT not caused by digitalis toxicity or WPW syndrome?**

Vagal maneuvers, adenosine, verapamil, or beta-blockers.

○ **Describe the key feature of Mobitz I (Wenckebach) second-degree AV block:**

A progressive prolongation of the PR interval until the atrial impulse is no longer conducted. If symptomatic, atropine and transcutaneous/transvenous pacing may be required.

○ **Describe the key feature of Mobitz II second-degree AV block:**

A constant PR interval in which one or more beats fail to conduct.

○ **What is the treatment for Mobitz II second-degree AV block?**

Atropine and transcutaneous/transvenous pacing, if symptomatic.

○ **Carotid massage or Valsalva maneuver is useful for slowing supraventricular rhythms. When is carotid massage contraindicated?**

With ventricular dysrhythmias, digitalis toxicity, stroke, syncope, seizures, known carotid artery disease, or in those with a carotid bruit.

○ **What are some common vagal maneuvers?**

Breath holding, Valsalva (bearing down as if having a bowel movement), stimulating of the gag reflex, squatting, pressure on the eyeballs, and immersing the face in cold water.

○ **What is more common: premature atrial beats or ventricular beats?**

Premature atrial beats. Palpitations that occur because of premature atrial beats are generally benign and asymptomatic. Reassurance is the only treatment. Less frequent but more serious causes of atrial premature beats include pheochromocytoma and thyrotoxicosis. Random unifocal PVCs are also benign but common in the general population. Runs of PVCs and/or associated symptoms of dyspnea, angina, or syncope require investigation and are most likely related to an underlying heart disease.

○ **How do the fixed-rate demand modes of pacemakers differ?**

Fixed-rate mode produces an impulse at a continuous specific rate, regardless of the patient's own cardiac activity. Demand mode detects the patient's electrical activity and triggers only if the heart is not depolarizing.

○ **What is the treatment for ventricular fibrillation in a patient with a pacemaker?**

Defibrillation, but be sure to keep the paddles away from the pacemaker.

○ **What is the average lifespan of a pacemaker battery?**

7 to 15 years.

○ **What are the most common causes of MAT (multifocal atrial tachycardia)?**

COPD with exacerbation is the most common cause, followed by CHF, sepsis, and methylxanthine toxicity. Treatment consists of treating the underlying disorder as well as the use of verapamil, magnesium, or digoxin for slowing the arrhythmia.

○ **What are the most common causes of atrial fibrillation?**

Coronary artery disease with myocardial ischemia and hypertensive heart disease are the most common causes. Other common causes are mitral or aortic valvular heart disease, cor pulmonale, dilated cardiomyopathy, hypertrophic cardiomyopathy (particularly the obstructive type), alcohol intoxication or "holiday heart syndrome," hypo- or hyperthyroidism, pulmonary embolism, sepsis, hypoxia, preexcitation syndrome, and pericarditis.

○ **How is atrial fibrillation treated?**

The treatment of atrial fibrillation consists of three major considerations:

1. Control of ventricular rate
2. Conversion, if possible or feasible, to sinus rhythm
3. Prevention of thromboembolic events, particularly CVA

Rate control is best managed with beta-adrenergic blocker or calcium channel blockers (diltiazem or verapamil), or less desirable, digoxin. Digoxin should be used in patients with poor LV systolic function and those with a contraindication to beta-blockers and calcium channel blockers. Digoxin provides good rate control at rest, but often suboptimal rate control during exertion. For conversion to sinus rhythm, in the stable patient with a duration of symptoms <48 hours, it is best managed, initially, with antiarrhythmic agents (amiodarone, ibutilide, propafenone, or procainamide). In the unstable patient or the patient with acute ischemia, hypotension or pulmonary edema, immediate synchronized electrical cardioversion, starting at 200 J should be performed without interruption of antiarrhythmic therapy. Patients with atrial fibrillation of 1 year duration or longer, or those with left atrial size of >5.0 cm on echocardiography cardioversion, are not recommended this therapy because of its low success rate. Patients with recent atrial fibrillation >2 days duration should be started on warfarin and anticoagulated to an INR between 2 and 3 for at least 3 weeks, before any attempt to cardiovert to sinus rhythm because of the significant risk for embolic CVA. Earlier cardioversion attempts could be considered if the patient is at adequate anticoagulation levels and no evidence of intrachamber thrombus by transesophageal echocardiography. Those patients with chronic atrial fibrillation should be on lifelong warfarin unless an absolute contraindication to warfarin exists or the patient cannot reliably take warfarin.

○ **What percentage of patients with atrial fibrillation converted to sinus rhythm will revert into atrial fibrillation?**

50% will revert to atrial fibrillation within 1 year of cardioversion, regardless of medical therapy.

○ **What is the risk of CVA in patients with atrial fibrillation, with or without anticoagulation?**

Patients with atrial fibrillation, not anticoagulated with warfarin, have a 25% incidence of CVA within 5 years (5% per year). Those patients anticoagulated to therapeutic levels have a 4% incidence of CVA within 5 years (0.8%). Aspirin is a clearly inferior substitute to warfarin, but is much more preferable to no anticoagulant or antithrombotic therapy.

○ **What is the key feature of Mobitz I second-degree AV block (Wenckebach)?**

A progressive prolongation of the PR interval until the atrial impulse is no longer conducted through to the ventricle, resulting in a dropped QRS. Almost always transient, atropine and transcutaneous/transvenous pacing is required for the rare instances of symptoms or cardiac stability.

○ **What is the feature of Mobitz II second-degree AV block?**

A constant PR interval until one sinus beat fails to conduct through the ventricle, resulting in a dropped QRS. Since this rhythm is indicative of His bundle damage, and 85% of patients with this rhythm eventually develop complete heart block, temporary pacing followed by permanent pacing is usually required.

○ **A 57-year-old man is scheduled for a total colectomy for ulcerative colitis. He has stable angina for several years and has hypertension. His pre-op EKG reveals NSR, LVH, and first-degree AV block. What is the likelihood of high-degree AV block occurring in the perioperative period?**

Patients with first-degree AV block have an extremely low incidence of developing high-degree AV block in the perioperative period. Thus, no temporary pacing in the perioperative period is required.

○ **A 26-year-old man presents to your clinic for an insurance physical. An EKG reveals Wolff-Parkinson-White syndrome. He is asymptomatic and has no history of palpitations or arrhythmia. What is the most appropriate management of this patient?**

No therapy or work-up is required at this time since there is no evidence that the risk of sudden death can be safely mitigated or that individuals with asymptomatic WPW can be reliably risk stratified with regard to sudden death.

○ **What is the most commonly occurring form of ventricular tachycardia?**

Ventricular tachycardia (VT) occurring in patients with healed myocardial infarction. Other causes include bundle branch reentry VT, VT of right ventricular outflow tract origin, idiopathic left ventricular tachycardia, drug-induced VT (proarrhythmia), and VT due to right ventricular dysplasia. Rare causes include long QT syndrome and lymphocytic myocarditis.

○ **A 48-year-old male patient with no history of angina, MI, or other cardiac symptoms is referred to you for evaluation of palpitations. A 24-hour Holter monitor reveals 4 three-beat runs of ventricular tachycardia without any symptoms. The patient has no risk factors for coronary artery disease, is not a smoker, and has a normal resting EKG. His echocardiogram is normal. What is the best management strategy for this patient?**

No therapy or further work-up is required. The patient should be reassured that the risk of sudden death is very low and that medical therapy will either worsen his arrhythmia or be of no significant benefit.

○ **A 28-year-old male patient with two previous episodes of palpitations and shortness of breath in the last year is brought in the emergency department by EMS presenting with severe palpitations, hypotension, and shortness of breath. His BP is 90/55 and HR is 195 bpm. A rhythm strip reveals narrow complex QRS tachycardia. A 12-lead EKG reveals what appears to be atrial fibrillation. Synchronized cardioversion is successful in terminating the arrhythmia, and the postcardioversion EKG reveals Wolff-Parkinson-White syndrome. What is the most appropriate management strategy in this patient?**

Electrophysiology testing with intracardiac mapping, followed by catheter ablation of the accessory conduction pathway.

○ **A 67-year-old woman with severe three-vessel coronary artery disease with very small distal vessels, deemed inoperable, is brought into the emergency department following a syncopal episode. The paramedics caught the final beats of what looked like a wide-complex QRS tachycardia on a rhythm strip and you confirm this on inspection of the tracing. She is now awake, alert, and breathing comfortably. An echocardiogram performed 1 month ago revealed a dilated left ventricle with poor systolic function (estimated ejection fraction is 20%–25%). What is the most appropriate management strategy for this patient?**

Empiric therapy with amiodarone.

○ **What medications, used to maintain sinus rhythm in a patient recently cardioverted from atrial fibrillation, should be avoided in patients with stress test proven myocardial ischemia?**

Class IC antiarrhythmics, such as flecainide and propafenone, and class IA agents, such as quinidine and procainamide. They can lead to lethal proarrhythmia in patients with active myocardial ischemia. Amiodarone, an agent that has anti-ischemic properties, is the preferred agent.

○ **What drugs can increase serum digoxin levels?**

Quinidine, procainamide, verapamil, and amiodarone.

○ **What are the end points in procainamide loading infusion for patient with unstable VT?**

Hypotension, QRS widened more than 50% of pretreatment width, arrhythmia suppression, or a total of 17 mg/kg.

○ **If a defibrillator is available, what is the immediate treatment of a patient with ventricular fibrillation?**

Unsynchronized countershock at 200 J (biphasic) or 360 J (monophasic).

○ **What is the differential diagnosis for pulseless electrical activity (PEA)?**
- Hypoxia/hypovolemia/hyper- or hypokalemia/hyperthermia
- Acute MI/acidosis
- Tension pneumothorax/tamponade/thrombosis (pulmonary)/tablets (drug overdose)

○ **What is the differential diagnosis of asystole?**

Drug overdose, acidosis, hyperkalemia, hypothermia, hypokalemia, and hypoxia.

○ **What is the treatment for unstable supraventricular tachycardia?**

Synchronized cardioversion.

○ **A patient in the emergency department suddenly demonstrates ventricular fibrillation on the monitor. The patient is alert and has a pulse. What should you do?**

Check the monitor leads.

○ **Inferior wall MIs commonly lead to what two types of heart block?**

First-degree AV block and Mobitz I second-degree AV block (Wenckebach). Sinus bradycardia can also occur. Progression to complete AV block is not common. The mechanism for this is damage to autonomic fibers in the atrial septum giving increased vagal tone impairing AV node conduction.

○ **Anterior wall MIs may directly damage intracardiac conduction. This may lead to which type of arrhythmias?**

A Mobitz II second-degree AV block that can suddenly progress to complete AV block.

○ **Which type of drug is contraindicated for the treatment of Torsades de pointes?**

Any drug that prolongs repolarization (QT interval). For example, class IA antiarrhythmics, such as quinidine and procainamide, are contraindicated for treating torsades de pointes. Other drugs that share this effect include TCAs, disopyramide, and phenothiazine.

○   **What is this cardiac arrhythmia shown in Figure 2-2?**

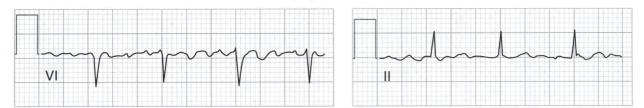

Figure 2-2   (Reproduced, with permission, from Fauci AS, Braunwald E, Kasper DL, et al., eds. *Harrison's Principles of Internal Medicine*. 17th ed. New York, NY: McGraw-Hill; 2008, Fig. 226-4A.)

Atrial fibrillation.

○   **What is the cardiac arrhythmia seen in Figure 2-3?**

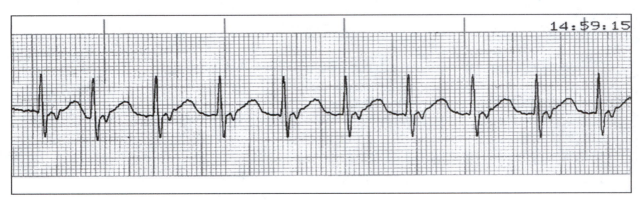

Figure 2-3

Accelerated junctional rhythm with retrograde P waves.

○   **What is the cardiac arrhythmia seen in Figure 2-4?**

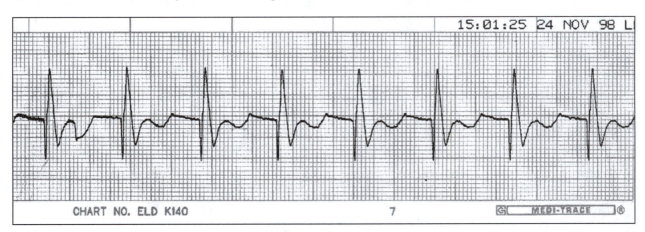

Figure 2-4

Ventricular pacemaker rhythm.

○ **What is the cardiac arrhythmia seen in Figure 2-5?**

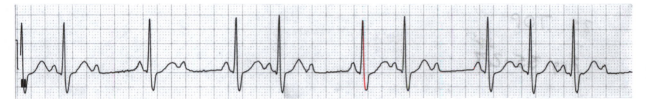

Figure 2-5 (Reproduced, with permission, from Stone CK, Humphries RL. *Current Diagnosis & Treatment Emergency Medicine.* 6th ed. New York, NY: McGraw-Hill, 2008, Fig. 33-28.)

Mobitz type II second-degree AV block.

○ **What is the EKG rhythm abnormality seen in Figure 2-6?**

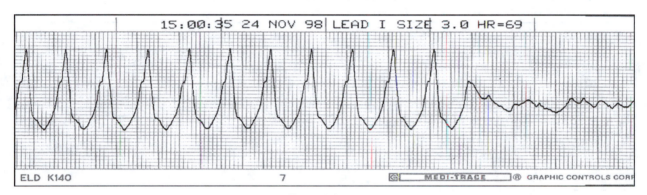

Figure 2-6

Ventricular tachycardia degrading into ventricular fibrillation.

○ **What is the cardiac arrhythmia seen in Figure 2-7?**

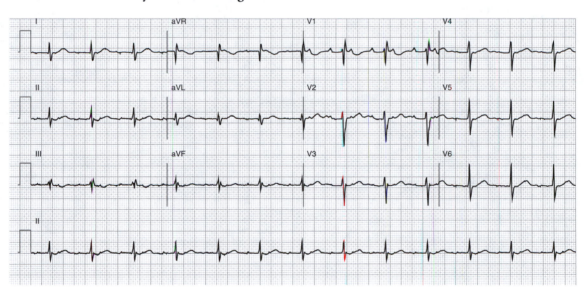

Figure 2-7 (Reproduced, with permission, from Fauci AS, Braunwald E, Kasper DL, et al., eds. *Harrison's Principles of Internal Medicine.* 17th ed. New York, NY: McGraw-Hill; 2008, Fig. e21-11.)

Atrial tachycardia with 2:1 conduction.

○   **What is the abnormality seen in the EKG in Figure 2-8?**

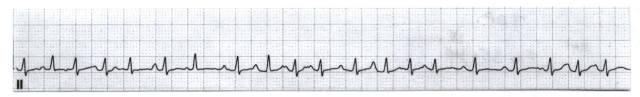

Figure 2-8 (Reproduced, with permission, from Stone CK, Humphries RL. *Current Diagnosis & Treatment Emergency Medicine.* 6th ed. New York, NY: McGraw-Hill; 2008, Fig. 33-15.)

Multifocal atrial tachycardia.

○   **What is the abnormality seen in the EKG in Figure 2-9?**

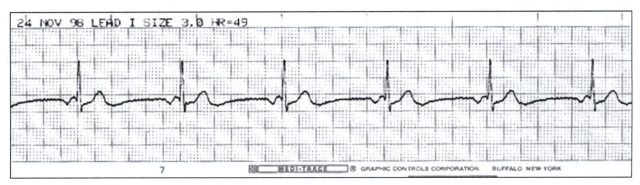

Figure 2-9

Junctional rhythm.

○   **What is the abnormality seen in the rhythm strip in Figure 2-10?**

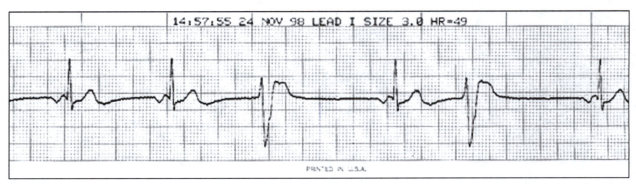

Figure 2-10

Junctional rhythm with escape ventricular beat.

○ **What is the abnormality seen in the rhythm strip in Figure 2-11?**

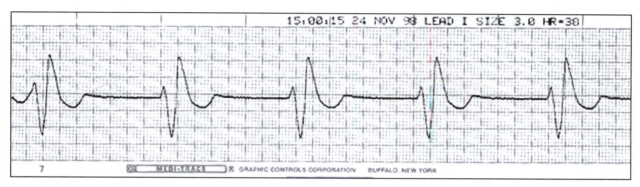

Figure 2-11

Idioventricular rhythm.

○ **What is the abnormality seen in the rhythm strip in Figure 2-12?**

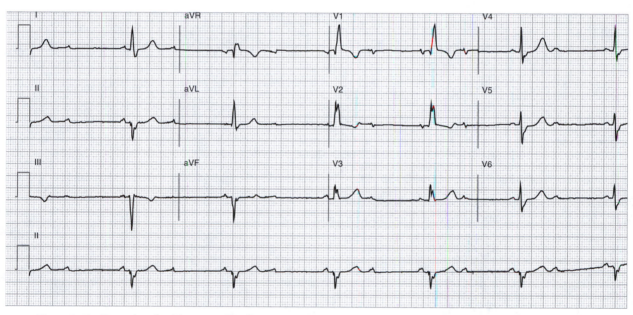

Figure 2-12 (Reproduced, with permission, from Fauci AS, Braunwald E, Kasper DL, et al., eds. *Harrison's Principles of Internal Medicine*, 17th ed. New York, NY: McGraw-Hill; 2008, Fig. e21-4.)

2:1 AV block.

○ · **What is the abnormality seen in the rhythm strip in Figure 2-13?**

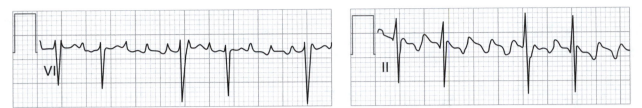

Figure 2-13 (Reproduced, with permission, from Fauci AS, Braunwald E, Kasper DL, et al., eds. *Harrison's Principles of Internal Medicine*, 17th ed. New York, NY: McGraw-Hill; 2008, Fig. 226-4B.)

Atrial flutter.

○   **What is the abnormality seen in the rhythm strip in Figure 2-14?**

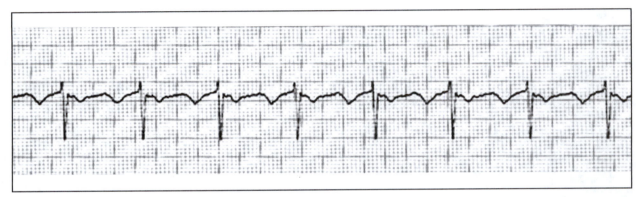

Figure 2-14

Rhythm strip erroneously mounted upside down. When viewed with right side up, it shows normal sinus rhythm.

○   **What is the abnormality seen in the rhythm strip in Figure 2-15?**

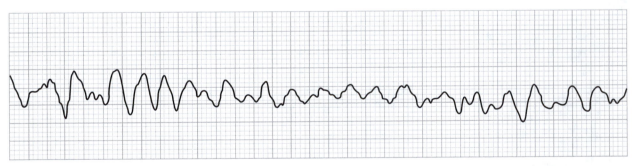

Figure 2-15 (Reproduced, with permission, from Gomella LG, Haist. Clinician's Pocket Reference, 11th ed. New York, NY: McGraw-Hill, 2007, Fig. 19.18.)

Ventricular fibrillation.

○ **What is the interpretation of the EKG shown in Figure 2-16?**

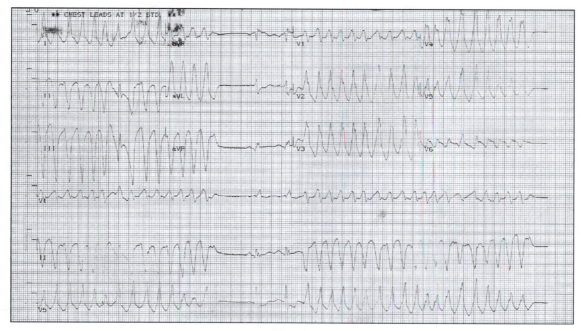

Figure 2-16

Ventricular tachycardia.

○ **What is the interpretation of the EKG shown in Figure 2-17?**

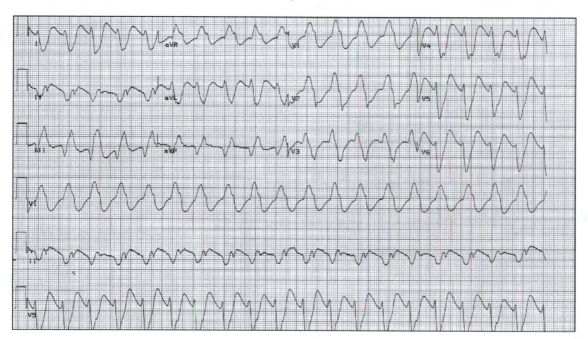

Figure 2-17

Ventricular tachycardia with hyperkalemia. Note the very wide QRS complex with the early stages of a "sine wave."

○   **What is the interpretation of the EKG shown in Figure 2-18?**

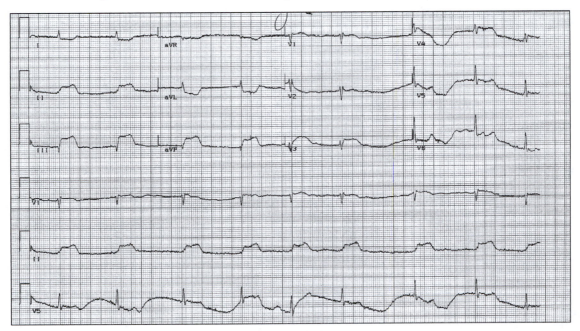

Figure 2-18

Acute inferior myocardial infarction with posterior wall involvement, and atrial fibrillation with slow ventricular rate.

○   **What is the interpretation of the EKG shown in Figure 2-19?**

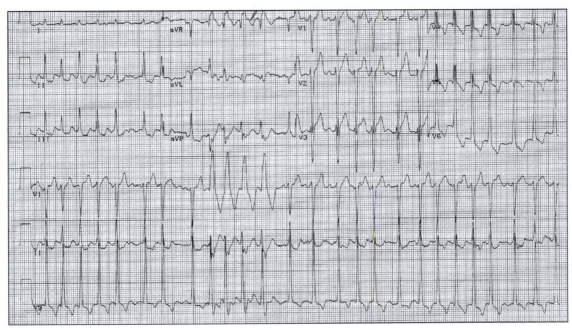

Figure 2-19

Atrial fibrillation with rapid ventricular rate of 155 bpm, LVH, and ischemic-type ST depression in the inferior and lateral leads.

○ **What is the interpretation of the EKG shown in Figure 2-20?**

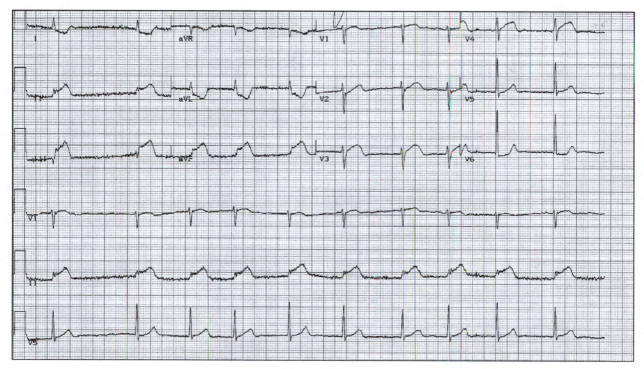

Figure 2-20

Acute inferior myocardial infarction and atrial fibrillation with slow ventricular rate.

○ **In the EKG shown in Figure 2-20, does the patient absolutely have myocardial ischemia?**

Not necessarily. Patients with supraventricular tachycardia of any type with ST depression can have "ischemic" appearing ST depression without having myocardial ischemia. The ST depression can be as a result of abnormal repolarization that occurs in any tachydysrhythmia. Nonetheless, it would be incorrect to automatically assume that this patient's ST depression is not due to myocardial ischemia.

○   **What is the interpretation of the EKG shown in Figure 2-21?**

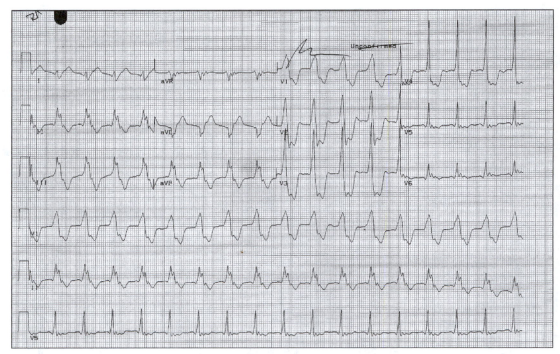

Figure 2-21

Ventricular tachycardia with a ventricular rate of 103 bpm. Note the VA conduction evidenced by the retrograde P waves, which occur in the early part of the ST segment.

○   **What is the interpretation of the EKG shown in Figure 2-22?**

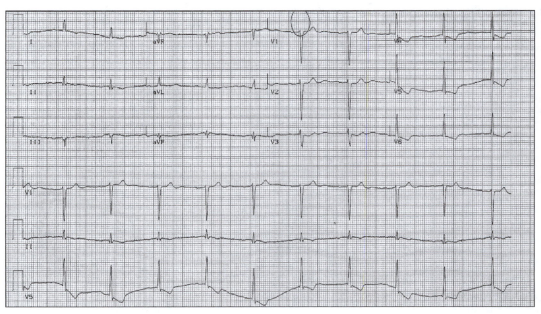

Figure 2-22

Ectopic atrial rhythm with an old inferior infarction and nonspecific ST-T abnormality.

○   **What is the interpretation of the EKG shown in Figure 2-23?**

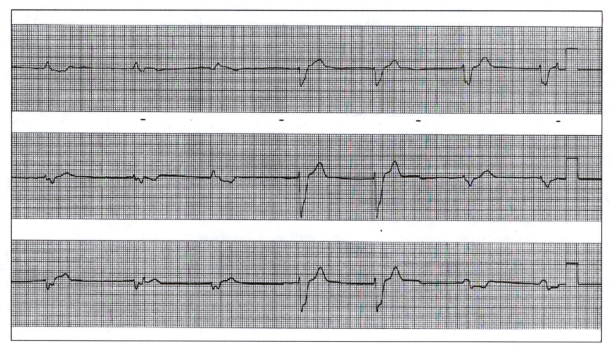

Figure 2-23

Idioventricular rhythm (rate of 40 bpm).

○   **What is the interpretation of the EKG shown in Figure 2-24?**

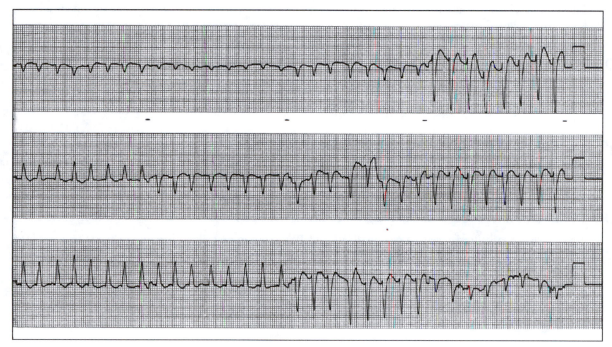

Figure 2-24

Supraventricular tachycardia.

○ **How do you treat ventricular fibrillation and pulseless ventricular tachycardia?**

Defibrillate at 360 J monophasic for the first and subsequent shocks. Continue CPR with an emphasis on chest compressions to respirations at a 30:2 ratio for 2 minutes between shocks. Epinephrine should be given at 1 mg IV/IO every 3 to 5 minutes or vasopressin 40 IU IV/IO × once and in place of the first two doses of epinephrine. Consider antidysrhythmic medications such as amiodarone 300 mg IV/IO or lidocaine (if amiodarone is not available) at 1 to 1.5 mg/kg.

○ **How do you treat pulseless electrical activity?**

Treat the underlying causes first (hypovolemia, hypoxia, hyper/hypokalemia, hypothermia, acidosis, acute MI, tamponade (cardiac), tension pneumothorax, thrombus (pulmonary), and drug overdose). If unknown cause or unsuccessful attempts to treat underlying cause, then give 1 mg of epinephrine IV/IO every 3 to 5 minutes or vasopressin 40 U IV/IO once and in place of the first two epinephrine doses. Atropine can be attempted for slow rates at 1 mg IV/IO every 3 to 5 minutes up to 3 mg maximum.

○ **How do you treat stable, narrow complex, paroxysmal supraventricular tachycardia?**

First attempt vagal maneuvers; but if there is no success, then use adenosine 6 mg rapid IV push (this can be repeated two more times up to 12 mg if needed). If adenosine fails and the ventricular function is preserved (EF >40), then use diltiazem. Other drugs could include beta-blockers, digoxin, DC cardioversion, procainamide, amiodarone, and sotalol. If the ventricular function is compromised (EF <40), then do not attempt cardioversion but attempt chemical conversion with diltiazem, amiodarone, or digoxin.

• • • CONGESTIVE HEART FAILURE • • •

○ **Which is the most common type of cardiac failure: high or low output?**

Low output failure. Reduced stroke volume, lowered pulse pressure, and peripheral vasoconstriction are all signs of low output failure.

○ **What is the most common cause of low output heart failure in the United States?**

Coronary artery disease. Other causes include congenital heart disease, cor pulmonale, dilated cardiomyopathy, hypertension, hypertrophic cardiomyopathy, infection, toxins, and valvular heart disease.

○ **Compare the mortality rate from CHF between men and women:**

Women fare slightly better. The 5-year mortality rate for women with CHF is 45% as compared to 60% for men. The majority of deaths from CHF result from ventricular dysrhythmias.

○ **Describe the three stages of chest radiographic findings in CHF:**

Stage I: Pulmonary arterial wedge pressure (PAWP) of 12 to 18 mm Hg. Blood flow increases in the upper lung fields (cephalization of pulmonary vessels).

Stage II: PAWP of 18 to 25 mm Hg. Interstitial edema is evident with blurred edges of blood vessels and Kerley B lines.

Stage III: PAWP >25 mm Hg. Fluid exudes into alveoli with the generation of the classic butterfly pattern of perihilar infiltrates.

○ **What do nitrates affect: preload or afterload?**

Predominantly preload.

○ **What does hydralazine affect: preload or afterload?**

Afterload.

○ **Do captopril, nifedipine, and prazosin affect afterload?**

Yes.

○ **When is dobutamine used in congestive heart failure?**

When heart failure is not accompanied with severe hypotension. Dobutamine is a potent inotrope with some vasodilation activity.

○ **When is dopamine selected in congestive heart failure?**

When a patient is in shock. Dopamine is a vasoconstrictor and a positive inotrope.

○ **What is the most common cause of right heart failure?**

Left ventricular heart failure.

○ **Match the sign or symptom with the most likely associated type of heart failure—left (L) or right (R):**

1. Hypotension
2. Hepatomegaly
3. Orthopnea
4. Cough
5. Dyspnea on exertion
6. Abdominal distention
7. Paroxysmal nocturnal dyspnea

8. Hemoptysis
9. S_3 gallop
10. Early satiety
11. Jugular venous distention
12. Ascites
13. Rales

(1) L, (2) R, (3) L, (4) L, (5) L, (6) R, (7) L, (8) L, (9) L, (10) R, (11) R, (12) R, (13) L.

• • • HYPERTENSION • • •

○ **What hypertensive medications should be used with caution in diabetic patients?**

Diuretics and beta-blockers should be used with caution because they may increase insulin resistance. If considered for the management of hypertension, they should not be a choice for first-line agent and be chosen only if there is a compelling indication such as heart failure or synergistic blood pressure management. ACE inhibitors and ARBs are the preferred first-line drugs of choice in diabetic patients.

○ **What antihypertensive class is most likely to present with a cough as a side effect?**

ACE inhibitors may cause a dry, persistent cough in up to 15% of patients who use them.

○ **What percentage of hypertension is secondary?**

Approximately 5%. Secondary hypertension should be suspected in patients younger than 35 years, those with sudden-onset hypertension, and those without a family history for hypertension.

○ **What is the most common cause of secondary hypertension?**

Renal parenchymal disease. In women, the most common cause is oral contraceptives. In patients older than 50 years, secondary hypertension can usually be contributed to renal artery stenosis. Other causes include pheochromocytoma, coarctation of the aorta, drugs (such as cocaine), hyperthyroidism, aldosteronism, and Cushing disease.

○ **What percentage of patients with aortic dissection are hypertensive?**

70% to 90%.

○ **What percentage of hypertensive patients are afflicted with left ventricular hypertrophy?**

50%. This is the primary reason that hypertension is a major risk factor for MI, CHF, and sudden death.

○ **What are the side effects of thiazide diuretics?**

Hyperglycemia, hyperlipidemia, hyperuricemia, hypokalemia, hypomagnesemia, and hyponatremia.

○ **Which drugs should be administered to lower the BP in a patient with thoracic aortic dissection?**

Sodium nitroprusside. A beta-blocker should also be used to reduce the dp/dt (propagation speed).

○ **A patient has a history of episodic blood pressure elevations. She complains of headache, diarrhea, and skin pallor. Probable diagnosis?**

Pheochromocytoma.

○ **What is the most common complication of nitroprusside?**

Hypotension. Thiocyanate toxicity accompanied by blurred vision, tinnitus, change in mental status, muscle weakness, and seizures is more prevalent in patients with renal failure or prolonged infusions. Cyanide toxicity is uncommon. However, this type of toxicity may occur with hepatic dysfunction, after prolonged infusions, and in rates greater than 10 mg/kg/min.

○ **Define a hypertensive emergency:**

In general, a blood pressure of $\geq 180/115$ with evidence of end organ dysfunction or damage.

○ **How quickly should a patient's blood pressure be lowered in a hypertensive emergency?**

Gradually over 2 to 3 hours to 140–160 systolic and 90–110 diastolic. To prevent cerebral hypoperfusion, the blood pressure should not be decreased by more than 25% of the mean arterial pressure.

○ **What drug is preferred for treatment of a hypertensive emergency?**

Sodium nitroprusside. It assists in relaxing smooth muscle tissue through the production of cGMP. As a result, there is decreased preload and afterload, decreased oxygen demand, and a slightly increased heart rate with no change in myocardial blood flow, cardiac output, or renal blood flow. The duration of action is 1 to 2 minutes. Sometimes, beta-blocker is required to treat rebound tachycardia.

○ **Define a hypertensive urgency:**

In general, a blood pressure of ≥180/115 without evidence of end organ dysfunction or damage. Blood pressure reduction in these individuals should be done gradually over 24 to 48 hours.

○ **What laboratory findings can assist in confirming end organ compromise in a hypertensive emergency?**
- Urinalysis: RBCs, red cell casts, and proteinuria
- BUN and CR: Elevated
- X-ray: Cardiomegaly, aortic dissection, pulmonary edema, or coarctation of aorta
- EKG: LVH and cardiac ischemia

○ **What are the signs of symptoms of hypertensive encephalopathy?**

Nausea, vomiting, headache, lethargy, coma, blindness, nerve palsies, hemiparesis, aphasia, retinal hemorrhage, cotton wool spots, exudates, sausage linking, and papilledema. Treat with labetalol or sodium nitroprusside and lower the mean arterial pressure to approximately 120 mm Hg.

○ **What is the first-line pharmacologic therapy for a 40-year-old obese white woman with uncomplicated mild hypertension?**

ACE inhibitors or a thiazide diuretic. Beta-blockers, ARBs, or calcium channel blockers could be considered if contraindications to ACEI or diuretics.

○ **What is the preferred choice of antihypertensive therapy for a 58-year-old white man with severe COPD and mild hypertension?**

Long-acting calcium channel blockers such as amlodipine, diltiazem, or nifedipine. These agents are particularly useful in patients with a likelihood of pulmonary hypertension. If pulmonary hypertension is suspected, verapamil should be avoided because of its significant negative inotropic effects.

○ **What is the agent of choice in diabetic patients with hypertension?**

ACE inhibitors or ARBs.

○ **Which agent is more likely to cause bradycardia: verapamil or diltiazem?**

Diltiazem. Diltiazem blocks conduction through both the SA and AV node, whereas verapamil blocks only the AV node.

○ **What antihypertensive agents are preferred agents to use in a 63-year-old obese, African American man?**

Calcium channel blockers. Diuretics and/or ACE inhibitors can be considered too.

○ **What is the most common side effect of esmolol, labetalol, and bretylium?**

Hypotension.

○ **What side effect can occur with a rapid infusion of procainamide?**

Hypotension. Other side effects include QRS/QT prolongation, ventricular fibrillation, and torsades de pointes.

○ **What is one of the most common side effect of antihypertensive medications that patients should be warned about?**

Orthostatic hypotension

○ **How long can ST and T *wave changes* persist after an episode of pain in unstable angina?**

Several hours.

○ **What are the diagnostic criteria for a Q wave?**

More than 0.04 seconds and at least one-quarter the size of the R wave in the same lead. Beware, EKGs can be normal in up to 10% of all acute MIs.

○ **What is the cause of Prinzmetal angina?**

Coronary artery vasospasm with or without fixed stenotic lesions. Prinzmetal angina is more often associated with ST segment elevation than with depression. Calcium channel blockers are the drugs of choice to treat this condition. Beta-blockers are contraindicated in patients with vasospasm without fixed stenotic lesions.

○ **Eighty to ninety percent of patients who experience sudden nontraumatic cardiac death are in what rhythm?**

Ventricular fibrillation. Early defibrillation is the key. In an acute MI, the infarction zone becomes electrically unstable. Ventricular fibrillation is most common during original coronary occlusion or when the coronaries begin to reperfuse.

○ **What is the rate of restenosis after percutaneous transluminal coronary angioplasty (PTCA)?**

20% to 30% within the first 6 months, but bare metal and drug-eluding stents have greatly reduced restenosis rates. PTCA is now rarely used by itself but commonly used prior to stent placement.

○ **What two drugs are commonly used to reduce thrombosis formation in a patient who has received an intracoronary stent?**

Aspirin and clopidogrel.

○ **What is the restenosis rate of coronary vessels following a coronary artery bypass graft (CABG)?**

When using venous grafts, there is a 50% restenosis rate within 5 to 10 years. When an artery is used, such as the internal mammary artery, the restenosis rate drops to 5% at 10 years. Occlusion of the grafts is caused by anastomy, trauma to the vessel, postoperative adhesions, or atherosclerosis.

○ **How are acute MI, angina pectoralis, and Prinzmetal angina differentiated?**

The pain is similar but typically differs in radiation, duration, provocation, and palliation. Obtaining an accurate history is the most important tool for diagnosing chest pain.

- Angina pectoralis is aggravated by exercise, cold, and excitement but is relieved with rest and nitroglycerin.
- Prinzmetal angina occurs at rest during normal activity, and generally at night or in the early morning. It lasts longer than angina pectoralis.
- Acute MIs produce pain with a greater radius of radiation that may last for hours.

○ **Which type of myocardial infarction is more often associated with thrombosis: transmural or subendocardial?**

Transmural. Thrombolytic therapy increases left ventricular ejection fraction post-MI, reduces the development of postinfarction CHF, and can reduce early MI mortality by 25%.

○ **How much aspirin should a post-MI patient take daily to reduce the incidence of reinfarction?**

75 to 150 mg daily.

○ **What is the most common cause of death during the first few hours of a MI?**

Cardiac dysrhythmias, generally ventricular fibrillation.

○ **When treating early MIs, beta-blockers decrease the risk of reinfarction. Which patients should not receive beta-blockers?**

Patients presenting with hypotension, congestive heart failure, severe left ventricular dysfunction, AV block, bradycardia, asthma, or other bronchospastic disease.

○ **How common are PVCs in post-MI patients?**

90% will have PVCs within the first few weeks. Concern arises if the PVCs are complex, which is the case in 20% to 40% of MI patients. Risk of sudden death in post-MI patients with complex PVCs increases two to five times.

○ **What percentage of the LV myocardium must be damaged to induce cardiogenic shock?**

40%. Twenty-five percent or greater damage to the heart typically results in heart failure.

○ **What percentage of MIs are clinically unrecognized?**

5% to 10%.

○ **A non–Q-wave infarction is usually associated with what?**

Subsequent angina or recurrent infarction. Non–Q-wave infarctions also have lower in-hospital mortality rate compared to Q-wave MIs.

○ **Why do T waves invert in an acute myocardial infarction?**

Infarction or ischemia causes a reversal of the sequence of repolarization, i.e., endocardial-to-epicardial as opposed to normally epicardial-to-endocardial.

○   **What EKG changes arise in a true posterior infarction?**

Large R wave and ST depression in V_1 and V_2.

○   **What conduction defects commonly occur in an anterior wall MI?**

The dangerous kind. Damage to the conducting system results in a Mobitz type II second- or third-degree AV block.

○   **How should PSVT be treated during an acute myocardial infarction?**

Adenosine, cardioversion, or vagal maneuvers could be attempted. Stable patients may be able to tolerate negative inotropes such as calcium channel blockers (verapamil) or even beta-blockers.

○   **A patient presents 1 day after discharge for an acute myocardial infarction with a new harsh systolic ejection murmur along the left sternal border and pulmonary edema. What is the diagnosis?**

Ventricular septal rupture. Diagnosis is made by either a Swan-Ganz catheterization or echocardiogram. These patients often present with cardiogenic shock.

○   **When does cardiac rupture usually occur in patients who have suffered acute MIs?**

50% arise within the first 5 days and 90% occur within the first 14 days post-MI.

○   **Which type of infarct commonly leads to papillary muscle dysfunction?**

Inferior wall MI. Signs and symptoms include a mild transient systolic murmur and pulmonary edema.

○   **A patient presents 2 weeks post–acute MI with chest pain, fever, and pleuropericarditis. A pleural effusion is detected on chest radiography. What is the diagnosis?**

Dressler (post–myocardial infarction) syndrome. This syndrome is caused by an immunologic reaction to myocardial antigens.

○   **What percentage of patients older than 80 years experience chest pain with an acute myocardial infarction?**

Only 50%. Twenty percent experience diaphoresis, stroke, syncope, and/or acute confusion.

○   **What three secondary processes resulting in myocardial deterioration occur following acute myocardial infarction?**

Ventricular remodeling, typically following Q-wave infarctions; infarct expansion, occurring most frequently from anteroapical infarctions and results in thinning of the left ventricular wall; and ventricular dilatation, an early and progressive response to acute myocardial infarction that is an important predictor of increased mortality following myocardial infarction.

○   **What is the most common cause of death related to acute myocardial infarction?**

Ventricular fibrillation, usually occurring within the first hour following symptoms.

○ **What percentage of patients with acute myocardial infarction develop cardiogenic shock?**

10%.

○ **What percentage of arteries successfully opened with thrombolytic therapy for acute myocardial infarction, reocclude?**

15% of arteries successfully opened reocclude during the first few days following thrombolytic therapy.

○ **What is the mortality benefit from aspirin alone in acute myocardial infarction with thrombolytic therapy and in subsequent reinfarction?**

Aspirin reduced mortality from acute myocardial infarction by 23% and reduced nonfatal reinfarction by 49%. When used with thrombolytic therapy, there was a 40% to 50% reduction in mortality from acute myocardial infarction.

○ **A 63-year-old man presents to the emergency department with moderate substernal chest pressure and lightheadedness for 90 minutes. His BP on admission is 80/40 and his HR is 110 bpm and regular. Physical examination reveals JVD to the angle of the jaw, a right parasternal S_3 gallop, an apical S_4 gallop, and clear lungs on auscultation. EKG reveals 2 mm ST elevation in leads II, III, and aVF with reciprocal ST depression in V_1 through V_3. What is the most likely diagnosis and what is the most appropriate initial therapy?**

Inferior wall myocardial infarction with right ventricular infarction. Initial therapy includes 160 to 325 mg of aspirin administration, thrombolytic therapy, and a large bolus of intravenous saline followed by a moderately high infusion rate of saline. If the patient remains hypotensive despite adequate infusion of saline (typically measured by development of lung congestion on auscultation), then intravenous dobutamine is indicated.

○ **A 70-year-old man is admitted to the hospital with chest pain of 3 hours duration. EKG demonstrates anterior ST elevation for which he is given aspirin, r-TPA, heparin, and intravenous nitroglycerin. His symptoms resolve. Serum chemistries reveal a peak CPK of 1800 and CK-MB fraction of 15%. The patient is eventually transferred out of the CCU and his hospitalization is uneventful until day 5, when he develops sudden, severe shortness of breath. BP is 110/75 and his pulse is 125 bpm and regular. Examination reveals a new systolic murmur. What would the most appropriate therapeutic intervention be?**

Intravenous sodium nitroprusside. This patient is most likely suffering from rupture of the left ventricular septum and subsequent defect—a not uncommon complication of MI. Afterload reduction is key to stabilization until surgical repair of the VSD can be performed, usually in about 8 to 12 weeks, after the infarct has healed. If nitroprusside fails to stabilize the patient, intra-aortic balloon counterpulsation and intravenous nitroglycerin should be employed.

○ **A 60-year-old patient suffers an acute inferior myocardial infarction. Three hours after he arrives in the hospital, he develops ventricular fibrillation and is successfully defibrillated back to normal sinus rhythm within 30 seconds. He makes a full recovery and has no further post-MI complications. What does his ventricular fibrillation episode indicate with regard to subsequent risk for sudden death?**

This episode has no bearing on his subsequent risk of sudden death. Ventricular fibrillation in the immediate setting of an acute myocardial infarction has no prognostic significance.

○ **A 65-year-old female patient presents to the hospital with sudden crushing chest discomfort and moderate shortness of breath. Her initial EKG reveals 2 mm ST depression in leads V_1 through V_4 and inverted T waves. She has bibasilar rales in the lower half of both lungs on auscultation. CXR reveals moderate pulmonary edema. Serial EKGs, CPKs, and troponins confirm a non–Q-wave myocardial infarction. With diuretics, her pulmonary edema resolves within 24 hours. What is the most appropriate management strategy at this point?**

Cardiac catheterization with coronary angiography. A non–Q-wave MI that results in pulmonary edema signifies a larger amount of myocardium at risk for reinfarction within the next year.

○ **What arrhythmias that occur in patients with acute myocardial infarction require temporary pacing?**

Complete heart block; new left bundle branch block; new bifascicular block; marked sinus bradycardia with ischemic pain, hypotension, CHF, frequent PVCs or syncope despite atropine; and Mobitz II second-degree AV block.

○ **A 54-year-old man, admitted 2 days ago with an acute anterolateral myocardial infarction, suddenly develops atrial fibrillation with a ventricular rate of 135 bpm. He subsequently complains of substernal chest discomfort. His BP is 135/70. What is the most appropriate immediate action to be taken?**

Synchronized DC cardioversion.

○ **What percentage of patients with acute myocardial infarction develop paroxysmal atrial fibrillation?**

10% to 15%.

○ **A 58-year-old man is admitted with an acute anteroseptal myocardial infarction. He is in pulmonary edema clinically, confirmed by chest radiography. His blood pressure is 122/76, his HR is 122. Despite two doses of 80 mg of intravenous furosemide, he remains in pulmonary edema. A Swan-Ganz pulmonary artery catheter is inserted and his initial hemodynamics reveal a cardiac output of 3.1 L/min and a pulmonary capillary wedge pressure of 27 mm Hg. What is the most appropriate pharmacologic agent in this setting?**

Intravenous dobutamine, at a dose of 5 to 20 μg/kg/min.

○ **What are the major complications of left ventricular aneurysms?**

LV thrombus formation (with subsequent risk of thromboembolic events), CHF, and ventricular arrhythmias.

○ **What is the current recommended therapy for patients with large anterior myocardial infarctions?**

Reperfusion therapy with thrombolytics, beta-blockers, intravenous nitroglycerin, and ACE inhibitors to limit and retard ventricular remodeling. Intravenous heparin in a sufficient dose to prolong the APTT to 1.5 to 2.0 times control should be started on admission and continued to discharge. In patients with large akinetic apical segments or mural thrombi, oral anticoagulation with warfarin is indicated for at least 6 months.

○ **What is the significance of pericarditis following acute myocardial infarction?**

Pericarditis occurs in about 20% of patients with acute myocardial infarction, more likely in Q-wave infarcts than non–Q-wave infarcts. Patients with pericarditis usually have significantly larger infarcts, lower ejection fractions, and a higher incidence of congestive heart failure. The presence of pericarditis and/or pericardial effusion following acute myocardial infarction is associated with higher mortality.

○ **A previously healthy 65-year-old man is admitted with an acute inferior myocardial infarction. Within several hours, he is hypotensive (BP 90/60) and oliguric. Insertion of a pulmonary artery catheter reveals the following pressure: pulmonary artery wedge pressure, 3 mm Hg; pulmonary artery, 21/3 mm Hg; and mean right atrial pressure, 11 mm Hg. What is the best treatment for this man?**

Fluids until his wedge pressure is between 16 and 20 mm Hg.

○ **A 60-year-old man with a recent syncopal episode is hospitalized with congestive heart failure and chest pain. His BP is 165/85 mm Hg, his pulse is 85 bpm, and there is a grade III/VI harsh systolic murmur at the apex and aortic area. An echocardiogram reveals a disproportionately thickened septum and anterior systolic motion of the mitral valve. What is this patient's diagnosis and what physical findings would most likely be present?**

Idiopathic obstructive hypertrophic cardiomyopathy (IHSS). The murmur typically decreases with handgrip and squatting and increases with Valsalva, vasodilators, standing, nitroglycerin, diuretics, and digoxin. Mitral regurgitation is frequent as a result of anterior systolic motion of the mitral valve. Congestive heart failure is present because of diastolic dysfunction, thus a S_4 gallop is common.

○ **In patients with coronary artery disease, which patients have been shown to benefit from revascularization with bypass grafting?**

Patients with left main coronary artery disease (>50% stenosis) and those with three vessel coronary artery disease (>70% stenosis) with depressed LV function (<40% EF).

○ **What are the classic EKG results associated with posterior MI?**

A large R wave in leads V_1 and V_2, ST depression in leads V_1 and V_2, Q waves in the inferior leads and, occasionally, ST elevation in the inferior leads.

○ **What is the most common complication of extracorporeal circulation?**

Stroke occurs in 1% to 2% of patients after open heart operations. Other postoperative complications are arrhythmias, bleeding, renal failure, and respiratory complications.

○ **What drug is used to reverse heparin after open heart surgery?**

Protamine.

○ **In 90% of the population, the right coronary artery terminates as the:**

Posterior descending artery.

○ **The left main coronary artery gives rise to which two coronary arteries?**

The left anterior descending artery and the left circumflex coronary artery.

○ **What is the vessel of preference in coronary bypass grafting?**

The internal mammary artery. Other artery grafts such as the radial artery are preferred too. Arterial grafts tend to have higher rates of patency at 10 years compared to venous grafts. Venous grafts are also more susceptible to atherosclerotic disease.

● ● ● **VASCULAR DISEASE** ● ● ●

○ **Are aortic aneurysms more common in men or women?**

Men (10:1 male-to-female ratio). Other risk factors include hypertension, atherosclerosis, diabetes, hyperlipidemia, smoking, syphilis, Marfan disease, and Ehlers-Danlos disease.

○ **A patient presents with sudden-onset chest and back pain. Further work-up reveals an ischemic right leg. What is your diagnosis?**

Suspect an acute aortic dissection when chest or back pain is associated with ischemic and/or neurologic deficits.

○ **What physical findings suggest an acute aortic dissection?**

Blood pressure and pulse differences between arms and/or legs, cardiac tamponade, and aortic insufficiency murmur.

○ **What CXR findings occur with a thoracic aortic aneurysm?**

Change in aortic appearance, mediastinal widening, hump in the aortic arch, pleural effusion (most commonly on the left), and extension of the aortic shadow.

○ **A 74-year-old male patient presents with acute-onset testicular pain. Ecchymosis is present in the groin and scrotal sac. What is the diagnosis?**

A ruptured aortic or iliac artery aneurysm.

○ **What X-ray study should be ordered for a patient with an abdominal mass and a suspected ruptured abdominal aortic aneurysm?**

None! The patient should go to the operating room immediately. About 60% of AAAs occur with calcification and appear on a lateral abdominal X-ray.

○ **What may an X-ray of a patient with an aortic dissection reveal?**

Widening of the superior mediastinum, a hazy or enlarged aortic knob, an irregular aortic contour, separation of the intimal calcification from the outer aortic contour that is greater than 5 mm, a displaced trachea to the right, and cardiomegaly.

○ **What is the most common symptom of aortic dissection?**

Interscapular back pain.

○ **Where do aortic dissections most often occur?**

Proximal ascending aorta (60%). Twenty percent of aortic dissections are found between the origin of the left subclavian and the ligamentum arteriosum in the descending aorta, and 10% are found in the aortic arch or the abdominal aorta. Dissection involves intimal tears propagated by hematoma formation.

○ **What aortic aneurysm diameter is generally considered to be an indication for surgery for an aneurysm in the (a) in the thorax and (b) in the abdomen?**

Those with a nondissecting thoracic aneurysm larger than 7 cm in diameter are candidates for surgery. However, surgery should be considered with smaller aneurysms for those with Marfan syndrome because of higher incidence of rupture. Nondissecting abdominal aortic aneurysms larger than 4 cm in diameter should be considered for surgical repair.

○ **Describe the Stanford classification of aortic dissections:**

Stanford type A: Always involves the ascending aorta but could include the descending aorta.

Stanford type B: Involves the descending aorta only.

○ **What dissections can be treated medically?**

Patients with Stanford type B and (type III) are eligible for medical, rather than, surgical treatment. Surgical treatment may be required for those with uncontrollable pain, aortic bleeding, hemodynamic instability, increasing hematoma size, or an impending rupture.

○ **What is the prognosis of an untreated aortic dissection?**

20% of afflicted individuals die within 24 hours, 60% within 2 weeks, and 90% within 3 months. With surgical treatment, the 10-year survival rate is 40%. Redissection occurs in 25% of these patients within 10 years of the original episode.

○ **Where is the most common site of peripheral aneurysms that develop from arteriosclerosis?**

The popliteal artery. Other sites include the femoral, carotid, and subclavian arteries.

○ **What artery is usually affected by arterial occlusive disease in diabetic patients?**

The popliteal artery. Because of diabetic neuropathy and the potential for the development of a necrotizing infection in a leg with compromised circulation, it is very important that patients with diabetes are knowledgeable about pedal hygiene.

○ **What is the Budd-Chiari syndrome?**

Thrombosis in the hepatic vein resulting in abdominal pain, jaundice, and ascites.

○ **Which arteries are most commonly involved in giant cell arteritis (chronic inflammation of the large blood vessels)?**

The carotid arteries and its branches. Treatment includes high doses of corticosteroids.

○ **What is the most common source of acute mesenteric ischemia?**

Arterial embolism (40%–50%). The source is usually the heart, generally from mural thrombus. The most common point of obstruction is the superior mesenteric artery.

○ **What laboratory results strongly suggest that a patient has mesenteric ischemia?**

Leukocytosis >15,000, metabolic acidosis (sometimes with anion gap), hemoconcentration, and elevated phosphate and amylase.

○ **Describe the Trendelenburg test for varicose veins:**

Raise the leg above the heart and then quickly lower it. If the leg veins become distended immediately after this test is performed, valvular incompetency is evident.

○ **A 68-year-old male patient with diabetes and a 60 pack-year history of smoking presents with sudden, severe substernal chest discomfort, radiating through the interscapular area. His BP is 158/80 mm Hg in the right arm and 135/65 mm Hg in the left arm. He complains of right arm numbness and weakness and you hear a grade II/VI diastolic murmur along the left sternal border. EKG reveals 1.5 mm ST elevation in the inferior leads. What is the diagnosis?**

Acute proximal thoracic aortic dissection, with involvement of the right coronary artery and brachiocephalic artery, as well as acute aortic regurgitation.

○ **In the patient described in the last question, what other life-threatening complication must one look for, both on auscultation and on chest radiograph?**

Pericardial effusion with cardiac tamponade. Listen for a pericardial rub on auscultation and look for marked cardiomegaly on CXR. Pulsus paradoxus of >10 mm Hg is virtually diagnostic of cardiac tamponade in this setting.

○ **What CXR findings occur with a dissecting thoracic aortic aneurysm?**

Tortuosity of the proximal aorta with an enlarged aortic knob, mediastinal widening, pleural effusion (most common on the left), extension of the aortic shadow, displaced trachea to the right, cardiomegaly, and separation of the intimal calcification from the outer contour that is greater than 5 mm.

○ **What is the prognosis for an untreated dissecting aortic aneurysm?**

25% die within 24 hours, 50% die within one week, 75% die within 1 month, and 90% die within 3 months. With surgical treatment, the 10-year survival is 50%, the 5-year survival is 75% to 80%. Redissection occurs in 25% of patients within 10 years of the original dissection.

○ **What is an ABI and why is it significant?**

An ankle/brachial index is the ankle systolic pressure (numerator) compared to the brachial systolic pressure (denominator). It is used as a screening tool for determining the presence of obstructive arterial disease of the lower extremities. A positive ABI is also considered an independent risk factor for coronary artery disease.

○ **What technical factors can affect the accuracy of the ABI?**

Probe pressure, rapid deflation of the BP cuff, arterial wall calcifications, and probe placement, which should be longitudinal to the vessel and at a 30- to 60-degree angle to the skin surface.

○ **Matching:**

1. Quinke pulse	a. Uvular pulsation during systole
2. Corrigan pulse	b. Head bobbing
3. de Musset sign	c. Visible pulsations in nail bed capillaries
4. Muller sign	d. Collapsing pulse
5. Duroziez sign	e. Drop in the systolic blood pressure >10 mm Hg with inspiration
6. Pulsus paradoxus	f. Femoral artery murmurs during systole if the artery is compressed proximally and during diastole if the artery is compressed distally

(1) c, (2) d, (3) b, (4) a, (5) f, and (6) e. These are all signs pertaining to aortic insufficiency.

• • • CONGENITAL HEART DISEASE • • •

○ **What are the more common symptoms of a child with an atrial septal defect (ASD)?**

In most cases, the patient is asymptomatic. In later teen to adult years, the patient may complain of mild fatigue or dyspnea. In rare cases, heart failure is present.

○ **What is the typical murmur that is heard in a patient with an ASD?**

A midsystolic crescendo–decrescendo over the left upper sternal border.

○ **A 5-month-old male infant is brought to the pediatrician's office because the mother is concerned about his feeding. She notes that the child appears to be short of breath, has poor weight gain, and his feeding is about half of what it should be. On physical examination, you note that his weight is in the 35th percentile, and a gallop is present on auscultation. There is also a slight murmur detected on the intrascapular region of the back on the left side. What is the most likely diagnosis?**

Coarctation of the aorta.

○ **What is the difference between the pressures of the upper half of the body compared to the lower in a patient with a coarctation of the aorta?**

The pulse pressures in the upper arms will be strong, while the lower extremities will be diminished or in some cases not detected by Doppler.

○ **What is the most common extracardiac congenital anomaly found in children?**

Patent ductus arteriosus (PDA).

○ **What is the most characteristic physical examination finding in an infant with a PDA?**

The infant will have a systolic thrill that is felt over the pulmonary artery and suprasternal notch. The child will also have a machine-like continuous murmur over the left upper sternal border.

○ **Name the four defects that are characteristic of tetralogy of Fallot:**

1. Ventricular septal defect (VSD)
2. Right ventricular hypertrophy
3. RV outflow obstruction from infundibular stenosis (pulmonary valve)
4. Overriding aorta (<50%); a right-sided aortic arch is seen in 25%

○ **What is the preferred test to determine if a child has tetralogy of Fallot?**

Echocardiogram.

○ **What is the most common congenital cardiac anomaly?**

Ventricular Septal Defect (VSD).

○ **Describe symptoms that can present in a child with a VSD:**

The size of the defect will determine the degree of symptoms. Small defects in children may not produce any symptoms, but clinical deterioration may occur at any time. In patients with a large defect, parents may describe grunting, sweating, failure to gain weight, tachypnea, and fatigue.

○ **What are some of the physical examination characteristics found in a patient with a VSD?**

The patient may have some respiratory distress, a thrill at the left lower sternal border (common), S_2 splits, S_3 is common, and a holosystolic murmur at the apex is common. Hepatic enlargement may also be present.

○ **What percentage of VSDs will resolve with conservative medical management?**

About 70% of small defects. Larger defects will either be monitored with symptoms and close examinations, or by surgical correction early in the child's life.

○ **What murmur is expected in patients with substantial aortic stenosis?**

A prolonged, harsh, loud (IV, V, or VI) systolic murmur.

○ **What is the most common cause of aortic regurgitation in adults?**

Mild aortic regurgitation frequently develops as a result of a bicuspid aortic valve. A severe aortic valve regurgitation is induced by rheumatic heart disease, syphilis, endocarditis, trauma, an idiopathic degeneration of the aortic valve, a spontaneous rupture of the valve leaflets, or aortic dissection.

○ **What are the signs and symptoms of acute aortic regurgitation?**

Dyspnea, tachycardia, tachypnea, and chest pain.

○ **What is the most common cause of aortic stenosis in patients younger than 50 years and older than 50 years?**

- Younger than 50: Calcification of congenital bicuspid aortic valves (1% of the population has congenital bicuspid valves).
- Older than 50: Calcification of degenerating leaflets.

○ **What triad of symptoms characterizes aortic stenosis?**

Syncope, angina, and left heart failure. As the disease progresses, systolic BP decreases and pulse pressure narrows.

○ **What are the findings in a patient with aortic stenosis?**

Angina, dyspnea on exertion, syncope, sustained apical impulse, narrow pulse pressure, parvus et tardus, systolic ejection crescendo–decrescendo murmur that radiates to the neck, systolic ejection click (not heard in severe cases when the valve is so stenosed that it is immobile), paradoxically split S_1 and soft S_2, and audible S_4.

○ **How does the heart murmur reflect the severity of aortic stenosis?**

A longer duration associated with an increase in intensity indicates severe aortic stenosis. The "loudness" of the murmur is not as important in assessing its severity.

○ **A patient presents to the hospital 1 month after placement of a mechanical prosthetic valve with fever, chills, and a leukocytosis. Endocarditis is suspected. Which bacterium is most commonly encountered in this situation?**

Staphylococcus aureus or *Staphylococcus epidermidis*.

O **What percentage of non-anticoagulated patients with mitral stenosis experience system emboli?**

About 25%. Patients with chronic atrial fibrillation or mitral stenosis should be chronically anticoagulated to prevent atrial mural thrombi.

O **What is the most common cause of mitral stenosis?**

Rheumatic heart disease. The most common initial symptom is dyspnea.

O **What physical findings may be associated with mitral stenosis?**

Prominent *a*-wave, early systolic left parasternal lift, loud and snapping first heart sound, and early diastolic opening snap with a low-pitched middiastolic rumble that crescendos into S_1.

O **A midsystolic click with a late systolic crescendo murmur is indicative of what cardiac disease?**

Mitral valve prolapse (MVP). This is the hallmark sign of MVP.

O **Is mitral valve prolapse more common among men or women?**

Women have a stronger genetic link to the disease. However, only 2% to 5% of the entire population has symptomatic MVP.

O **What age group typically develops MVP syndrome?**

Patients in their twenties and thirties. Most patients with MVP are asymptomatic. MVP syndrome is symptomatic with chest pain, fatigue, palpitations, postural syncope, and dizziness.

O **Rheumatic heart disease is the most common cause of stenosis of what three heart valves?**

Mitral, aortic (along with congenital bicuspid valve), and tricuspid.

O **What is the most frequent cause of mitral stenosis?**

Rheumatic fever. Far less common causes include congenital, malignant carcinoid, SLE, rheumatoid arthritis, infective endocarditis with large vegetation, and the mucopolysaccharidoses of the Hunter-Hurley phenotype.

O **What percentage of patients with rheumatic heart disease have pure mitral stenosis?**

25%. An additional 40% have combined MS and MR.

O **What are the principal symptoms in mitral stenosis?**

Dyspnea is the most common. Patients with severe mitral stenosis can experience orthopnea, hemoptysis, chest pain, and frank pulmonary edema, often precipitated by exertion, fever, URI, sexual intercourse, pregnancy, or the onset of rapid atrial fibrillation.

O **What are two most serious complications of mitral stenosis?**

Thromboembolism, most often occurring in the setting of atrial fibrillation, and pulmonary edema.

○ **What maneuvers can one do to differentiate the opening snap of mitral stenosis from a split S_2 sound?**

Sudden standing widens the A_2-opening snap interval whereas a split S_2 narrows on standing. Progressive narrowing of the A_2-opening snap interval on serial examinations suggests an increase in the severity of mitral stenosis.

○ **What is the most accurate noninvasive technique for quantifying the severity of mitral stenosis?**

Doppler echocardiography.

○ **What is the medical management strategy of rheumatic mitral stenosis?**

- Penicillin prophylaxis for beta-hemolytic streptococcal infections and prophylaxis for infective endocarditis
- Aggressive and prompt treatment of anemia and infections
- Avoidance of strenuous exertion
- Oral diuretics and sodium restriction in symptomatic patients
- Beta-blockers to reduce heart rate
- Cardioversion of atrial fibrillation
- Aggressive slowing of refractory atrial fibrillation
- Anticoagulant therapy in patients who have experienced one or more thromboembolic episodes, or who have mechanical prosthetic valves

○ **What is the symptomatic period after an attack of rheumatic fever in patients with mitral stenosis?**

In temperate zones, such as the United States and Europe, about 15 to 20 years. In tropical and subtropical areas and in underdeveloped areas, about 6 to 12 years.

○ **What is the indication for mitral valve surgery or balloon valvuloplasty in patients with mitral stenosis?**

Moderate symptoms (class II) or greater in a patient with moderate to severe mitral stenosis (mitral valve orifice size of less than 1.0 cm^2 per square meter BSA or less than 1.5 to 1.7 cm^2 mitral valve area in normal adults).

○ **A 28-year-old Hispanic woman is referred to you for evaluation of dyspnea and palpitations. She has a diastolic murmur consistent with mitral stenosis. Echocardiography confirms severe, noncalcific mitral stenosis with trivial mitral regurgitation, with a mitral valve area of 0.8 cm^2. EKG reveals atrial fibrillation. What is the most appropriate course of therapy for this patient?**

Open mitral valvotomy (commissurotomy) followed by cardioversion to normal sinus rhythm. This is palliative, obviates the need for anticoagulation for the immediate future, and results in at least 5 to 10 years of symptom-free life for over half of the patients.

○ **What is the most common cause of mitral regurgitation?**

Rheumatic fever. It is more frequent in men than women. Other causes include infective endocarditis, mitral valve prolapse, ischemic heart disease, trauma, SLE, scleroderma, hypertrophic cardiomyopathy, dilated cardiomyopathy involving the left ventricle, and idiopathic degenerative calcification of the mitral annulus.

○ **What are the physical findings of patients with chronic mitral regurgitation?**

Harsh, pansystolic murmur heard best at the apex, radiating to the axilla or the base. The murmur is diminished by maneuvers that decrease preload or afterload, such as amyl nitrate inhalation, Valsalva, or standing, and increases with maneuvers that increase preload or afterload, such as squatting, handgrip, or phenylephrine administration.

○ **What are the most common causes of acute mitral regurgitation?**

Acute myocardial infarction with papillary muscle dysfunction (15% of acute MI results in acute mitral regurgitation) or papillary muscle rupture (3% of acute MI), infective endocarditis, chordate tendinea rupture secondary to chest trauma, rheumatic fever, mitral valve prolapsed, and hypertrophic cardiomyopathy with rupture of chordate tendinea.

○ **Which is the best test to assess the detailed anatomy of rheumatic mitral valve disease and determine whether mitral valve replacement is necessary or whether reconstruction is feasible?**

Transesophageal echocardiography.

○ **What is the appropriate medical management of mitral regurgitation?**

Vasodilator therapy with ACE inhibitors is the hallmark of therapy, even in patients who are asymptomatic. Diuretics are used in patients with severe MR. Cardiac glycosides, such as digoxin, are indicated in patients with severe MR and clinical evidence of heart failure. Endocarditis prophylaxis is indicated in all patients with MR. Anticoagulation should be given to all patients in atrial fibrillation.

○ **A 33-year-old female patient comes to you for a physical examination and you notice a harsh systolic murmur at the apex that is also heard at the base. The murmur increases on standing and Valsalva and decreases with handgrip. What is the most likely finding on echocardiography?**

Mitral valve prolapse. The murmur of pure mitral regurgitation decreases with Valsalva and standing and increases with handgrip or squatting.

○ **A 46-year-old male patient with a history of rheumatic fever at age 12 is admitted with an acute myocardial infarction. The patient's post-MI course is complicated by congestive heart failure. Echocardiogram reveals severe mitral regurgitation with rupture of one of the papillary muscles and prolapsed posterior mitral valve leaflet without apparent calcification. Systolic function by echocardiogram is mildly reduced. What is the appropriate course of action in this patient?**

Mitral valve reconstruction and repair of the papillary muscle.

○ **What is the classic triad of symptoms of aortic stenosis?**

Syncope (often exertional), angina, and heart failure.

○ **What is the most common cause of aortic stenosis in patients younger than 65 years?**

Calcification of congenitally bicuspid aortic valves (50%) followed by rheumatic heart disease (25%).

○ **What is the most common cause of aortic stenosis in patients older than 65 years?**

Calcific degeneration of the aortic leaflets.

○ **Once patients with aortic stenosis become symptomatic, what is their average survival without valve replacement?**

From the onset of syncope and/or angina, the mean survival is 2 to 3 years. From the onset of congestive heart failure, the mean survival is 1.5 years.

○ **How does the heart murmur reflect the severity of aortic stenosis?**

The longer the duration of the murmur and the greater the increase in intensity of the murmur, the more severe the aortic stenosis. The degree of loudness of the murmur is not as important in assessing severity.

○ **What is the best pharmacologic agent for patients with asymptomatic aortic stenosis?**

Without contraindications, beta-blockers are the best agents as they are the most useful in treating left ventricular hypertrophy and its sequelae that develop as a result of aortic stenosis.

○ **A 68-year-old female patient with severe asymptomatic aortic stenosis suddenly complains of dyspnea and palpitations. On EKG, she is found to be in atrial fibrillation with a ventricular rate of 130 bpm. What is the most appropriate action to be taken?**

Immediate DC cardioversion followed by a search for previously unrecognized mitral valve disease. Once stabilized, the patient should be referred for cardiac catheterization and aortic valve replacement.

○ **What is a mitral valve prolapsed syndrome?**

A symptom complex consisting of palpitations, chest pain, easy fatigability, exercise intolerance, dyspnea, orthostatic phenomena, and syncope or presyncope in patients with mitral valve prolapsed, predominately related to autonomic dysfunction.

○ **What disorders are seen with increased frequency in patients with MVP syndrome?**

Graves disease, asthma, migraine headaches, sleep disorders, fibromyositis, and functional gastrointestinal syndromes.

○ **What is the most common cause of isolated severe aortic regurgitation?**

Aortic root dilatation resulting from medial disease. Other common causes include congenital (bicuspid) aortic valve, previous infective endocarditis, and rheumatic heart disease.

○ **What is the survival rate of chronic aortic regurgitation after diagnosis?**

The 5-year survival, after diagnosis, is 75%. The 10-year survival is 50%. Once symptoms begin, without surgical treatment, death occurs within 4 years after the development of angina, 2 years after the development of CHG.

○ **What is the preferred pharmacologic agent in patients with asymptomatic chronic aortic regurgitation?**

Nifedipine or ACE inhibitors. Both have major improvements in LVEF and major reduction in LV end-diastolic volume and mass with significantly lower incidence of the need for aortic valve replacement at 5 years.

○ **What is the most common cause of acute tricuspid regurgitation and what is the preferred management of this situation?**

Tricuspid valve endocarditis, often as a result of intravenous drug abuse. The preferred management is complete removal of the valve with immediate or eventual replacement of the valve. Antibiotic therapy usually is futile in preventing valve surgery.

○ **A 38-year-old female patient with known mitral valve prolapse is scheduled for dental cleaning. Her dentist calls for you asking recommendations for endocarditis prophylaxis. She is not allergic to penicillin. What are your recommendations?**

No antibiotic prophylaxis is necessary for patients with only the diagnosis of mitral valve prolapse. Antibiotic prophylaxis is recommended for those with prosthetic heart valves, history of infective endocarditis, and other specific congenital heart defects or congenital heart defect repairs utilizing prosthetic material.

○ **A 55-year-old man who underwent a 4-vessel CABG 3 years ago and has mild mitral and tricuspid regurgitation is scheduled for a colonoscopy for rectal bleeding. What recommendations regarding endocarditis prophylaxis would you give this surgeon?**

No antibiotic prophylaxis is needed in this setting.

○ **Which valve is most commonly injured during blunt trauma?**

The aortic valve.

○ **What is the abnormality seen in the M-mode echocardiogram shown in Figure 2-25?**

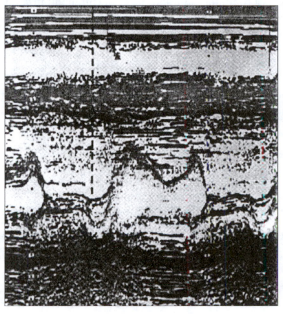

Figure 2-25

Prolapse of the posterior leaflet of the mitral valve.

● ● ● OTHER HEART DISEASE AND CONDITIONS ● ● ●

○ **What are some adverse drug effects of lidocaine?**

Drowsiness, nausea, vertigo, confusion, ataxia, tinnitus, muscle twitching, respiratory depression, and psychosis.

○ **In CPR, what is the ventilation to compression ratio for one or two rescuers?**

One and two rescuers should perform 2 breaths to 30 compressions at a rate of 100 compressions per minute. (New guidelines emphasize compressions over ventilations during the first several minutes of a cardiac arrest.)

○ **What are the most common causes of myocarditis in the United States?**

Viruses. Other causes include post–viral myocarditis, an autoimmune response to recent viral infection, bacteria (diphtheria and tuberculosis), fungi, protozoa (Chagas disease), and spirochetes (Lyme disease).

○ **A 25-year-old patient presents with splinted breathing and sharp, precordial chest pain that radiates to the back. The pain increases with inspiration and is mildly relieved by placing the patient in a forward sitting position. What might the EKG show?**

The patient probably has pericarditis. The EKG may reveal intermittent supraventricular tachycardias, ST-segment depression in leads aVR and VI with ST segment elevation in all of the remaining leads. PR depression and T-wave inversion may also arise.

○ **What is the most common cause of pericarditis?**

Idiopathic. Viral pericarditis is a common cause and the most common infectious etiology. Other causes are myocardial infarction, post–viral syndrome, aortic dissection that has ruptured into the pericardium, malignancy, radiation, chest trauma, connective tissue disease, uremia, and drugs, i.e., procainamide or hydralazine.

○ **What physical findings indicates acute pericarditis?**

Pericardial friction rub. The rub is heard best at the left sternal border or apex with the patient in a forward sitting position. Other findings include fever, tachycardia, and pleuritic chest pain.

○ **What will be the appearance of a pericardial effusion on an X-ray?**

A water bottle silhouette.

○ **What is the treatment for pericarditis without effusion?**

A 2-week treatment of 650 mg aspirin every 4 hours, if no contraindications exist. Ibuprofen, indomethacin, or colchicines are other alternatives. The use of corticosteroids is controversial because recurrent pericarditis is common as the dose is tapered.

○ **What is the 1-year recurrence rate for patients who have been resuscitated from sudden cardiac death?**

30%.

○ **Splinter hemorrhages, Osler nodes, Janeway lesions, petechiae, and Roth spots can be indications of what process?**

They are physical signs associated with infective endocarditis.

○ **True/False: Osler nodes are usually nodular and painful:**

True. In contrast, the macular Janeway lesions are painless.

○ **What percentage of patients with infective endocarditis display peripheral manifestations of the disease?**

50%.

○ **What is bacterial endocarditis?**

An infectious process where bloodborne bacteria that attach onto damaged or abnormal heart valves or on the endocardium near anatomical defects.

○ **How is bacterial endocarditis diagnosed?**

By evidence of valvular vegetations on echocardiogram combined with a positive blood culture. The Duke criteria is often utilized as a diagnostic tool for infectious endocarditis.

○ **Who is at high risk for developing endocarditis?**

People with prosthetic heart valves, persons with previous incidents of endocarditis, persons with complex congenital heart disease, intravenous drug user, and persons with surgically devised systemic pulmonary shunts.

○ **What are the risk factors for endocarditis?**

Risk factors include intravenous drug use, prosthetic valves, acquired valvular heart disease, hypertrophic cardiomyopathy, hemodialysis, peritoneal dialysis, indwelling venous catheters, post–cardiac surgery, rheumatic heart disease, and uncorrected congenital conditions. It is controversial as to whether mitral valve prolapsed with significant regurgitation is a moderate risk factor.

○ **What are the most common organisms associated with endocarditis?**

Streptococcus viridians, Staphylococcus aureus, Enterococcus, and fungal organisms. Staph. aureus is responsible for 75% of disease in IVDAs.

○ **What is more common in the general population: left-sided or right-sided endocarditis?**

Left-sided (aortic and mitral involvement).

○ **What is more common in intravenous drug abusers: left-sided or right-sided structural disease?**

Right-sided (60%) is most common.

○ **How is infective endocarditis treated?**

Intravenous antibiotics for 4 to 6 weeks. Close follow-up is necessary and the patient should have a series of two separate negative blood cultures to demonstrate resolution of the condition. If resolution of the infections does not occur promptly, embolization occurs, or fulminant CHF ensues and surgical valve replacement is indicated.

○ **What are the EKG changes associated with pericarditis?**

Concave upward ST elevation in at least seven leads except V_1 and aVR. PR segment depression may also be present.

○ **What is the most frequently reported bacterial isolate in patients with myocardial abscesses?**

Staphylococcus aureus.

○ **What is the clinical picture of myocardial abscesses?**

Low grade fevers, chills, leukocytosis, conduction system abnormalities, nonspecific EKG changes, and signs and symptoms of acute MI.

○ **What is mural endocarditis?**

Inflammation and disruption of the nonvalvular endocardial surface of the cardiac chambers.

○ **What are the risk factors for mural endocarditis?**

Usually, mural endocarditis is from seeding of an abnormal area of endocardium during bacteremia or fungemia. Infectious thrombi from pulmonary veins, ventricular aneurysms, mural thrombi, chordal friction lesions, pacemaker lead insertion sites, idiopathic hypertrophic subaortic stenosis, jet lesions from ventriculoseptal defects, and other congenital defects are other factors. Immunocompromised patients are also at increased risk.

○ **What is the clinical presentation of prosthetic vascular graft infection?**

Erythema, skin breakdown, or purulent drainage. Other symptoms may be thrombosis of the graft, fluid around the graft, or pseudoaneurysm formation.

○ **What are the complications from arterial catheterization?**

Thrombosis (19%–38%), infection (4%–23%), pseudoaneurysm, and rupture.

○ **How many deaths per year in the United States are due to cardiovascular disease?**

864,480 in 2005 or 35.3% of all deaths. CVD death rates have declined with a 26.4% drop between 1995 and 2005.

○ **A radial pulse on examination indicates a BP of at least what level?**

80 mm Hg.

○ **A femoral pulse on examination indicates a BP of at least what level?**

70 mm Hg.

○ **A carotid pulse on examination indicates a BP of at least what level?**

60 mm Hg.

● ● ● **REFERENCES** ● ● ●

Crawford MH *Current Medical Diagnosis and Treatment: Cardiology*. 3rd ed. New York, NY: McGraw-Hill; 2009.

Fauci AS, Braunwald E, Kasper DL, et al., eds. *Harrison's Principles of Internal Medicine*, 17th ed. New York: McGraw-Hill; 2008. http://www.accessmedicine.com

Fuster Valentin OR-W. *Hurst's The Heart*. 12th ed. New York, NY: McGraw-Hill; 2008.

McPhee SJ, Papadakis MA, eds. *Current Medical Diagnosis and Treatment 2009*. New York, NY: McGraw-Hill; 2009.

McPhee SJ, Ganong WF. *Pathophysiology of Disease: An Introduction to Clinical Medicine*. 5th ed. New York, NY: McGraw-Hill; 2006.

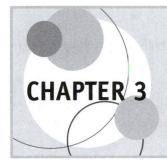

CHAPTER 3 Pulmonary

Daniel Thibodeau, MHP, PA-C

● ● ● **INFECTIOUS DISORDERS** ● ● ●

○ **What are the main symptoms of individuals with acute bronchitis?**

Persistent cough for more than 3 weeks, fever, and constitutional symptoms.

○ **What is the main causative agent of acute bronchitis?**

Viral pathogen. Most of the time, adenovirus, rhinovirus, and influenza are the agents. In some cases, *H. influenza*, *M. pneumoniae*, and *C. pneumoniae* can be the causative agents.

○ **Name some diseases that can mimic acute bronchitis:**

Asthma and allergic bronchospasm can present with the same symptoms of acute bronchitis. Other causes can be congestive heart failure, bronchogenic tumors, and reflux esophagitis can all present with respiratory symptoms similar to that of bronchitis.

○ **Is the use of antibiotics indicated for an acute case of bronchitis?**

No.

○ **What are the treatment options for patients with acute bronchitis?**

Supportive care. If the patient presents with wheezing on examination, the use of albuterol is supported. If, however, the patient presents only with a cough, bronchodilators are not indicated.

○ **What percentage of cigarette smokers develop chronic bronchitis?**

10% to 15%. Chronic bronchitis generally develops after 10 to 12 years of smoking.

○ **What are the signs and symptoms of patients with acute bronchiolitis?**

Fever, cough, rhinorrhea, wheezing, tachypnea, and respiratory distress.

49

○ **Describe the typical findings of a chest X-ray in a patient with acute bronchiolitis:**

They are nonspecific but can include increased interstitial marking, peribronchial cuffing, and hyperinflation and in some cases segmental atelectasis.

○ **How do you confirm a case of bronchiolitis?**

Most cases can be diagnosed on history and physical examination alone. Nasal washings to look for RSV may be done. Laboratory results are nonspecific and may show mild leukocytosis.

○ **Which is the most common type of pathogen in bronchiolitis?**

RSV. It generally affects children younger than 2 years. Bronchiolitis rarely develops in adults. Second most common pathogen is adenovirus.

○ **What is the treatment for severe RSV documented bronchiolitis?**

Ribavirin.

○ **A 24-year-old female patient has a high fever, hoarseness, and increased stridor of 3 hours duration. She also has a low fever and sore throat. Examination shows an ill-appearing woman with a temperature of 40°C, inspiratory stridor, drooling, and mild intercostal retractions. She prefers to sit up. What is the most likely diagnosis?**

Epiglottitis.

○ **What pathogen is responsible for most cases of epiglottitis?**

Group A *streptococcus*. It is followed by *S. pneumoniae, Haemophilus parainfluenzae,* and *S. aureus.* Usually, viruses are not the causative agents.

○ **What is the narrowest part of the adult airway?**

The glottic opening.

○ **What is the "thumb print sign"?**

A soft tissue inflammation of the epiglottis seen on a lateral X-ray of the neck. The epiglottis, normally long and thin, appears swollen and flat at the base of the hypopharynx in patients with epiglottitis.

○ **What is the treatment of choice for acute epiglottitis?**

Maintaining the airway is of paramount importance. If the airway is stable, treatment with a cephalosporin is indicated. Ampicillin/sulbactam is the preferred treatment for 7 to 10 days. Cefuroxime, cefotaxime, or ceftriaxone is appropriate for β-lactam allergic patients.

○ **A 2-year-old child presents with wheezing, rhonchi, inspiratory stridor, and a sudden harsh cough, which worsens at night. What is the diagnosis?**

Croup, also known as laryngotracheitis. This condition is usually preceded by a URI and is frequently caused by the parainfluenza virus.

○ **What age group usually contracts croup?**

6 months to 3 years. Croup is characterized by cold symptoms; a sudden, barking cough; inspiratory and expiratory stridor; and a slight fever.

○ **What is the difference between the cough of croup and the cough of epiglottitis?**

Croup has a seal-like barking cough, while epiglottitis is accompanied by a minimal cough. Children with croup have a hoarse voice, while those with epiglottitis have a muffled voice.

○ **What is the most common pathogen that causes croup?**

Parainfluenza type virus. Other pathogens include influenza, RSV, adenovirus, and in some cases *Mycoplasma pneumoniae*.

○ **What is the "steeple sign"?**

Subglottic edema, which creates a symmetrically tapered configuration in the subglottic portion of the trachea when imaged in a frontal soft tissue X-ray of the neck. This is consistent with croup.

○ **A 3-year-old male child is woken in the middle of the night with a barking seal-like cough and signs and symptoms that are consistent with croup. On examination, the child's respirations are 35/min and oxygen saturation is 95% on room air. There is no evidence of stridor on examination and his lungs are clear. What is the recommended treatment for this patient?**

Supportive care, fluids, and observation at home. If oxygen saturation is down, oxygen therapy is indicated. In all cases, inhalable racemic epinephrine by nebulizer is warranted.

○ **What if the child presented with stridor on examination?**

Administer dexamethasone 0.6 mg/kg IM one-time dose along with all the other therapies mentioned above.

○ **A 34-year-old woman wakes up with a history of sudden onset of fever, body aches, malaise, chills, cough, and a sore throat. She reports that several other members at home have the same symptoms, as do some of her coworkers. On examination, her temperature is 101°F, pulse 100, respiratory rate 18, and BP 122/86. Her throat appears to be moist without any abnormalities, lungs are clear, and the rest of the examination is unremarkable. What is the most probable cause of this illness?**

Influenza.

○ **Which strain of influenza is considered to cause more pandemic outbreaks?**

Influenza A.

○ **Which syndrome can be caused by an outbreak of influenza B virus?**

Reyes syndrome.

○ **What is the main method of transmission for the influenza virus?**

It spreads via aerosol by cough and sneeze and via hand-to-hand contact.

○ **What is the most common type of pneumonia seen in influenza patients?**

Viral. A secondary bacterial pneumonia can be caused by *Streptococcus pneumoniae, Staphylococcus aureus,* and *Haemophilus influenza.*

○ **What method is used to detect a positive influenza illness?**

Throat, nasopharyngeal, or sputum samples with a rapid influenza A or B test.

○ **What is the treatment of choice for a patient with influenza B virus?**

Oseltamivir orally or Zanamivir inhaled. However, these medications must be started within 24 to 26 hours of onset of the illness for them to be effective.

○ **Name some other therapies that are helpful in symptomatic relief of an influenza illness:**

Supportive care with fluids, analgesics such as acetaminophen for body aches, myalgias, and fever. A cough suppressant with or without codeine may be helpful also.

○ **Which patients should be vaccinated with the influenza vaccine?**

Children between the ages of 6 and 59 months, pregnant women (during flu season), children and adults with chronic disorders of the cardiovascular and pulmonary systems, nursing home and chronic care facility patients, any care workers who are at risk of exposure, and health care workers.

○ **What age group is usually afflicted by pertussis?**

Infants younger than 2 years of age.

○ **What are some of the hallmark symptoms of a patient with pertussis?**

Initially, the patient has the same types of symptoms as in common cold. Within 1 to 2 weeks of the illness progressing, the patient develops a cough that evolves into a paroxysmal phase with more frequent and spasmodic bursts of 5 to 10 at a time. This can also have the sound of a terminal audible whoop. Posttussive vomiting may also occur.

○ **What is the main pathway for infection leading to pneumonia?**

Aspiration via the oropharynx.

○ **Describe the different presentations of bacterial and viral pneumonia:**

Bacterial pneumonia is typified by a sudden onset of symptoms, including pleurisy, fever, chills, productive cough, tachypnea, and tachycardia. The most common bacterial pneumonia is pneumococcal pneumonia.

Viral pneumonia is characterized by the gradual onset of symptoms, no pleurisy, chills or high fever, general malaise, and a nonproductive cough.

○ **What is the leading identifiable cause of acute community-acquired pneumonia in adults?**

Streptococcus pneumoniae.

○ **Name the risk factors for community-acquired pneumonia:**

Alcoholism, asthma, immunosuppression, ≥70 years of age.

○ **Name the risk factors for pneumococcal pneumonia:**

Dementia, seizure disorder, alcoholism, smoking, COPD, and HIV.

○ **A young infant patient who you suspect has pneumonia is ordered to have a chest X-ray performed. When you view the results, you note the presence of pneumatoceles on the film. What pathogen is likely responsible for this type of finding?**

Staphylococcus aureus.

○ **A 24-year-old male patient has had fevers, chills, and a productive cough with dark green sputum for the last week. On physical examination, his temperature is 101.3°F, P 90, R 22, and BP 124/85. There is coryza with moist mucous membranes and a regular rhythm on cardiac examination. Lung sounds reveal an area of crackles with a mild expiratory wheeze at the right lower base of the lung fields. Based on this history and physical examination, what is the treatment of choice for this patient?**

A macrolide antibiotic (clarithromycin or azithromycin) for the treatment of community-acquired pneumonia.

○ **If this patient required inpatient treatment of pneumonia but without ICU admission, what is the class of antibiotics that would be indicated? What if the patient needed to be in the ICU?**

Fluoroquinolone for non-ICU patients (moxifloxacin, levofloxacin, and gemifloxacin).

For ICU patients, ceftriaxone, ampicillin-sulbactam, **plus** azithromycin or fluoroquinolone.

○ **What are some of the more common complications associated with community-acquired pneumonia?**

Respiratory failure, shock, worsening of comorbid diseases, especially metastatic infection, lung abscess, and complicated pleural effusion.

○ **Which bacterial pneumonias frequently cause frank hemoptysis?**

Pseudomonas aeruginosa, Klebsiella pneumoniae, and *Staphylococcus aureus.*

○ **What bacteria are associated with pneumonia following influenza?**

Streptococcus pneumoniae, Staphylococcus pneumoniae, and *Hemophilus influenza.*

○ **What two underlying medical conditions are associated with *Hemophilus influenzae* pneumonia?**

Chronic obstructive lung disease and HIV infection.

○ **What is the most common etiologic agent of atypical pneumonia?**

Mycoplasma pneumoniae.

○ **What is considered to be the second most common cause of atypical pneumonia?**

Chlamydia pneumoniae.

○ **Of the following organisms, which is commonly spread by person-to-person contact:** *Legionella pneumoniae* **or** *Mycoplasma pneumoniae?*

Mycoplasma pneumoniae.

○ **What three X-ray findings are associated with a poor outcome in patients with pneumonia?**

Multilobar involvement, a cavitary lesion, and pleural effusions.

○ **What is the most common cause of pneumonia in children?**

Viral pneumonia. Infecting viruses include influenza, parainfluenza, RSV, and adenoviruses.

○ **Match the pneumonia with the treatment:**

1. *Klebsiella pneumoniae*	a. **Erythromycin, tetracycline, or doxycycline**
2. *Streptococcal pneumonia*	b. **Penicillin G**
3. *Legionella pneumophila*	c. **Cefuroxime and clarithromycin**
4. *Haemophilus influenza*	d. **Erythromycin and rifampin**
5. *Mycoplasma pneumoniae*	

(1) c, (2) b, (3) d, (4) c, and (5) a.

○ **Empyema is most often caused by what organism?**

Staphylococcus aureus, and in most cases methicillin-resistant *S. aureus* (MRSA). Gram-negative organisms and anaerobic bacteria may also cause empyema.

○ **What is the chest X-ray finding that suggests a right middle lobe pneumonia?**

Loss of the right heart border.

○ **What is the chest X-ray finding of a patient with a left upper lobe consolidation?**

Infiltrate seen on the AP to the lower lung field without obstruction of the diaphragm, with confirmation on the lateral film.

○ **What are the most common causes of staphylococcal pneumonias?**

Drug use and endocarditis. This pneumonia produces high fever, chills, and a purulent productive cough.

○ **What are the extrapulmonary manifestations of mycoplasma?**

Erythema multiforme, pericarditis, and CNS disease.

○ **What is the most frequent etiology of nosocomial pneumonia?**

Pseudomonas aeruginosa. There is a high mortality associated with pneumonia caused by *Pseudomonas.* It most frequently occurs in immunocompromised patients or patients on mechanical ventilation.

○ **A 67-year-old alcoholic man was found in an alley, covered in his own vomit and beer. Upon examination, he is shaking, has a fever of 103.5°F and is coughing up currant jelly sputum. What is the diagnosis?**

Pneumonia induced by *Klebsiella pneumoniae*. This is the most probable etiology in alcoholics, the elderly, the very young, and the immunocompromised patients. Other gram-negative bacteria, such as *E. coli* and other Enterobacteriaceae, may cause pneumonia in alcoholic patients who have aspirated.

○ **Describe the classic chest X-ray finding associated with *Legionella* pneumonia:**

Dense consolidation and bulging fissures. Expect elevated liver enzymes and hypophosphatemia. The patient with *Legionella* pneumonia classically presents with a relative bradycardia.

○ **A 43-year-old man presents with pleurisy, sudden onset of fever and chills, and rust-colored sputum. What is the probable diagnosis?**

Pneumococcal pneumonia caused by *Streptococcus pneumoniae*; it is the most common community-acquired pneumonia. It is a consolidating lobar pneumonia and can be treated with penicillin G or erythromycin.

○ **A 20-year-old college student is home for winter break and presents complaining of a 10-day history of a nonproductive dry hacking cough, malaise, a mild fever, and no chills. What is a probable diagnosis?**

Mycoplasma pneumoniae, also known as walking pneumonia. Although this is the most common pneumonia that develops in teenagers and young adults, it is an atypical pneumonia and most frequently occurs in close contact populations, i.e., schools and military barracks.

○ **A 56-year-old smoker with COPD presents with chills, fever, green sputum, and extreme shortness of breath. An X-ray shows a right lower lobe pneumonia. What is expected from the sputum culture?**

Haemophilus influenza. This organism is generally found in pneumonia and bronchitis patients with underlying COPD. The next most common organism detected in this patient population is *Moraxella catarrhalis*.

Ampicillin/clavulanate (Augmentin) is the drug of choice, but patients at high risk should have yearly influenza vaccinations.

○ **If a patient has a patchy infiltrate on a chest X-ray and bullous myringitis, what antibiotic should be prescribed?**

Erythromycin for mycoplasma.

○ **In what season does *Legionella* pneumonia most commonly occur?**

Summer. *Legionella pneumophila* thrives in environments such as the water-cooling towers that are used in large buildings and hotels. Staphylococcal pneumonias also occur more frequently in summer.

○ **An older patient with GI symptoms, hyponatremia, and a relative bradycardia probably has which type of pneumonia?**

Legionella.

○ **What is the most common cause of pneumonia in sickle cell disease?**

Streptococcus pneumoniae.

○   **Which type of pneumonia is often associated with cold agglutinins?**

Mycoplasma pneumoniae.

○   **Name four antibiotics known to have in vitro activity against anaerobic bacteria in virtually all cases:**

1. Metronidazole
2. Chloramphenicol
3. Imipenem
4. Beta-lactam/beta-lactamase inhibitors

○   **What is the drug of choice for pneumonias acquired in the outpatient setting due to anaerobic bacteria?**

Clindamycin.

○   **What is the recommended duration of antibiotic therapy for necrotizing anaerobic pneumonia, lung abscess, or empyema?**

4 to 8 weeks.

○   **What anaerobic respiratory infection is associated with slowly enlarging pulmonary infiltrates, pleural effusions, rib destruction, and fistula formation?**

Actinomycosis.

○   **What proportion of the patients with pneumonia develop pleural effusions?**

40%.

○   **What is the definition of nosocomial pneumonia?**

Pneumonia occurring in patients who have been hospitalized for at least 72 hours.

○   **What are the two most important routes of transmission of nosocomial bacterial pneumonia?**

Person-to-person transmission via health care workers and contaminated ventilator tubing.

○   **Describe the chest X-ray image of mycoplasma pneumonia:**

Patchy densities involving the entire lobe. Pneumatoceles, cavities, abscesses, and pleural effusions can occur but are uncommon. Treat with erythromycin.

○   **Which type of bacterial pneumonia commonly occurs secondary to viral illness?**

Staphylococcal infection.

○   **What two types of pneumonia are often contracted during the summer months?**

Staphylococcal and *Legionella* pneumonia.

○ **Describe the chest X-ray image of *Legionella* pneumonia:**

Dense consolidation and bulging fissures. Expect elevated liver enzymes and hypophosphatemia. Relative bradycardia is evident upon physical examination.

○ **What are the potential, often rare, complications of Mycoplasma pneumonia?**

- Nonpulmonary: Hemolytic anemia, aseptic meningitis, encephalitis, Guillain-Barré syndrome, pericarditis, and myocarditis.
- Pulmonary: ARDS, atelectasis, mediastinal adenopathy, pneumothorax, pleural effusion, and abscess.

○ **Describe a patient with chlamydial pneumonia:**

Chlamydial pneumonia is usually seen in infants 2 to 6 weeks of age. The patient is afebrile and does not appear toxic.

○ **In which type of patients is staphylococcal pneumonia likely?**

Patients who are hospitalized, debilitated, or abusing drugs.

○ **What pathogen is suggested by pneumonia with a single rigor?**

Pneumococcus.

○ **Where is the most common site of aspiration pneumonitis?**

Right lower lobe.

○ **A patient with currant jelly sputum is likely to have which type of pneumonia?**

Klebsiella or type 3 pneumococcus.

○ **Under what conditions should staphylococcal pneumonia be considered as a possible diagnosis?**

Although staphylococcal pneumonia accounts for only 1% of bacterial pneumonias, it should be considered in patients with sudden chills, hectic fever, pleurisy, and cough (especially following a viral illness, such as measles or influenza).

○ **Where does aspiration generally occur as revealed by chest X-ray?**

The lower lobe of the right lung. This is the most direct path for foreign bodies into the lung.

○ **Describe the classic chest X-ray findings in a patient with mycoplasma pneumonia:**

Patchy diffuse densities involving the entire lung. Pneumatoceles, cavities, abscesses, and pleural effusions can occur but are uncommon. Treat the patient with erythromycin.

○ **What three findings should be present to consider a sputum sample adequate?**

1. >25 PMNs
2. <10 squamous epithelial cells per low-powered field
3. A predominant bacterial organism

○ **What degree of leukocytosis is considered a risk factor for poor outcome among patients with bacterial pneumonia?**

Greater than 30,000 cells/mm^3.

○ **At what age should the pneumococcal vaccine be administered to healthy adults with no comorbid conditions?**

Age 65 or older.

○ **A patient has a staccato cough and a history of conjunctivitis in the first few weeks after birth. What type of pneumonia would this patient have?**

Chlamydial pneumonia.

○ **What are the two most common ventilator associated pneumonia?**

Pseudomonas aeruginosa and MRSA.

○ **What percentage of people in the Ohio and the Mississippi valleys are infected with histoplasmosis?**

100% in endemic areas. However, only 1% of these individuals develop the active disease. The spores of *H. capsulatum* can remain active for 10 years. For unknown reasons, bird and bat feces promote the growth of the actual fungus. The disease is transmitted when the spores are released and inhaled.

○ **How is the diagnosis of histoplasmosis made?**

By bronchoalveolar lavage or by tissue biopsy and blood cultures.

○ **What does the chest X-ray of a patient with histoplasmosis look like?**

Interstitial pneumonitis, patchy alveolar infiltrates, and mediastinal adenopathy may be present.

○ **What is the treatment of choice for a histoplasmosis pneumonia?**

Itraconazole for 6 to 12 weeks duration.

○ **Where in the United States is coccidioidomycosis most prevalent?**

The southwest. If severe, treat the afflicted patient with amphotericin B.

○ **A 46-year-old man with a history of HIV has been diagnosed with coccidioidomycosis pneumonia. His examination and vital signs are stable. What is the initial treatment plan for this patient?**

Most of these immunocompromised patients do not require specific therapy. Close follow-up and monitoring of symptoms are enough to ensure that the illness is resolving.

○ **Which type of fungal pneumonia seen in immunocompromised patients, is highly invasive into the lung parenchyma?**

Aspergillosis.

○ **What is characteristic of the chest X-ray of aspergillosis pneumonia?**

Usually a bilateral upper lobe infiltrate. In some cases, a fungal ball with a cavitary lesion can be seen on CT scan.

○ **What is the primary treatment for aspergillosis pneumonia?**

Itraconazole.

○ **What is the best method for detecting adenovirus pneumonia?**

Detectiing adenovirus pneumonia is difficult because it appears quite similar to CAP; but if suspected, the PCR from respiratory secretions, blood, urine, and solid tissues is used.

○ **What is the mortality rate of adenovirus pneumonia?**

Around 30%, and up to 50% in immunocompromised patients.

○ **How does a human get infected and develop pneumonia by the hantavirus?**

This is by rodent-to-human contact or by cleaning up after a rodent. The virus enters via the respiratory epithelium.

○ **Hantavirus occurs most commonly in what geographic location?**

Southwestern United States, especially in areas with deer mice.

○ **Name the antiviral medications that are used for viral pneumonia:**

Amantadine and Flumadine for influenza A, and ribavirin for RSV, adenovirus, and hantavirus pneumonia. Oseltamivir and Zanamivir can both be used for influenza A and B pneumonia.

○ **A 67-year-old female patient presents with a 4-day history of fevers, malaise, cough, and a generalized vesicular rash that started on the scalp and then spread to arms and legs. The cough and respiratory symptoms have been correlating to the rash on the legs in timing. The chest X-ray reveals patchy diffuse infiltrates and there is also a small right pleural effusion. What is the etiology of this illness?**

Varicella pneumonia. This type of pneumonia can also be at risk for immunocompromised, pregnant, and postpartum patients.

○ **What is the treatment for varicella pneumonia?**

Acyclovir for 7 to 10 days.

○ **What secondary bacterial infection often occurs following a viral pneumonia?**

Staphylococcal pneumonia.

○ **What is the pathogen that is responsible for HIV-/AIDS-related pneumonia?**

Pneumocystis jirovecii.

○ **What is the difference between PCP pneumonia and *P. jirovecii* pneumonia?**

PCP is transmitted through animal contact and does not transmit to humans. P. jeroveci is the human form.

○ **Name five HIV-related pulmonary infections:**

PCP, TB, histoplasmosis, Cryptococcus, and CMV.

○ **Describe the chest X-ray of a patient with PCP:**

A reticular or miliary pattern ranging from fine to course, ill-defined patchy areas, segmental and subsegmental consolidation; 5% to 10% of PCP pneumonias will have a normal chest X-ray.

○ **What laboratory tests aid in the diagnosis of PCP?**

A rising LDH or a LDH > 450 and an ESR > 50. A low albumin implies a poor prognosis.

○ **The initial therapy for PCP includes what antibiotic?**

Trimethoprim-sulfamethorazole (Bactrim).

○ **What other medication should be prescribed to a patient with PCP?**

Corticosteroids when the Po_2 is <70 mm Hg or an oxygen saturation of <90%.

○ **What two drugs are used as prophylactic treatment to prevent PCP in HIV patients?**

Aerosolized pentamidine (Pentam) or trimethoprim/sulfamethoxazole (Bactrim).

○ **What is the most common cause of community-acquired bacterial pneumonia among patients infected with HIV?**

Streptococcus pneumoniae.

○ **What is the recurrence rate of PCP for those patients who do not receive prophylaxis?**

30%.

○ **What is the typical time of year that RSV has an outbreak?**

During late winter and early spring.

○ **What are the usual cases that present with an RSV infection?**

Pneumonia, tracheobronchitis, and bronchiolitis.

○ **What are some of the common presenting symptoms of RSV?**

Fever (low grade), tachypnea, and wheezing are all signs. Apnea is a common symptom. In children, RSV can also cause acute and recurrent otitis media.

○ **What is the treatment of an RSV illness?**

Supportive care, which includes hydration, humidified air, and fever reduction with acetaminophen. In very serious cases, ribavirin can be used.

○ **What are the classic signs and symptoms of TB?**

Night sweats, fever, weight loss, malaise, cough, and greenish yellow sputum most commonly observed in the mornings.

○ **What are the three stages of TB infections?**

Primary, active, and latent.

○ **What is the most common complaint of individuals with TB?**

Cough.

○ **What is the main transmission of TB to humans?**

Airborne spread through respiratory droplets that are infected with tuberculosis.

○ **Which population is at greatest risk for tuberculosis?**

Patients who have had recent infections, fibrotic lesions, and comorbidities such as HIV, silicosis, chronic renal failure, diabetes, IV drug use, immunosuppressive therapy, and gastrectomy, as well as posttransplantation patients.

○ **What age group is most affected by the tuberculosis mycobacterium? And what gender?**

Age group: 25 to 34 years; women more than men. As the age becomes older, the gender changes to men. The reasons are unknown.

○ **What do chest X-rays reveal in cases of tuberculosis?**

Cavitation of the right upper lobe. Lower lung infiltrates, hilar adenopathy, atelectasis, and pleural effusion are also common.

○ **What is a Gohn lesion?**

It is a spontaneously healed TB lesion and presents on chest X-ray as a small calcified lesion.

○ **What is the range of time that results in an immune response to occur?**

2 to 10 weeks.

○ **A positive TB test is which type of reaction?**

Type 4. Cells are mediated, hypersensitivity is delayed, and neither complements nor antibodies are involved.

○ **What laboratory test is used to detect TB microscopically?**

Acid-fast bacillus smear.

○ **What is the best method to yield a positive TB samples?**

Needle biopsy, pleural fluid analysis, and needle biopsy of the pleura together gives a 90% diagnosis rate. Individually, each test alone produces a much lower yield.

○ **Right upper lobe cavitation with parenchymal involvement is a classic indicator for what?**

TB. Lower lung infiltrates, hilar adenopathy, atelectasis, and pleural effusion are also common.

○ **Does latent TB transmit to other humans?**

No, and the disease is not active.

○ **Name the first-line treatment drugs for TB in patients who are HIV negative:**

Isoniazid, rifampin, pyrazinamide, and ethambutol for 2 months daily. After the initial 2-month regimen, INH and rifampin can be continued for 4 months.

○ **What is the treatment for HIV-positive patients with TB?**

Similar to the non–HIV class with exception to adding an additional 6 months of treatment for a total of 12 months duration. Resistance to isoniazid will cause a longer treatment plan with the other primary medications.

○ **What are the side effects of INH?**

Neuropathy, pyridoxine loss, lupus-like syndrome, anion-gap acidosis, and hepatitis.

○ **What percentage of tuberculosis cases are drug resistant?**

About 15%. The rate is highly dependent upon geographic location.

○ **Name some common extrapulmonary TB sites:**

The lymph nodes, bone, GI tract, GU tract, meninges, liver, and the pericardium.

○ **True/False: Patients younger than 35 years of age with positive TB skin tests should undergo at least 6 months of isoniazid chemoprophylaxis:**

True.

○ **What are the typical roentgenographic features of a tuberculous pleural effusion?**

They are usually unilateral, small to moderate, and more commonly on the right side. Two-thirds of these can be associated with coexisting parenchymal disease (which may not be apparent on chest radiograph). They are commonly associated with primary disease. The incidence of loculations may be up to 30%.

○ **Is the tuberculin skin test a reliable test for active TB?**

No. It has a low sensitivity and specificity to detect active or latent disease.

○ **In which patients should you reserve caution in prescribing INH, rifampin?**

Patients with renal failure.

○ **What is the relapse rate for TB?**

It is less than 5%; the main cause for this is noncompliance.

○ **Hoarseness can herald far greater problems than viral laryngitis. At what point is a more thorough work-up indicated?**

If hoarseness persists for over 6 to 8 weeks or is accompanied by a mass, chest pain, weight loss, aspiration dyspnea, or any other signs of malignancy. Be suspicious of smokers with chronic cough or hoarseness if there is a change in either.

○ **What percent of upper respiratory infectious agents are nonbacterial?**

Nonbacterial agents account for more than 90% of pharyngitis, laryngitis, tracheal bronchitis, and bronchitis.

○ **In treating a patient with a common cold, you prescribe an oral decongestant. Is it necessary to also suggest an antitussant?**

No. Most coughs, arising from a common cold, are caused by the irritation of the tracheobronchial receptors in the posterior pharynx as a result of postnasal drip. Postnasal drip can be relieved with decongestant therapy, thus eliminating the need for cough suppressant therapy.

○ **What are the most common etiologies of a chronic cough?**

Postnasal drip (40%), asthma (25%), and gastroesophageal reflux (20%). Other etiologies include bronchitis, bronchiectasis, bronchogenic carcinoma, esophageal diverticula, sarcoidosis, viruses, and drugs.

○ **What age group is afflicted with the most colds per year?**

Kindergartners win the top billing with an average of 12 colds/year. Second place goes to preschoolers with 6 to 10 colds/year. School children contract an average of 7 colds/year. Adolescents and adults average only 2 to 4 colds/year.

○ **What is the duration of a common cold?**

3 to 10 days (self-limited).

○ **What antibiotic is the most effective for treating uncomplicated lung abscesses?**

Clindamycin.

○ **True/False: Flora of lung abscesses are usually polymicrobial:**

True.

○ **Which gram-negative aerobes are known to cause lung abscess?**

Pseudomonas and *Klebsiella*.

○ **What are the two major risk factors for the development of anaerobic lung infection?**

Periodontal disease and predisposition to aspiration.

○ **Empyema in the absence of parenchymal lung infiltrate suggests what underlying process?**

Subphrenic or other intra-abdominal abscess.

○ **What are the two most important risk factors for the development of anaerobic lung abscess?**

Poor oral hygiene and a predisposition toward aspiration.

○ **What organisms are most commonly present in a pulmonary abscess?**

Mixed anaerobes.

○ **Which general group of bacteria is most commonly found in lung abscesses?**

Anaerobic bacteria.

○ **How do retropharyngeal abscesses arise?**

Lymphatic spread of infections in the nasopharynx, oropharynx, or external auditory canal.

● ● ● **NEOPLASTIC DISEASE** ● ● ●

○ **What is the most common cancer in the United States?**

Lung cancer, which accounts for 29% of all cancer deaths.

○ **What is the average age range for a patient with lung cancer?**

55 to 65 years.

○ **What are some of the symptoms that are present in patients with lung cancer?**

Cough, hemoptysis, wheeze and stridor, dyspnea, and postobstructive pneumonitis (fever and productive cough) are a few complaints.

○ **Which form of lung cancer is the most common?**

Adenocarcinoma followed by squamous cell, then small cell (oat cell) carcinoma.

○ **What percentage of effusions are associated with malignancy?**

25%.

○ **What routine program is recommended for screening lung cancer in the adult population?**

None. Screening programs for lung cancer have not demonstrated a decrease in morbidity or mortality. Practitioners must be aware of the signs and symptoms associated with lung cancer, including chronic nonproductive cough, increased sputum production, hemoptysis, dyspnea, recurrent pneumonia, hoarseness, pleurisy, weight loss, shoulder pain, SVC syndrome, exercise fatigue, and anemia. Incidental findings on a chest X-ray should also be investigated.

○ **Where do the following cancers most commonly develop within the lung: adenocarcinoma and large cell carcinomas and squamous and small cell carcinomas?**

Adenocarcinoma and large cell carcinomas are usually located peripherally, while squamous and small cell carcinomas are located centrally. These four malignancies account for 88% of all lung cancers.

○ **What type of lung cancer is commonly associated with hypercalcemia?**

Squamous cell carcinoma. The production of parathormone-related peptide can produce hypercalcemia even without bony metastases.

○ **What type of lung tumors can cause excessive ACTH production and Cushing syndrome?**

Small cell carcinoma and carcinoid tumors.

○ **Second-hand cigarette smoke exposure is a risk factor for the development of what two major lung diseases?**

Lung cancer and COPD.

○ **The incidence of lung cancer is increasing in the USA among members of which gender?**

Women.

○ **What percentage of lung cancers are a result of smoking, either active or former smokers?**

85%.

○ **What is the relative risk for first-degree family members getting lung cancer?**

Two- to three-fold risk.

○ **What accounts for this increase?**

Increased cigarette smoking prevalence.

○ **Which vitamin has been associated with a protective effect against the development of lung cancer?**

Vitamin A.

○ **Bilateral periostitis, typically affecting the long bones and associated with lung cancer, is known as what other disease?**

Hypertrophic osteoarthropathy (HPO).

○ **What myopathic syndrome is associated with lung cancer?**

Eaton-Lambert syndrome.

○ **What is the initial diagnostic test in a clinically stable patient suspected of having lung cancer?**

Sputum cytologic examination.

○ **What is the 5-year survival of all patients diagnosed with primary lung cancer?**

~15%.

○   **Which primary lung cancer is most likely to cavitate?**

Squamous cell carcinoma.

○   **Which lung cancer is the most prevalent in nonsmoking women?**

Adenocarcinoma.

○   **What percentages of patients that have lung cancer are asymptomatic?**

5% to 15%.

○   **The increase in death rate from lung cancer among smokers, as opposed to nonsmokers, is how high?**

8- to 20-fold.

○   **Do low tar cigarettes decrease the risk of lung cancer?**

No.

○   **The risk of lung cancer following smoking cessation approaches that of lifelong nonsmokers after how many years?**

15.

○   **The incidence of lung cancer among urban residents is how many times higher than among rural residents?**

About 1.5 times higher among urban residents.

○   **The most common malignancy associated with asbestos exposure is which of the following: esophageal carcinoma, primary lung cancer, mesothelioma, or gastric carcinoma?**

Primary lung cancer.

○   **What is the incidence of pleural effusion associated with malignancy?**

Malignant pleural effusions are the second most common exudative effusions after parapneumonic effusions. The most common malignancies are lung and breast cancer.

○   **What are the conditions associated with malignant transudative effusions?**

Lymphatic obstruction, endobronchial obstruction, and hypoalbuminemia due to the primary malignancy.

○   **What type of effusions are suggestive of malignancy?**

Massive effusions, large effusions without contralateral mediastinal shift, or bilateral effusions with normal heart size suggest malignancy.

○   **What percentage of lung cancer is related to smoking?**

80%.

○ **What other exposures are also factors contributing to the development of bronchogenic carcinoma?**

Radon, uranium, nickel, arsenic, bis (chloromethyl) ether, ionizing radiation, vinyl chloride, mustard gas, polycyclic aromatic hydrocarbons, and chromium.

○ **What is the major indication for laser bronchoscopy in the treatment of bronchogenic carcinoma?**

Tumor obstruction of large airways.

○ **What is Pancoast syndrome?**

Tumor of the apex of the lung that gives rise to Horner syndrome and shoulder pain. The tumor invades the bronchial plexus.

○ **Which primary lung cancer is most frequently associated with paraneoplastic syndromes?**

Small cell undifferentiated carcinoma.

○ **What finding indicates emergent radiation therapy for superior vena cava syndrome?**

Cerebral edema.

○ **The best 5-year survival for non–small cell carcinoma of the lung is achieved by what therapy modality?**

Surgical resection.

○ **Are carcinoid tumors related to smoking?**

No.

○ **What are the clinical features of carcinoid syndrome?**

Flushing and diarrhea is the most common. Other symptoms include salivation, lacrimation, diaphoresis, diarrhea, and hypotension.

○ **What is the treatment for a nonmetastatic carcinoid tumor?**

Surgery is the only option and may improve the symptoms.

○ **What cancers generally metastasize to the lungs?**

Breast, colon, prostate, and cervical cancers.

○ **What is the description of a solitary pulmonary nodule?**

It is defined as a density that is sharply marginated and surrounded by lung tissue that ranges in size on average of 1 to 6 cm in size.

○ **What percentage of pulmonary nodules is malignant?**

35%.

○ **Radiographic stability for what period is assumed to indicate benign origin of a solitary pulmonary nodule?**

2 years.

○ **A 27-year-old female nonsmoker is found to have a 2-cm nodule found on a chest X-ray during a preop screening film. The patient is asymptomatic and is otherwise healthy. What is the standard of care in monitoring this nodule?**

For patients younger than 35 years of age, 3-month serial CT scans of the chest for 1 year are required. If the patient is older than 35 years of age and is a smoker, an immediate evaluation of the tissue is required.

○ **A solitary pulmonary nodule in an HIV-infected patient may represent which of the following: PCP, histoplasmosis, cryptococcosis, or bronchogenic carcinoma?**

All of the above.

● ● ● OBSTRUCTIVE PULMONARY DISEASE ● ● ●

○ **What is the peak age of asthma?**

3 years of age.

○ **What is the gender ratio of asthmatic patients in childhood and adults?**

There is a 2:1 male-to-female ratio in childhood, but evens in numbers in adult populations.

○ **What are some categories of risk factors for those with asthma and what are some of those factors?**

There are three categories:

- **Endogenous**: Gender, atopy, hyperresponsiveness, and genetic predisposition.
- **Triggers**: Allergens, URI viral infections, exercise, cold air, β-blockers, aspirin, stress, and irritants.
- **Environmental**: Indoor/outdoor allergens, occupational, passive smoking, and respiratory infections.

○ **What blood cell is known to cause the initial inflammatory changes that result in asthma?**

Mast cells.

○ **Which blood cell is proliferated during an allergen response?**

Eosinophils.

○ **What extrinsic allergens most commonly affect asthmatic children?**

Dust and dust mites.

○ **What are the common symptoms that present in asthma?**

Cough, shortness of breath, pain between the scapula, itching under the chin (sometimes), and a nonproductive cough especially in children (aka variant asthma cough).

○ **What is the "best" pulmonary function test for the diagnosis of asthma?**

FEV1/FVC. This test determines the amount of air exhaled in 1 minute compared to the total amount of air in the lung that can be expressed. A ratio under 80% is diagnostic of asthma. Peak flow monitors are helpful in monitoring asthma at home or during an acute exacerbation.

○ **Is wheezing an integral part of asthma?**

No; 33% of children with asthma will only have cough variant asthma with no wheezing.

○ **What X-ray markings may be observed in a patient with a long history of bronchial asthma?**

Increased bronchial wall markings and flattening of the diaphragm. The bronchial wall markings are caused by epithelial inflammation and thickening of the bronchial walls.

○ **Patients with exercise-induced asthma will most likely trigger their asthma with what kind of exercise?**

High intensity exercise for more than 5 to 6 minutes.

○ **What is the first-line treatment for asthma?**

Use of β_2-agonist bronchodilators, specifically albuterol in either metered dose inhaler (MDI) or nebulized.

○ **Are anticholinergics medications (i.e., ipratropium bromide) alone effective for the treatment of asthma?**

No. They are effective only with use of albuterol as the first-line treatment and if the first-line treatment is not effective on its own.

○ **What is the clinical indication for the use of theophylline?**

It is indicated for use in patients with severe asthma who require additional bronchodilators.

○ **What are some of the common side effects of theophylline?**

Nausea, vomiting, and headaches.

○ **What is the most effective medication for reduction of inflammation in the treatment of asthma?**

Inhalable corticosteroids.

○ **Is there a need to administer a tapering dose of steroids?**

No. In cases of steroid regimens of 5 to 10 days duration, a tapering dose is not needed.

○ **Is the sole use of antileukotrienes effective for the suppression of asthma symptoms?**

No, they are useful in conjunction with inhalable corticosteroids but are not effective as a stand-alone treatment.

○ **At what point do you need to consider adding more therapy above the normal albuterol regimen so as to control asthma? What is the treatment of choice when you must administer an additional medication?**

When rescue inhaler is used three or more times in a week, and inclusion of inhalable corticosteroids will be the next medication added to the regimen.

○ **Which is more effective for relieving an acute exacerbation of bronchial asthma in a conscious patient: nebulized albuterol or albuterol MDI administered via an aerosol chamber?**

They are both equally effective.

○ **What are the positive effects of administering β-agonists in the treatment of asthma?**

Relaxation of smooth muscle, inhibition of mast cells, inhibition of airway edema, increase in mucociliary clearance, increase mucus production, and decrease in cough.

○ **What are the chances that a child born to two asthmatic parents will also have asthma?**

Up to 50%.

○ **Are there any contraindications to administering a topical β₂-blocker for glaucoma (i.e., timolol) to a patient with asthma?**

Yes, there is evidence that even a topical β-blocking agent may exacerbate asthma symptoms.

○ **What treatment should be initiated for an acute asthmatic patient who does not improve with humidified O₂, albuterol nebulizers, steroids, or anticholinergics?**

Subcutaneous epinephrine, 0.3 cm³ administered every 5 minutes.

○ **Asthmatic patients will most likely have a family history of what?**

Asthma, allergies, or atopic dermatitis.

○ **What are the recommended therapeutic serum theophylline levels?**

10 to 15 mg/L.

○ **What medications should be avoided for an asthmatic patient who is pregnant?**

Epinephrine and parenteral β-adrenergic agonists.

○ **A 23-year-old woman who has a history of asthma is 29 weeks pregnant. She is having an asthma attack and is receiving treatment in the emergency room with an albuterol nebulizer. Given this scenario, is this patient a candidate for oral or parenteral steroids?**

Yes. If steroids are indicated for this condition, then one should not hold back from giving them.

○ **What is a normal peak expiratory flow rate in adults?**

Men: 550 to 600 L/minute. Women: 450 to 500 L/minute. However, this varies somewhat with body size and age.

○ **Which β-adrenergic receptors primarily control bronchiolar and arterial smooth muscle tone?**

β-2-adrenergic receptors.

○ **Terbutaline is administered subcutaneously for asthma in what dose?**

0.01 mL/kg of 1 mg/mL terbutaline up to 0.25 mL, i.e., 0.25 mg, which may be repeated once in 20 to 30 minutes.

○ **Is theophylline useful in the emergency management of a severely asthmatic pediatric patient?**

No. It has not been shown to affect further bronchodilatation in patients fully treated with β-adrenergic agents. However, theophylline can be used successfully for inpatient management of asthma and may be started in the hospital.

○ **If corticosteroids are prescribed for acute asthma exacerbation, how should prednisone be dosed?**

1 to 2 mg/kg/day in two divided doses. Tapering is not necessary if the duration of therapy is 5 days or less.

○ **What is the appropriate parenteral dose of methylprednisolone (Solu-Medrol) to administer to a pediatric patient with status asthmaticus?**

1 to 2 mg/kg every 6 hours.

○ **Can beta-adrenergic agonists result in tolerance?**

Yes. Repeated administration of beta agonist bronchodilators can result in hyposensitization of the receptors, but this should not preclude their use. Glucocorticoids have been shown to restore the depressed receptor responsiveness.

○ **True/False: Cardioselective beta-blockers avoid precipitation of bronchospasm in asthmatic individuals:**

False.

○ **What is the therapeutic drug of choice for beta-blocker–induced bronchospasm?**

Inhalable ipratropium bromide. If severe, parenteral glucagon can reverse effects.

○ **How do steroids function in the treatment of asthma?**

Steroids increase cAMP, decrease inflammation, and aid in restoring the function of β-adrenergic responsiveness to adrenergic drugs.

○ **What is the most common cause of refractory asthma?**

Medical noncompliance.

○ **What is bronchiectasis?**

Bronchiectasis is an abnormal dilatation of the proximal medium-sized bronchi greater than 2 mm in diameter. It occurs due to the destruction of the muscular and elastic components of their walls and is usually associated with chronic bacterial infection and foul smelling sputum.

○ **Which gender is more affected by bronchiectasis?**

Women.

○ **What are the symptoms of bronchiectasis?**

Chronic cough, purulent sputum, fever, weakness, weight loss, dyspnea in some patients, and hemoptysis. Hemoptysis is generally mild, originates from bronchial arteries, and is seen in 50% to 70% of all cases.

○ **What are the main causative agents of bronchiectasis?**

Adenovirus and influenza.

○ **What are the most common complications of bronchiectasis?**

Recurrent attacks of pneumonia, empyema, pneumothorax, and lung abscess.

○ **A chest X-ray shows honeycombing, atelectasis, and increased bronchial markings. What is the diagnosis?**

Bronchiectasis, an irreversible dilation of the bronchi that is generally associated with infection. Bronchography shows dilations of the bronchial tree, but this method of diagnosis is not recommended for routine use.

○ **Bronchiectasis occurs most frequently in patients with what conditions?**

Cystic fibrosis, immunodeficiencies, lung infections, or foreign body aspirations.

○ **Which lung segments are most frequently involved in bronchiectasis?**

Posterior basal segments of the left or right lower lobes.

○ **What are the most common causes of upper lobe bronchiectasis?**

Tuberculous endobronchitis and allergic bronchopulmonary aspergillosis (ABPA).

○ **What is the mainstay of treatment of bronchiectasis?**

Antibiotics.

○ **What are the adjunctive treatment measures that may be beneficial in patients with bronchiectasis?**

Chest physiotherapy, nutritional support, inhalable indomethacin (shown to decrease bronchial hypersecretion by inhibiting neutrophil recruitment), bronchodilators, supplemental oxygen, immunoglobulin administration for immunoglobulin deficiency, replacement treatment for patients with alpha-1-anti-trypsin deficiency, and recombinant DNAase to reduce sputum viscosity in patients with cystic fibrosis (CF).

○ **What is the definition of chronic bronchitis?**

A productive cough for 3 months out of each year for 2 years straight.

○ **What is the definition of emphysema?**

Emphysema is a pathologic diagnosis of the destruction of terminal bronchioles with air trapping and enlargement of the air spaces. Coupled with chronic bronchitis, these two diseases make up COPD.

○ **What is the hallmark symptom of COPD?**

Exertional dyspnea.

○ **What is a "blue bloater"?**

An overweight patient with COPD, bronchitis, and central cyanosis. These individuals have normal lung capacity and are hypoxic.

○ **What is a "pink puffer"?**

A patient with COPD and emphysema. These patients are generally thin and noncyanotic. They have an increased total lung capacity and a decreased FEV1.

○ **What percentage of all COPD patients have either smoked or had a significant exposure to cigarette smoke?**

80%.

○ **Other than smoking, what are the risk factors for COPD?**

Environmental pollutants, recurrent URIs (especially in infancy), eosinophilia or increased serum IgE, bronchial hyperresponsiveness, a family history of COPD, and protease deficiencies.

○ **Is there any hope for patients with COPD who quit smoking?**

Yes. Symptomatically speaking, coughing stops in up to 80% of these patients, and 54% of COPD patients find relief from coughing within a month of quitting.

○ **If a patient with chronic bronchitis suffers an acute exacerbation of illness, such as dyspnea, cough, or purulent sputum, what type of O_2 therapy should be initiated?**

In the case of acute exacerbation of bronchitis, oxygen therapy should be guided by Po_2 levels. Adequate oxygen must be maintained at a Po_2 above 60 mm Hg. This should be accomplished with the minimal amount of oxygen necessary. The Po_2 must be kept above 60 mm Hg even if the patient loses the drive to breathe.

○ **What are the more common pathogens that are found in the sputum of COPD patients?**

Streptococcus pneumoniae, H. influenzae, or *Moraxella catarrhalis.*

○ **Are there any changes to the EKG if the patient has COPD?**

Yes, there can be several. Sinus tachycardia can be seen as well as RVH and LVH. Supraventricular arrhythmias (MAT, A-fib/flutter) as well as ventricular irritability can also be present.

○ **Which pulmonary function test shows an increase in COPD?**

Residual volume. All other tests (FEV_1, FEV_1/FVC, and $FEV_{25\%-75\%}$) indicate decreases and diffusion capacity.

○ **Which part of the lung is affected by emphysema? By chronic bronchitis?**

Emphysema: Terminal bronchi
Chronic bronchitis: Large airways

○ **What is the typical appearance of a chest X-ray in a patient with emphysema?**

Increased inflation from cephalo to caudal, with flattening of the diaphragm. In some patients, bullae can develop.

○ **What is the risk of placing a patient with COPD on a high FIO_2?**

Suppression of the hypoxic ventilatory drive.

○ **What are some potential complications related to COPD?**

Pneumonia, cor pulmonale, bronchitis, pulmonary thromboembolism, and left-sided heart failure.

○ **What is the single most important therapy for patients with COPD?**

Smoking cessation.

○ **What pharmacologic agents are used for the initial treatment of COPD?**

Bronchodilators are the mainstay treatment.

○ **Are there any other therapies in addition to bronchodilators?**

Yes, corticosteroids (usually inhaled) are a second-line treatment. This is followed by theophylline as a third-line therapy.

○ **Are there any changes to therapy for COPD patients who require admission to the hospital?**

Yes, the addition of ipratropium as well as of broad-spectrum antibiotic and oxygen is indicated. Chest PT is also helpful in clearing secretions for those patients who may be developing mucous plugging.

○ **What parameters should make you consider initiating "home oxygen" therapy for a patient with COPD?**

If the patient has a resting Po_2 less than 55 mm Hg, or if the patient has a Po_2 of less than 60 mm Hg with evidence of tissue hypoxia. O_2 desaturation with exercise may also require home O_2. Home O_2 therapy, 18 h/day, may increase the life span of a patient with COPD by 6 to 7 years.

○ **What nonpharmacologic therapies are indicated for the treatment of COPD?**

Aside from smoking cessation, respiratory therapy to increase the clearing of secretions is helpful. Aerobic exercise is also helpful to increase exercise capacity.

○ **What are some late-stage diseases that are caused by COPD?**

Cor pulmonale, pulmonary hypertension, pneumonia, and chronic respiratory failure.

○ **What is the most common lethal, inheritable disease among the Caucasian population?**

Cystic fibrosis, an autosomal recessive disease that occurs in 1 in 3200 births, and 1 in 25 is a carrier.

○ **A newborn presents with poor weight gain, steatorrhea, and a GI obstruction arising from thick meconium ileus. What test should be performed?**

The sweat test, which detects electrolyte concentrations in the sweat. The infant may have cystic fibrosis, an autosomal recessive defect that affects the exocrine glands, producing higher electrolyte concentrations in the sweat glands.

○ **What condition must be ruled out when childhood nasal polyps are found?**

Cystic fibrosis (CF).

○ **What is the classic triad of cystic fibrosis?**

- COPD
- Pancreatic enzyme deficiency
- Abnormally high concentration of sweat electrolytes

○ **What are the diagnostic criteria for cystic fibrosis?**

Primary Criteria:

- Characteristic pulmonary manifestations and/or
- Characteristic gastrointestinal manifestations and/or
- A family history of CF

Plus

- Sweat Cl (concentration >60 mEq/L) [repeat measurement if sweat Cl is 50–60 mEq/L].

Secondary Criteria:

- Documentation of dual CFTR mutations and
- Evidence of one or more characteristic manifestations

○ **What are the immunological defects in cystic fibrosis?**

Patients with have low levels of serum IgG in the first decade of life, which increase dramatically once chronic infection is established. T-lymphocyte numbers are adequate. With advancing severity of pulmonary disease, lymphocytes proliferate less briskly in response to *P. aeruginosa* and other gram-negative organisms. Deficient opsonic activity of alveolar macrophages are seen in patients with established *P. aeruginosa* infection. Major IgG subclass in serum and lungs in CF patients is IgG.

○ **Pathology in cystic fibrosis is confined predominantly to what part of the lung?**

The conducting airways.

○ **What is the most common site of nonpulmonary pathology in cystic fibrosis?**

The GI tract, with striking changes seen in the exocrine pancreas. Islets of Langerhans are spared.

○ **What are the reproductive abnormalities in cystic fibrosis?**

- *In men:* The vas deferens, tail and body of the epididymis, and the seminal vesicles are either absent or rudimentary.
- *In women:* Uterine cervical glands are distended. The mucous and cervical canals are plugged with tenacious mucous secretions. Endocervicitis also seen.

○ **What are the most frequent respiratory pathogens in patients with cystic fibrosis?**

Staphylococcus aureus and *Pseudomonas aeruginosa.*

○ **What are the various radiographic manifestations of cystic fibrosis?**

Hyperinflation, peribronchial cuffing, mucous impaction in airways seen as branching fingerlike shadows, bronchiectasis, subpleural blebs, (most prominent along the mediastinal border), and prominent pulmonary artery segments with advanced disease.

○ **What is the immediate mortality with massive hemoptysis?**

~ 10%.

○ **What are the conditions associated with an elevated sweat chloride?**

CF, hypothyroidism, pseudohypoaldosteronism, hypoparathyroidism, nephrogenic diabetes insipidus, type I glycogen storage disease, mucopolysaccharidosis, malnutrition, PGE administration, hypogammaglobulinemia, and pancreatitis.

○ **What are some of the more common pulmonary complications of Cystic Fibrosis How do you manage them?**

Pulmonary Complication	Management
Right-sided heart failure	Improve oxygenation through intensive pulmonary therapy.
Respiratory failure	Vigorous medical therapy of the underlying lung disease and infection.
Atelectasis	Aggressive antibiotic therapy and frequent chest physiotherapy.
Pneumothorax	Conservative if <10% and patient asymptomatic. Pleurodesis to avoid recurrence.
Small-volume hemoptysis	Aggressive treatment of lung infection.
Persistent massive hemoptysis	Bronchial artery embolization along with aggressive treatment of the lung infection.

○ **What two vaccinations should be given to all cystic fibrosis patients?**

Pneumococcal and influenza vaccines.

○ **What is the only definitive treatment for advanced cystic fibrosis?**

Double lung transplant.

○ **What is the life expectancy of a patient with cystic fibrosis?**

The median survival age is over 35 years of age.

○ **Prior steroid administration can precipitate adrenal insufficiency under conditions of stress. How long can these effects last?**

Up to 1 year.

• • • PLEURAL DISEASES • • •

○ **Differentiate between transudate and exudate:**

- *Transudate:* Systemic factors that influence the formation and shift of fluid into the pleural space.

  Pleural: Serum protein <0.5

  Pleural: Serum LDH is <0.6

  Most common with heart failure from LV dysfunction (most common), renal disease, and liver disease.

- *Exudate:* Local factors that influence the formation and absorption of fluid into the pleural space.

  Pleural: Serum protein >0.5

  Pleural: Serum LDH >0.6

  Most common with pneumonia, malignancy, pulmonary embolism, and trauma.

○ **What are the clinical features associated with pleural effusion?**

A pleural rub (may be the only finding in the early stages), pleuritic chest pain due to involvement and inflammation of parietal pleura, cough (distortion of lung), dyspnea (mechanical inefficiency of respiratory muscles stretched by outward movement of chest wall and downward movement of diaphragm), diminished chest wall movements, dull percussion, decreased tactile and vocal fremitus, decreased breath sounds, and whispering pectoriloquy. With large amounts, there may be contralateral shift of the mediastinum.

○ **Where does pain from pleurisy radiate?**

The shoulder, as a result of diaphragmatic irritation.

○ **What is the minimum amount of pleural liquid that can be detected roentgenographically?**

Approximately 250 mL in upright views of the chest. A lateral decubitus film taken with the patient lying on the affected side can detect as little as 50 mL of liquid.

○ **What are the indications for the chest tube placement in parapneumonic effusion?**

Presence of a complicated parapneumonic effusion, as evidenced by presence of fever, presence of loculations, gross appearance of fluid purulent (pus), increased WBC count and low glucose (usually <40 mg/dL), a decreased pH (less than 7.0 or 0.15 less than the arterial pH), and elevated LDH (>1000 IU/L) are usually considered indications for placement of chest tube for drainage.

○ **What are the characteristic features of a tuberculous pleural effusion?**

Pleural fluid is exudative with a protein content >0.5 g/L, >90% to 95% lymphocytes (in the acute phase, there may be a polymorphonuclear response).

○ **What is the treatment of tuberculous pleural effusion?**

A 9-month course of isoniazid 300 mg and rifampin 600 mg, daily. A therapeutic thoracentesis is recommended only to relieve dyspnea. Corticosteroids can decrease the duration of fever and the time required for fluid absorption, but do not decrease the amount of pleural thickening at 12 months after treatment is initiated. They are therefore recommended only for patients who are markedly symptomatic and only after institution of appropriate antimicrobial therapy.

○ **What are the common features of pleural effusions associated with congestive heart failure?**

Bilateral effusion, more commonly right-sided, associated with cardiomegaly. Fluid is transudate, serous, <1000 mononuclear cells, pH >7.4, and pleural fluid glucose levels same as serum.

○ **What are the radiological features of pleural effusion associated with cirrhosis?**

They are small to massive right-sided effusion in 70%, left-sided effusion in 15%, and bilateral effusions in 15% with normal heart size.

○ **What is the mechanism of pleural effusions associated with atelectasis?**

Atelectasis leads to decreased perimicrovascular pressure, resulting in a pressure gradient. Fluid moves from the parietal pleural interstitium into the pleural space due to decreased perimicrovascular pressure.

○ **What is the primary mechanism of pleural effusion in nephritic syndrome?**

Decreased plasma oncotic pressure due to hypoalbuminemia.

○ **What factors play a role in the pathogenesis of pleural effusions associated with pulmonary embolism?**

Effusions are present in 40% to 50% of cases of pulmonary embolism. Increased capillary permeability, due to ischemia and leak of protein rich fluid into pleural space, are the main factors. Atelectasis may contribute to transudate and lung necrosis can lead to hemorrhage.

○ **What are the characteristics of a pleural effusion associated with chronic pancreatitis?**

Pleural effusions associated with chronic pancreatitis are usually large or massive unilateral effusions that occur rapidly after thoracentesis. The pleural fluid can have very high amylase content (>200,000 IU/L). Direct fistulous communications from the pancreatic bed are responsible. Failure of conservative treatment is an indication for the surgical intervention, such as drainage (up to 50%).

○ **What are the characteristic features of pleural fluid in patients with lupus?**

LE cells in the pleural fluid. A ratio of pleural fluid/serum ANA of >1.0 is suggestive of lupus.

○ **What are some drugs reported to be associated with pleural effusion?**

Procainamide, nitrofurantoin, Dantrolene, Methysergide, procarbazine, methotrexate, Amiodarone, mitomycin, and Bleomycin.

○ **What pathological process is suggested by an air–fluid level in the pleural space?**
Bronchopleural fistula.

○ **What is the profile of a classic patient with a spontaneous pneumothorax?**
Male, athletic, tall, slim, and 15 to 35 years of age.

○ **What is the recurrence rate of spontaneous pneumothoraces?**
50%.

○   **What is the main cause for a patient to develop a pneumothorax?**

The most common reason is rupture of a bleb.

○   **A 20-year-old male patient presents with pleuritic chest pain with shortness of breath that has worsened over the last 24 hours after he had a violent cough. In general, the patient is healthy and has no medical problems. On examination, he is afebrile, has a pulse of 100, respirations of 22, and blood pressure is 122/83. Head and neck is normal, and the patient has decreased breath sounds on the right with hyperresononant percussion. What is the likely diagnosis?**

Primary spontaneous pneumothorax.

○   **Which types of pneumonia are commonly associated with pneumothorax?**

Staphylococcal, TB, Klebsiella, and PCP.

○   **What therapy may increase the body's absorption of a pneumothorax or pneumomediastinum?**

A high F_{IO_2}.

○   **Do all pneumothoraces need to have a chest tube or surgical intervention?**

No. A small pneumothorax that is <25% with mild to minimal symptoms can be observed as an outpatient with serial chest X-rays to observe reinflation.

○   **A 26-year-old man has been diagnosed with a primary spontaneous pneumothorax, which has been treated and now has a reoccurrence. What is the treatment for this patient?**

Surgical pleurodesis. This procedure should completely resolve the condition.

○   **What is the definition of a secondary pneumothorax?**

It is a pneumothorax that is caused by COPD, typically by an emphysematous bleb. This tends to be more life-threatening due to the underlying lung disease present.

○   **Is therapy for secondary pneumothorax different from a primary pneumothorax?**

Yes, the initial treatment is with a chest tube to re-inflate the lung, then surgical intervention with pleurodesis. If required, a blebectomy or stapling is indicated.

○   **What are some of the more common techniques for pleurodesis?**

Mechanical abrasion of the chest wall, chemical application with multiple agents (tetracycline, urea, mechlorethamine, iodoform, and hypertonic glucose), or pleural staple ling are used. Talc has been implemented in the past but is a controversial technique. It is still used in some places.

○   **What is the indication for a chest tube in a patient with a pneumothorax?**

Over 20% to 25% pneumothorax or a clinical indication, such as respiratory distress or enlarging pneumothorax.

○   **What are the most common reasons for a traumatic pneumothorax?**

Insertion of a transthoracic needle, thoracentesis, and central line placement.

○ **What is the most important cause of hypoxia in a patient with flail chest?**

Underlying lung contusion.

○ **Signs of tension pneumothorax on a physical examination include:**

Tachypnea, unilateral absent breath sounds, tachycardia, pallor, diaphoresis, cyanosis, hyperresonant percussion on affected side, tracheal deviation, hypotension, and neck vein distention.

○ **What is the most significant finding on a chest X-ray in a patient with a tension pneumothorax?**

Shift of the mediastinum away from the effected side.

○ **What is the initial treatment for a tension pneumothorax?**

Large bore IV catheter placed in the anterior second intercostal space (not a chest tube).

○ **What are the risk factors of pneumothorax?**

Pneumothorax (risk factors):

Tall stature
Thin body mass
Twenties of age
Tobacco smoking
Trauma
Tumors

● ● ● PULMONARY CIRCULATION ● ● ●

○ **What does normal ventilation with decreased lung perfusion suggest?**

Pulmonary embolus.

○ **What are the most common signs and symptoms of PE?**

In order from most to least common: tachypnea, CP, dyspnea, anxiety tachycardia, fever, DVT, hypotension, and syncope.

○ **What percentage of patients with a symptomatic PE will also have a DVT present in the lower extremities?**

50% to 70%.

○ **What is the most common type of substance that forms a pulmonary embolus?**

A thrombus.

○ **Are there any other substances that can cause the formation of an embolus?**

Yes, there are several which include air from a surgery or a central venous line, amniotic fluid, fat embolus, foreign bodies, parasites, septic emboli, and tumor cells.

○ **Name some risk factors that can predispose a patient to a PE:**

Venous stasis (immobility, obesity, stroke), injury to the vascular wall (prior embolus, trauma, and orthopedic surgery), and hypercoagulability (Virchow triad).

○ **What is Virchow triad?**
- Injury to the endothelium of the vessels
- Hypercoagulable state
- Stasis

These represent risk factors for pulmonary embolus.

○ **Most pulmonary embolisms arise from what veins?**

The iliac and femoral veins.

○ **What is the most common hypercoagulability genetic disorder in white patients?**

Factor V Leiden, which is a resistance to protein C.

○ **Name some other hypercoagulable states predisposing individuals to thrombosis and pulmonary embolism:**

Deficiencies of protein S and antithrombin III, antiphospholipid syndrome, malignancy particularly adenocarcinoma, nephritic syndrome, protein losing enteropathy, extensive burns, paroxysmal nocturnal hemoglobinuria, and oral contraceptives.

○ **What historical findings suggest an embolus as opposed to a thrombosis in a lower extremity?**
- *Embolus*: Associated with a history of arrhythmia, valvular disease, MI, no skin changes from chronic arterial insufficiency, and no symptoms in the opposite extremity.
- *Thrombosis*: Opposite extremity shows evidence of chronic arterial occlusive disease with history of rest pain, claudication, etc.

○ **What three syndromes are associated with the various degrees of pulmonary embolism?**

1. Acute cor pulmonale: Occurs with massive embolism that obstructs over 60% of the pulmonary circulation.
2. Pulmonary infarction: Occurs with embolization to the distal branches of the pulmonary circulation.
3. Acute dyspnea: Milder obstruction not enough to warrant infarction.

○ **What is the equation for the A–a gradient?**

$$\text{A–a} = (713 \text{ mm Hg} \times F_{IO_2}) - P_{CO_2} - P_{O_2}/0.8)$$

The normal A–a gradient is 5 to 15 mm Hg (though it increases with age). The A–a gradient increases with PE and diffusion defects (i.e., pulmonary edema and right to left cardiac shunts).

○ **Can a patient with a PE have a P_{O_2} greater than 90 mm Hg?**

Yes, but rarely (5%).

○ **What are the most common CXR findings in PE?**

Pleural effusions, atelectasis, and pulmonary infiltrates.

○ **What are two relatively specific CXR findings in PE?**

1. Hampton hump: Area of lung consolidation with a rounded border facing the hilus.
2. Westermark sign: Dilated pulmonary outflow tract proximal to the emboli with decreased perfusion distal to the lesion.

   While both of these findings are specific to PE, they are not seen much.

○ **What test is considered the gold standard for the diagnosis of DVT? For the diagnosis of PE?**

- DVT: venography.
- PE: pulmonary angiography.

○ **What changes to an EKG are commonly seen in patients with a PE?**

Sinus tachycardia is the most common, followed by nonspecific ST-T changes. These will be seen in about 40% of patients.

○ **When treating DVT/PE, when should warfarin therapy be initiated?**

On the first or second day after initiation of heparin therapy. Although heparin should be administered immediately, it can be discontinued when the PTT is 1.5 to 1.8 times normal for at least 3 days.

○ **How long should chronic warfarin therapy, as a prophylaxis for DVT, be given?**

Warfarin should be administered for at least 3 to 6 months after a DVT to maintain an INR at two to three times the normal.

○ **What is the anticoagulant treatment schedule for a PE?**

IV heparin until PTT is 2 to 2.5 times normal. After 1 day of treatment, warfarin is added until the INR is greater than 2.0. If clots recur, consider a Greenfield filter in the IVC. Pulmonary embolectomy is only necessary in cases of massive embolisms. Lovenox may also be used instead of heparin.

○ **What is the risk factor for PE in a patient with an axillary or subclavian vein thrombus?**

About 15%.

○ **What test is most sensitive for evaluating a PE?**

Ventilation–perfusion scan is the most sensitive test. However, it is not as specific as a pulmonary angiogram; 5% of normal volunteers will have an abnormal scan and virtually any pulmonary pathology will produce an abnormal scan (i.e., pneumonia).

○ **What is the preferred test to detect a PE in a pregnant patient?**

V/Q scan. The IV dye load during pregnancy is not ideal. When performing a V/Q scan, make sure to insert a Foley catheter in the bladder to remove the radioactive material from the bladder so that it does not expose the fetus.

○ **What is the major etiology of pulmonary hypertension?**

Chronic hypoxia, most commonly from COPD.

○ **What are the major mechanisms that cause pulmonary hypertension to occur?**

- **Reduction of the cross section of the pulmonary bed,** such as in hypoxemia, emphysema, interstitial lung disease, parasitic infections, and sickle cell disease.
- **Increase in pulmonary venous pressure** as in LV failure, mitral stenosis, restrictive pericarditis, or left atrial myxoma.
- **Increase in pulmonary venous flow** such as a congenital left to right shunt.
- **Increase in blood viscosity** (polycythemia).
- **Other conditions** such as HIV, and HTN related to cirrhosis, and portal hypertension.

○ **What are the common symptoms related to pulmonary hypertension?**

Dyspnea, fatigue, chest pain, and syncope on exertion.

○ **Primary pulmonary hypertension is most common in what population?**

Young women. PPH is rapidly fatal within a few years.

○ **What heart sounds accompany pulmonary hypertension?**

A splitting of the second heart sound and a louder P2.

○ **What could you expect to see on an ECG in a patient with pulmonary HTN?**

Right ventricular strain or hypertrophy, and right atrial enlargement.

○ **What is the most effective method in measuring pulmonary venous pressures in cases of suspected pulmonary hypertension?**

Right-sided heart catheterization.

○ **Which noninvasive method can be done to measure pressures?**

Echocardiography with Doppler flow.

○ **What is the main treatment plan for patients with secondary pulmonary hypertension?**

Treat the underlying disorder that is causing the hypertension.

○ **What is the 2-year survival rate in patients with pulmonary hypertension?**

50%.

○ **What is cor pulmonale?**

It is the dilation and hypertrophy of the right ventricle in response to changes within the pulmonary vascular and parenchymal system.

○ **What are the two leading conditions that predispose a patient to developing cor pulmonale?**

COPD and chronic bronchitis, which leads to pulmonary hypertension.

○   **What is the most common symptom of patients with cor pulmonale?**

Dyspnea.

○   **What is the effect of brain natriuretic peptide (BNP) levels in patients with cor pulmonale?**

They are usually markedly elevated chronically.

○   **What is the treatment for cor pulmonale?**

Treat the underlying cause of the reason for the disease being present.

○   **What are the pulmonary manifestations in Paget disease?**

High output cardiac failure with pulmonary edema, impaired respiratory control from bony involvement at base of skull, vertebral fractures leading to kyphosis, and restrictive lung disease.

○   **What are the pulmonary manifestations of polycythemia?**

Pulmonary embolism related to hyperviscosity and pulmonary hemorrhage related to an increased bleeding tendency.

○   **What is the classic presentation of venous air embolism?**

Sudden hypotension with a mill wheel murmur audible over the precordium.

○   **What is the preferred patient position in suspected venous air embolism?**

Left lateral decubitus and Trendelenburg.

● ● ● RESTRICTIVE PULMONARY DISEASE ● ● ●

○   **What are some of the signs and symptoms of idiopathic pulmonary fibrosis (IPF)?**

Exertional dyspnea, nonproductive cough, inspiratory crackles, and digital clubbing on examination.

○   **What are some expected findings on chest X-rays and lung scans in patients with IPF?**

Basilar, and subpleural reticular opacities. These are associated with bronchiectasis and honeycombing.

○   **Name some illnesses that can accelerate the disease and overall prognosis of patients with IPF:**

Infections (pneumonia, bronchitis), pulmonary embolism, pneumothorax, and heart failure.

○   **What is the survival rate of a patient with IPF who is intubated?**

Only 25% of patients make it off the vent and survive.

○   **Is there a recommended therapy for patients with an exacerbation of IPF?**

No. There is no one therapy that is recommended. Symptomatic treatment is done. The only other option is lung transplantation for those patients who qualify.

○ **Name the four major groups of pneumoconiosis and the more common types within those groups:**

1. Metal dusts: siderosis, stannosis, and baritosis.

2. Coal dusts: coal dust from mining.

3. Inorganic dusts: free silica from mining

4. Silicate dusts: asbestosis, talcosis, kaolin (sands), and Shaver disease (from aluminum production).

○ **What is the major mechanism that these dusts are routed into the lungs?**

By inhalation.

○ **How do these products injure the lungs?**

They cause an initial inflammatory reaction and then over time create a fibrosis to the lung tissue.

○ **Upper lobe nodules and eggshell hilar node calcification are displayed on X-rays of an individual with what disease?**

Silicosis.

○ **What is the average exposure time necessary for the development of silicosis following silicon dioxide inhalation?**

20 to 30 years. Employees in mining, pottery, soap production, and granite quarrying are at risk. This population also has a higher chance of acquiring TB.

○ **A 14-year-old adolescent boy was exposed to asbestos for 3 days has a nonproductive cough and chest pain. Does this boy have asbestosis?**

No. Although a nonproductive cough and pleurisy are symptoms of asbestosis, other signs, such as exertional dyspnea, malaise, clubbed fingers, crackles, cyanosis, pleural effusion, and pulmonary hypertension, should be displayed before making a diagnosis of asbestosis. In addition, asbestosis does not develop until 10 to 15 years after regular exposure to asbestos.

○ **Asbestosis increases the risk of what two diseases?**

Lung cancer and malignant mesothelioma.

○ **Exposure to what mineral, used as insulation, greatly enhances the carcinogenic potential of exposure to cigarette smoke?**

Asbestos.

○ **What parts of the pulmonary system are affected by asbestosis?**

The pleura and peritoneum. Asbestosis increases the risk of mesotheliomata. It also causes pneumoconioses that invade the lungs.

○ **What age population and race is the most prevalent in the United States for sarcoidosis?**

Patients in the age groups of 30 to 40 years, black, women more than men.

○ **What are the usual presenting symptoms in patients with sarcoidosis?**

They are usually nonpulmonary. They include symptoms of the skin, eyes, and peripheral nerves. Some patients will have quick onset of malaise, fever, and dyspnea. Erythema nodosum, parotid enlargement, lymphadenopathy, and hepatomegaly are also common findings.

○ **What are the three stages of findings in the chest X-ray of a sarcoidosis patient?**
- Stage I: bilateral hilar adenopathy alone
- Stage II: hilar adenopathy and parenchymal involvement
- Stage III: parenchymal involvement alone

○ **What is the best method of test to determine pulmonary sarcoidosis?**

Transbronchial biopsy.

○ **What is the treatment for patients with sarcoidosis?**

Oral steroids (prednisone) 0.5 to 1.0 mg/kg/day to suppress the symptoms.

○ **What are some advanced pulmonary disease complications related to sarcoidosis?**

Advanced fibrosis, bronchiectasis, cavitation, pneumothorax, hemoptysis, and respiratory failure.

• • • OTHER PULMONARY DISEASES AND CONDITIONS • • •

○ **What is ARDS?**

Acute respiratory distress syndrome is a syndrome of rapid dyspnea, hypoxia, and pulmonary infiltrates, which lead to respiratory failure. This can be a result of a direct or indirect insult on the lungs.

○ **What are some direct and indirect illnesses that can cause ARDS?**
- Direct: Pneumonia, near drowning, toxic inhalation
- Indirect: Sepsis, trauma, drug overdose, pancreatitis

○ **What is the most common cause of ARDS?**

Sepsis and pneumonia.

○ **What are the three phases of ARDS progression?**

Exudative, proliferative, and fibrotic phase.

○ **What is the goal of management in patients with ARDS?**

There is little that can be done for these patients. However, by maintaining a low left atrial filling pressure, higher pressures can be prevented from developing into the pulmonary system, thus reducing the chance of increased permeability of fluid into the extravascular space. Mechanical ventilation is helpful in patients whose respiratory drive is failing and can no longer oxygenate themselves.

○ **What is the mortality range in patients with ARDS?**

Anywhere from 41% to 65%.

○ **A preterm infant is breathing rapidly and grunting. Intercostal retractions, nasal flaring, and cyanosis are noted. Auscultation shows decreased breath sounds and crackles. What is the diagnosis?**

Newborn respiratory distress syndrome, also known as hyaline membrane disease. X-rays show diffuse atelectasis. Treatment involves artificial surfactant and O2 administration through CPAP.

○ **At what age is the preterm infant more likely to have hyaline membrane disease?**

When the infant is around 26 to 28 weeks old.

○ **How is fetal lung maturity assessed?**

By measuring the ratio of lecithin to sphingomyelin (L/S). An L/S ratio greater than 2 and the presence of phosphatidyl glycerol confirm that the fetal lungs are mature.

○ **Other than avoiding prematurity, what can be done to prevent newborn respiratory distress syndrome?**

If the fetus is older than 32 weeks, administer betamethasone 48 to 72 hours before delivery to augment surfactant production.

○ **If newborn hyaline membrane disease is present, what is the treatment for these patients?**

In addition to intravenous surfactant, oxygen with or without nasal CPAP long-term is indicated. This is done until the lung maturity has reached an acceptable level.

○ **What factor determines the magnitude of injury in gastric acid aspiration?**

The gastric pH. A pH less than 3 produces the most severe injury.

○ **Under what circumstances is aspiration of vomitus, oral secretions, or foreign material likely?**

Anything producing an altered level of consciousness (e.g., alcohol, overdose, general anesthesia, stroke), impaired swallowing or abnormal gastrointestinal motility, or disruption of the esophageal sphincters predisposes to aspiration.

○ **What are the signs of a large obstructing foreign body in the larynx or trachea?**

Respiratory distress, stridor, inability to speak, cyanosis, loss of consciousness, and death.

○ **What are the symptoms of a smaller (distally lodged) foreign body?**

Cough, dyspnea, wheezing, chest pain, and fever.

○ **What is the procedure of choice for foreign body removal?**

Rigid bronchoscopy. Fiberoptic bronchoscopy is an alternate procedure in adults, not in children. If bronchoscopy fails, thoracotomy may be required.

○ **What are the common radiographic findings in foreign body aspiration?**

Normal film, atelectasis, pneumonia, contralateral mediastinal shift (more marked during expiration), and visualization of the foreign body.

○ **What are the common directly toxic (noninfected) respiratory tract aspirates?**

Gastric contents, alcohol, hydrocarbons, mineral oil, and animal and vegetable fats. All of these produce an inflammatory response and pneumonia. Gastric contents are the most common offender.

○ **What are the consequences of aspirating acid?**

The response is rapid, with near-immediate bronchitis, bronchiolitis, atelectasis, shunting, and hypoxemia. Pulmonary edema may occur within 4 hours. The clinical manifestations are dyspnea, wheezing, cough, cyanosis, fever, and shock.

○ **Under what circumstances are antibiotics used in aspiration?**

Aspiration of infected material, intestinal obstruction, immune compromised host, and evidence of bacterial superinfection after a noninfected aspirate (new fever, infiltrates, or purulence after the initial 2 to 3 days).

○ **What are the radiographic manifestations of acid aspiration?**

Varied, may be bilateral diffuse infiltrates, irregular "patchy" infiltrates, or lobar infiltrates.

○ **What outcomes occur in patients who do not rapidly resolve gastric acid aspiration pneumonitis?**

ARDS (adult respiratory distress syndrome), progressive respiratory failure, and death; bacterial superinfection.

○ **At what percentage of an airway obstruction will inspiratory stridor become evident?**

70% occlusion.

○ **A foreign body is suspected in the lower airways. What will plain films show?**

Air trapping on the affected side. Inspiration and expiration views demonstrate mediastinal shift away from the affected side.

○ **What is the most common cause of death among infants 1 to 12 months old?**

Sudden infant death syndrome.

○ **Where in the airway are foreign bodies usually lodged in children older than 1 year?**

In the lower airway.

○ **Stridor is observed in what phase of respiration?**

Inspiratory.

○ **What is stridor due to?**

With extrathoracic airway obstruction, the pressure inside the extrathoracic part of the airway is much more negative relative to atmospheric pressure. This results in further narrowing of the larynx during inspiration and therefore, stridor.

○ **Grunting is observed during what phase of respiration?**

Expiratory. Exhalation against a closed glottis.

○ **In the diagnosis of a radiolucent foreign body lodged in the right mainstem bronchus, producing incomplete obstruction, inspiratory and expiratory films will show air-trapping and increased lucency of the lung on the involved side. This phenomenon is due to:**

Ball-valve air trapping. Air enters around the foreign body during inspiration, but is trapped as the airway closes around the foreign body during expiration, preventing emptying of that side.

○ **You are at a restaurant and the person at the table next to you begins coughing loudly. She stands up and begins wheezing between coughs, but she is still able to eke out a "Help! I'm choking." How should you help?**

Encourage her to cough deeper and keep breathing. Do not interrupt her spontaneous attempts at expulsion if she still has good air exchange, as evidenced by her state of consciousness and the degree of coughing and wheezing. Should she display severe respiratory difficulty with a weakening cough and the inability to talk, perform the Heimlich maneuver.

○ **What should be done if this patient above is markedly obese and in severe respiratory distress?**

The normal Heimlich maneuver will not be as effective. Instead of positioning your fists above the patient's navel, place your cupped fist on the patient's chest and deliver swift thrusts. This is also the method of choice for pregnant women.

○ **True/False: Pulse oximetry is a reliable method for estimating oxyhemoglobin saturation in a patient suffering from CO poisoning:**

False. COHb has light absorbance that can lead to a falsely elevated pulse oximeter transduced saturation level. The calculated value from a standard ABG may also be falsely elevated. The oxygen saturation should be determined by using a co-oximeter that measures the amounts of unsaturated O_2Hb, COHb, and metHb.

○ **What is the indication for long-term tracheostomy?**

When intubation is expected to exceed 3 weeks.

○ **What are the potential mechanisms of cardiorespiratory collapse?**

Mechanical obstruction of pulmonary vasculature, alveolar capillary leak, pulmonary edema from LV failure, and anaphylaxis.

○ **What are the indications for intubation and ventilation after near drowning?**

Apnea, pulselessness, altered mental status, severe hypoxemia, and respiratory acidosis.

○ **Calculate the alveolar–arterial oxygen (A-aO_2) gradient given the following arterial blood gas obtained at sea level: pH 7.24, PaCO_2 60, PaO_2 45:**

30 mm Hg.

To calculate the alveolar–arterial oxygen gradient, first calculate the expected alveolar partial pressure of oxygen (PaO_2) using the alveolar gas equation: $P_{AO_2} = P_{IO_2} - P_{aCO_2}/R$, where P_{IO_2} is the partial pressure of oxygen in the inspired gas and R is the respiratory exchange ratio, commonly estimated at 0.8. P_{IO_2} is calculated as follows: $P_{IO_2} = F_{IO_2} (P_B - P_{H_2O})$, where F_{IO_2} is the inspired concentration of oxygen (0.21 at sea level), P_B is the atmospheric pressure (760 mm Hg at sea level), and P_{H_2O} is the partial pressure of water (47 mm Hg). At sea level, P_{IO_2} is equal to 150 mm Hg. Thus, for this example, $P_{AO_2} = 150 - 60/0.8$ or 75 mm Hg.

The A-aO_2 gradient is $P_{AO_2} - P_{aO_2}$. Therefore, in this example, the A-aO_2 gradient is $75 - 45$ or 30 mm Hg.

○ **What is the age-related decline in PaO_2?**

The PaO_2 declines by 2.5 mm Hg per decade. Given that a PaO_2 of 95 to 100 mm Hg is normal for a 20-year-old, a PaO_2 of 75–80 would be normal for a 80-year-old.

○ **What are the four principal mechanisms that lead to hypoxemia?**

Hypoventilation, diffusion limitation, shunt, and ventilation–perfusion inequality. A fifth mechanism, low inspired oxygen concentration, is important only at altitudes above 8000 feet.

○ **Which of the four above mechanisms is the most common?**

Ventilation–perfusion inequality.

○ **What are the three major mechanisms of hypoventilation and what clinical conditions are associated with each?**

1. Failure of the central nervous system ventilatory centers: drugs (narcotics, barbiturates) and stroke.
2. Failure of the chest bellows: chest wall diseases (kyphoscoliosis), neuromuscular diseases (amyotrophic lateral sclerosis), and diaphragm weakness.
3. Obstruction of the airways: asthma and chronic obstructive pulmonary disease.

○ **How can hypoxemia secondary to hypoventilation alone be distinguished from the other causes of hypoxemia?**

If the hypoxemia is from hypoventilation alone, the $A\text{-}aO_2$ gradient is normal. It is elevated in all other causes.

○ **What are the most common clinical conditions in which shunt is the primary mechanism for hypoxemia?**

Alveolar filling with fluid (pulmonary edema) and pus (pneumonia) are the most commonly seen clinically. Any condition that fills or closes the alveoli preventing gas exchange can lead to shunt.

○ **How can shunt be distinguished from the other causes of hypoxemia?**

If given 100% oxygen, the hypoxemic patient with shunt will not have a significant increase in their PaO_2. There will be a significant increase in PaO_2 when 100% oxygen is given to patients with hypoventilation or ventilation–perfusion inequality.

○ **A leftward shift in the oxyhemoglobin dissociation curve indicates an increased or decreased hemoglobin affinity for oxygen?**

Ventilation-increased.

○ **Changes in temperature, $PaCO_2$ or pH, or the level of 2,3-diphosphoglycerate (2,3-DPG) cause a shift in the oxyhemoglobin dissociation curve. To cause a rightward shift, what are the changes that must occur?**

Increased temperature, increased $PaCO_2$, decreased pH, and increased 2,3-DPG level. An easy way to remember this is that these conditions are often associated with decreased tissue oxygen levels. By right-shifting the curve, more oxygen is released from the hemoglobin to the tissues.

○ **How does the shape of the oxyhemoglobin dissociation curve effect the oxygen content of blood?**

Since SaO_2 does not increase significantly if the PaO_2 >60 mm Hg, the oxygen content of blood will increase significantly above this level only by increasing the hemoglobin concentration.

○ **What are the determinants of oxygen delivery to the peripheral tissues?**

Oxygen content of the blood (CaO_2) and cardiac output. An increase in either will increase oxygen delivery to the tissues.

○ **What is the difference between anatomic and physiologic dead space?**

Dead space refers to areas of lung that are ventilated but not perfused. Anatomic dead space refers to the conducting airways (trachea, bronchi, and bronchioles) where there is no gas exchange because there are no alveoli. Physiologic dead space includes the anatomic dead space and any diseased lung in which there is ventilation but no perfusion.

○ **What is the normal dead space in an average 70 kg subject?**

150 mL.

○ **Which pulmonary diseases are most associated with an increased physiologic dead space?**

Asthma and chronic obstructive pulmonary disease (COPD).

○ **How is the minute ventilation related to alveolar and dead space ventilation?**

Minute ventilation (V_E) is the product of tidal volume multiplied by breathing frequency

($V_E = V_T \times f$). Alveolar ventilation (V_A) is that portion of the minute ventilation that contributes to gas exchange, whereas dead space ventilation (V_D) is that portion that does not contribute to gas exchange. Thus, $V_E = V_A + V_D$.

○ **What is the effect of increased alveolar ventilation (V_A) on $PaCO_2$?**

$PaCO_2$ will decrease as V_A increases.

○ **Why do asthmatic patients eventually have an increased $PaCO_2$ if untreated?**

As the asthma attack continues untreated, the work of breathing will continue to increase. Eventually, the diaphragm fatigues and the patient hypoventilates. The hypoventilation, in association with the increased dead space and increased CO_2 production, increases the $PaCO_2$.

○ **What is the normal $PaCO_2$ and does it vary with age?**

Normal $PaCO_2$ is 35 to 45 mm Hg and does not vary with age.

○ **What is the normal expected change in pH if there is an acute change in the $PaCO_2$?**

The pH will increase or decrease 0.8 units for every 10 mm Hg decrease or increase (respectively) in $PaCO_2$.

○   **What are the consequences of hypercapnia?**

Acute hypercapnia has physiologic consequences due to the increased $Paco_2$ itself and the decreased pH. Physiologic effects of the $Paco_2$ increase include:

- increases in cerebral blood flow.
- confusion, headache ($Paco_2$ >60 mm Hg), obtundation and seizures ($Paco_2$ >70 mm Hg).
- depression of diaphragmatic contractility.

The primary consequences of the decreased pH are on the cardiovascular system with changes in cardiac contractility (decreased), the fibrillation threshold (decreased), and vascular tone (predominantly vasodilatation).

○   **What are the consequences of hypocapnia?**

Acute hypocapnia has physiologic consequences due to the decreased $Paco_2$ itself and the increased pH. Physiologic effects of the $Paco_2$ decrease include:

- decreases in cerebral blood flow. This reflex is used in the management of neurologic disorders with high intracranial pressures as a short-term measure to decrease the increased intracranial pressure.
- confusion, myoclonus, asterixis, loss of consciousness, and seizures.

The primary consequences of the increased pH are, again, primarily on the cardiovascular system with increased cardiac contractility and vasodilatation.

○   **What is the cause of the hypoxemia?**

Hypoventilation is one cause. However, since the $A\text{-}ao_2$ gradient is elevated, there is another cause in addition to the hypoventilation. In an obese patient, both ventilation–perfusion inequality and shunt (secondary to atelectasis) can contribute to the development of hypoxemia.

○   **A 50-year-old woman presents with a pneumonia in the right lower and middle lobes. On 50% oxygen by facemask, her Pao_2 is 75 mm Hg. Should the patient be positioned right side down or up?**

Right side up. Blood flow is gravity dependent. If the patient is positioned right side down, blood flow will preferentially go to the right side. However, because of the pneumonia, this will increase the amount of shunt, lowering the Pao_2 further.

○   **True/False: If a patient presents with a $Paco_2$ of 75, he/she should be emergently intubated:**

False. There is no $Paco_2$ level at which a patient must be intubated. Intubation is based upon the total clinical condition of a patient, not just upon a blood gas result.

○   **A 45-year-old patient presents to the emergency department after being rescued from a fire. The patient is dyspneic and cyanotic. Sao_2 on 50% mask is 84%. The blood gas, however, reveals a Pao_2 of 125 mm Hg. Why the discrepancy?**

A fire victim is likely to have carbon monoxide poisoning. The carbon monoxide has converted the hemoglobin to carboxyhemoglobin, which decreases the binding of oxygen to hemoglobin and prevents an accurate pulse oximetry reading. However, carbon monoxide does not affect dissolved oxygen, which is what is measured in the arterial blood gas.

○   **What is the treatment for carbon monoxide poisoning?**

100% oxygen, which increases carbon monoxide clearance by competing for binding to hemoglobin. If there is no significant response to 100% oxygen, hyperbaric oxygen (oxygen provided at higher than atmospheric pressure) is an alternative therapy.

○ **A 25-year-old woman with a history of mitral valve prolapse presents with "nervousness," chest tightness, hand numbness, and mild confusion. Arterial blood gas reveals pH 7.52, $PaCO_2$ 25 mm Hg, and PaO_2 108 mm Hg. What is the diagnosis?**

Acute anxiety attack. She is hyperventilating.

○ **Why is the PaO_2 elevated?**

Because the lower $PaCO_2$ means a higher PAO_2 (see alveolar gas equation above).

○ **What is the treatment?**

The acute hyperventilation can be terminated by having the patient breathe in and out of a bag. Anxiolytics can also be provided.

○ **True/False: Oxygen should never be given to a hypoxemic patient with COPD who has chronic CO_2 retention:**

False. Oxygen should always be given to a patient who is hypoxemic.

○ **Adequacy of alveolar ventilation is reflected by which component of arterial blood gas analysis?**

$PaCO_2$.

○ **Patients on mechanical ventilation can develop hypoventilation based on what factors?**

Increased dead space (including length of ventilator circuit proximal to the "Y" piece separating the inspiratory and expiratory limbs), decreased tidal volume, overdistention of lung, air leaks, and massive pulmonary embolism.

○ **What is the principal mechanism of increased $PaCO_2$ with increased FIO_2?**

Worsening V/Q mismatch and the Haldane effect.

○ **How does malnutrition contribute to respiratory failure?**

Increase in the oxygen cost of breathing and respiratory muscle weakness.

○ **How can the work of breathing with mechanical ventilation associated with intrinsic PEEP be reduced?**

Add CPAP, reduce tidal volume, reduce inspiratory time, and increase expiratory time.

○ **Through what mechanism does PEEP decrease cardiac output?**

Reduced preload.

○ **Through what mechanism does positive pressure ventilation increase cardiac output?**

Decreased afterload.

○ **How can compliance of the lung/chest wall be approximated from airway pressure measurements during mechanical ventilation?**

Compliance = tidal volume/(inspiratory plateau pressure − end expiratory pressure).

○ **What are the primary determinants of the work of breathing?**

Minute ventilation, lung/chest wall compliance, and presence of intrinsic PEEP.

○ **When may end-tidal carbon dioxide detectors prove inaccurate?**

In patients with very low blood flow to the lungs, or in those with a large dead space (i.e., following a pulmonary embolism).

○ **What is the most common complication of endotracheal intubation?**

Intubation of a bronchus. Other complications include lacerations of the lip, tongue, pharyngeal or tracheal mucosa resulting in bleeding, hematoma, or abscess. Tracheal rupture, avulsion of an arytenoid cartilage, vocal cord injury, pharyngeal–esophageal perforation, intubation of the pyriform sinus, aspiration of vomitus, hypertension, tachycardia, or arrhythmias can also occur.

○ **What oxygen concentration will be supplied by nasal cannula with a flow rate of 1 L/min?**

24%. For each 1 L/min increase in flow, a 4% increase in oxygen concentration will occur; 6 L/min produces a 44% oxygen concentration.

○ **What oxygen flow rate is recommended for face mask ventilation?**

At least 5 L/min. Recommended flow is 8 to 10 L/min, which will produce oxygen concentrations as high as 40% to 60%.

○ **What oxygen concentration can be supplied with a face mask and oxygen reservoir?**

6 L/min provides approximately 60% oxygen concentration, and each liter increases the concentration by 10%; 10 L/min is almost 100%.

○ **A pulmonary embolism causes which type of cyanosis?**

Central cyanosis. However, secondary shock and right-sided heart failure can lead to peripheral cyanosis.

○ **What are the two most common errors made in the intubation of a neonate?**

1. Placing the neck in hyperextension; this moves the cords even more anteriorly.

2. Inserting the laryngoscope too far.

○ **Name the two primary causes of peripheral cyanosis with a normal SaO$_2$:**

Decreased cardiac output and redistribution (may be secondary to shock, DIC, hypothermia, vascular obstruction).

○ **As Pco_2 increases, pH will decrease. How much is the pH expected to decrease for every 10 mm Hg increase in Pco_2?**

pH decreases by 0.08 U for each 10 mm Hg increase in Pco_2.

○ **Describe Kerley A and B lines:**

Kerley A lines are straight, nonbranching lines in the upper lung fields. Kerley B lines are horizontal, nonbranching lines at the periphery of the lower lung fields.

○ **A patient presents with cough, lethargy, dyspnea, conjunctivitis, glomerulonephritis, fever, and purulent sinusitis. What is the probable diagnosis?**

Wegener granulomatosis. This is a necrotizing vasculitis and pulmonary granulomatosis that attacks the small artery and veins. Treat the patient with corticosteroids and cyclophosphamide.

○ **What serological test is diagnostic for Wegener granulomatosis?**

c-ANCA in association with appropriate clinical evidence. A renal, lung, or sinus biopsy may also be helpful in making the diagnosis.

○ **What is the typical time period during which acute radiation pneumonitis develops?**

Within the first eight weeks after radiation.

○ **What laboratory finding distinguishes patients with primary SLE and drug-induced lupus?**

Drug-induced lupus has a positive ANA, but a *negative* ds-DN

○ **The chest X-ray reveals no pulmonary parenchymal lesions but does show prominent hila and an enlarged right ventricle. What diagnostic test should be performed?**

The patient has no pulmonary parenchymal lesions to cause a shunt; therefore, she most likely has an intracardiac right-to-left shunt (most likely a previously undiagnosed atrial septal defect). An echocardiogram should be performed.

○ **Of the following, which pattern of calcification of a solitary pulmonary nodule is most likely to be associated with a malignant lesion: lamellar (onion skin), popcorn, eccentric, or central?**

Eccentric.

○ **What happens to minute ventilation at submaximal work rates in Interstitial lung disease?**

It increases due to increased dead space ventilation. As the respiratory rate increases, tidal volume decreases.

○ **What is the incidence of post-operative respiratory complications in patients with COPD?**

50% or more.

○ **Which neuromuscular diseases and spinal diseases can lead to ventilatory insufficiency?**

Muscular dystrophy, polymyositis, myotonic dystrophy, polyneuritis, Eaton Lambert syndrome, myasthenia gravis, amyotrophic lateral sclerosis, injury, Guillain-Barre syndrome, multiple sclerosis, Parkinson disease, and stroke.

○ **What are some clinical disorders associated with increased capillary permeability causing exudative pleural effusion?**

Pleuropulmonary infections, circulating toxins, systemic lupus erythematosus, rheumatoid arthritis, sarcoidosis, tumor, pulmonary infarction, and viral hepatitis.

○ **What is the incidence of pleural involvement in systemic lupus erythematosus?**

50% to 75% of patients with systemic lupus erythematosus develop pleural effusion or pleuritic pain during the course of their disease.

○ **What are the clinical features of lupus pleuritis?**

Pleuritic chest pain is the most common presentation. Other features are cough, dyspnea, pleural rub, and fever. An episode of pleuritis usually indicates exacerbation of lupus.

○ **What percentage of elderly have sleep apnea?**

40%.

○ **What is the most common cause of sleep apnea in adults?**

An upper airway obstruction, generally by the tongue or enlarged tonsils. A medulla that is not responsive to CO_2 buildup is the most common cause in children. Obstruction by the tongue or enlarged tonsils also induces sleep apnea.

○ **What is a complication of central sleep apnea in children?**

SIDS. Affected children develop morning cyanosis. However, children can be treated with theophylline.

○ **Under what conditions does neurogenic pulmonary edema occur?**

Neurogenic pulmonary edema is commonly associated with increased intracranial pressure. It is commonly seen with head trauma, subarachnoid hemorrhage, and even with seizures.

○ **Is a nonsmoker who has lived with a smoker for 25 years at greater risk of lung cancer than a nonsmoker who has not lived with a smoker?**

Of course. The risk is 1.34 times as great as a person living in a smoke-free environment.

○ **What percentage of smokers who quit lapse back into their smoking habits?**

85%.

● ● ● **REFERENCES** ● ● ●

Brunton Laurence L, L. J. (2006). *Goodman and Gilman's the Pharmacological Basis of Therapeutics.* 11th ed. New York, NY: McGraw-Hill.

Fauci Anthony S, B. E. (2008, 7 1). Harrisons Online. New York.

Hall JB, Schmidt G, Wood LD. *Principles of Critical Care.,* 3rd ed. New York, NY: McGraw-Hill; 2005.

McPhee Stephen J, PM. *Current Medical Diagnosis and Treatment 2009.* New York, NY: McGraw-Hill; 2009.

McPhee SJ, Ganong WF. *Pathophysiology of Disease—An Introduction to Clinical Medicine.* 5th ed. New York, NY: McGraw-Hill; 2006.

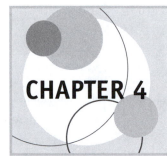

CHAPTER 4   **Endocrine**

Jacqueline Jordan Spiegel, MS, PA-C

● ● ● **DISEASES OF THE THYROID GLAND** ● ● ●

○ **At what cervical level is the thyroid located?**

It is located at the level of the fourth cervical vertebra.

○ **What are the etiologies associated with a GOITER?**

Graves or Hashimoto disease

Oral contraceptives or other medications

Infection

Tumors

Environmental (iodine deficiency)

Receptor defects (resistance to thyroxin)

○ **Which medications are commonly found to result in sporadic goiters?**

Oral contraceptives, lithium, amiodarone, and iodide-containing asthma inhalers.

○ **What are the main etiologies for elevated thyroid-binding globulin (TBG) levels?**

- Pregnancy
- Infancy
- Estrogens (oral contraceptives/HRT)
- Heroin

○ **What is thyrotoxicosis?**

A hypermetabolic state occurring secondary to excess circulating thyroid hormone.

○ **What are the etiologies for thyrotoxicosis?**

- Thyroid hormone overdose
- Thyroid hyperfunction
- Thyroid inflammation

○ **What is the most common cause of hyperthyroidism?**

Grave disease (toxic diffuse goiter).

○ **What is a thyrotropin receptor stimulating antibody (TSH receptor antibodies)?**

An antibody commonly found in Grave disease, which binds to the TSH receptor leading to thyroid stimulation, excessive thyroid hormone production, and goiter.

○ **Which HLA is associated with Grave disease?**

HLA-DR3. The association of this HLA type represents a sevenfold relative risk for Grave disease.

○ **Is Grave disease more common in men than in women?**

Women are affected five times more often than men.

○ **What are the classical signs and symptoms of Grave disease?**

Emotional lability, autonomic hyperactivity, exophthalmos, tremor, increased appetite, weight loss, diarrhea, and a goiter in nearly all affected individuals.

○ **How is Grave disease confirmed by laboratory testing?**

Increased free T3 and T4 levels with decreased TSH. Frequently, thyroid peroxidase and TSH receptor stimulating antibodies are present.

○ **What treatment options exist for patients with Grave disease?**

Patients can be managed medically with propylthiouracil (PTU) or methimazole, surgically with a subtotal thyroidectomy, or with radioiodine therapy (RAI).

○ **Which of the treatment options for Grave disease is considered definitive?**

Radioactive iodine therapy is the definitive treatment of choice.

○ **What drug blocks the uptake of radioactive iodine and should be stopped prior to radioactive iodine scanning or therapy?**

Potassium iodine.

○ **What are the three largest concerns with surgical management of Grave disease?**

1. Hyper- or hypothyroidism depending on the amount of tissue removed
2. Vocal cord paralysis
3. Hypoparathyroidism

○ **What is the most common precipitant of thyroid storm?**

Infections (usually pulmonary).

○ **What signs and symptoms are helpful for diagnosing thyroid storm?**

History of hyperthyroidism, widened pulse pressure, tachycardia, hypertension, a palpable goiter, tachycardia, fever/hyperthermia, diaphoresis, increased CNS activity (tremors), emotional lability, delirium or coma, and heart failure.

○ **How do you manage acute thyrotoxicosis (thyroid storm)?**

- Support and hydration.
- IV propylthiouracil 1 g to block thyroid production and effects.
- Propranolol at 10 mg/kg IV over 10 to 15 minutes for hypertension and cardiac arrhythmias.
- Lugol iodide, five drops PO every 8 hours or sodium iodide 125 to 250 mg/dl IV over 24 hours will stop thyroxine production.
- Oral dexamethasone at 0.2 mg/kg or oral hydrocortisone 5 mg/kg is another measure that can be taken to further reduce peripheral conversion of T4 to T3.

○ **What is the most common cause of non-iatrogenic hypothyroidism?**

Autoimmune Hashimoto thyroiditis.

○ **What are the clinical manifestations of acquired hypothyroidism?**

Cold intolerance, constipation, low-pitched voice, menstrual irregularities, mental and physical slowing, dry skin, coarse brittle hair, and decreased energy level with increased need for sleep.

○ **How can primary hypothyroidism be distinguished from secondary hypothyroidism?**

Primary hypothyroidism (source is thyroid): TSH levels are high, free T4 and T3 levels are low, and possible presence of antibodies.

Secondary hypothyroidism (source is pituitary): TSH levels are low or normal, free T4 and T3 levels are low, and no antibodies.

○ **What drugs may worsen hypothyroidism?**

Propranolol and phenothiazine.

○ **What is the recommended treatment for hypothyroidism?**

Thyroxine (T4) hormone replacement.

○ **When initiating thyroid hormone replacement therapy, what is the recommended replacement dose?**

1 to 2 μg/kg/day. The initial dose should take into account patient's age, weight, and cardiac status. Average starting dose is typically 50 μg. Dosage adjustments are made in increments of 25 to 50 μg until at therapeutic level.

○ **What is the recommended monitoring of thyroid hormone replacement therapy?**

The therapy should be monitored using serum TSH and plasma-free T4 levels: Initially, every 4 to 6 weeks until at therapeutic dose, every 6 months thereafter, and at 4 to 6 weeks following any adjustment in dose.

○ **What are the hallmark clinical features of myxedema coma?**

Hypothermia (75%), bradycardia, and coma.

○ **What is the recommended treatment for myxedema coma?**

Thyroxine (T4) administered as an IV bolus at dose of 50 to 100 μg every 6 to 8 hours until replete thyroid hormone reserves and then followed by oral dosing. Triiodothyronine (T3) is NOT recommended in the treatment of myxedema coma.

Supportive measures, correction of hypothermia, ventilatory support, and hydration with normal saline are also indicated.

○ **What is the most common clinical manifestation of lymphocytic thyroiditis?**

The appearance of a goiter.

○ **Of hypothyroid, euthyroid, and hyperthyroid, which is the most common presentation of patients with lymphocytic thyroiditis?**

The majority will be euthyroid. However, many patients will eventually become hypothyroid, while only a few will manifest the symptoms of hyperthyroidism.

○ **What is DeQuervain disease?**

A subacute, nonsuppurative thyroiditis. Its clinical manifestations involve a tender thyroid, fever, and chills, usually remitting within several months.

○ **What is the etiology of DeQuervain thyroiditis?**

Most likely due to a viral infection such as mumps or Coxsackie virus.

○ **Which types of nodules are more likely to be malignant on a thyroid scan, hot or cold?**

Cold. This procedure should not be considered confirmatory. Cysts and benign adenomas can also read as cold. Some types of thyroid cancers will read as "warm" and thus be dismissed. Use caution when interpreting results.

○ **What test should be performed to distinguish a benign cystic nodule from a malignant nodule?**

Fine needle aspiration biopsy and cytological evaluation.

○ **What is a solitary thyroid nodule most likely to be?**

A nodular goiter (50%). Other possibilities to consider include carcinoma (20%), adenoma (20%), cyst (5%), or thyroiditis (5%).

○ **If fine needle aspiration of a thyroid nodule reveals parafollicular cells, what type of carcinoma should be suspected?**

Medullary carcinoma of the thyroid.

○ **What combination of disorders account for multiple endocrine neoplasia type IIA?**

Medullary carcinoma of the thyroid, adrenal medullary hyperplasia or pheochromocytoma, and hyperparathyroidism.

○ **Define sick euthyroid syndrome:**

Altered thyroid function in the setting of an acute nonthyroidal illness; no true thyroid dysfunction is present; often seen in critically ill patients.

○ **What changes in thyroid function are seen in a sick euthyroid syndrome?**

Most common change is a fall in plasma T3 levels typically due to decrease in the deiodinase activity, which converts T4 to T3 in the peripheral tissue.

Also seen is low plasma total T4 concentrations. This is due to decrease in binding of T4 to thyroid binding globulin.

Finally, plasma TSH levels can be both suppressed (due to high levels of corticosteroids in setting of critical illness) or elevated in response to drops in circulating T4 and T3.

● ● ● DISEASES OF THE PARATHYROID GLAND ● ● ●

○ **What is the most common cause of hypercalcemia?**

Hyperparathyroidism. This condition accounts for 60% of ambulatory hypercalcemic patients.

○ **Is the pituitary gland responsible for parathyroid regulation?**

No. Unlike the thyroid gland, the parathyroids are not regulated by the pituitary gland, but rather, by circulating calcium levels.

○ **What is pseudohypoparathyroidism?**

An autosomal recessive disorder characterized by kidneys' unresponsiveness to PTH, shortened fourth and fifth metacarpals and metatarsals, and short stature, all occurring without evidence of parathyroid dysfunction.

○ **What other mineral must be considered in a patient who appears hypocalcemic?**

Magnesium. Giving calcium in the setting of low magnesium will not correct the problem. However, magnesium administration will correct both calcium and magnesium levels.

○ **What is the difference between primary and secondary hyperparathyroidism?**

In primary hyperparathyroidism, the defect is in the parathyroid gland, (i.e., an adenoma or hyperplasia). While in secondary hyperparathyroidism, the elevated PTH is a physiologic response to a low calcium level, usually a result of renal disease.

○ **What are the diagnostic laboratory findings seen in hyperparathyroidism?**

Elevated serum calcium and elevated intact PTH with concomitant decreased phosphorous levels.

○ **What is von Recklinghausen disease?**

Hyperparathyroidism, leading to cystic changes in bone due to osteoclastic resorption with fibrous replacement, thus forming nonneoplastic "brown tumors."

○ **What are the clinical features of hypercalcemic crisis?**

Anorexia

Belly pain

Coma

Delirium

Emesis

Fatigue/weakness

○ **What is a positive Chvostek sign?**

Facial grimacing as a result of repeated contractions of the facial muscles when percussion (with the tip of index or middle finger) is applied to the facial nerve (at the top of the cheek just below the zygomatic bone in front of the ear). Chvostek maneuver generally indicates hypocalcemia. It may be present in approximately 10% to 30% of normal individuals.

○ **What is Trousseau sign and when is it exhibited?**

A carpal spasm induced when the blood pressure cuff on the upper arm maintains an above-systolic pressure for approximately 3 minutes. Fingers become spastically extended at the interphalangeal joints and flexed at the metacarpophalangeal joints. It is typically present in latent tetany because of hypocalcemia, hypomagnesemia, severe alkalosis, and strychnine poisoning.

○ **Which is a more reliable physical examination finding of hypocalcemia, Trousseau sign or Chvostek sign?**

Trousseau sign; 10% of normal people have a positive Chvostek sign, and studies reveal approximately 29% of hypocalcaemia may result in a false negative Chvostek sign; therefore, this test a poor discriminator. On the other hand, Trousseau sign is relatively specific for hypocalcaemia—94%of hypocalcaemic patients display a positive sign, comparedwith 1% of normocalcaemic people.

○ **What is the most common cause of hyperparathyroidism?**

Parathyroid adenoma (85%).

○ **What are the treatment options for hyperparathyroidism?**

Definitive treatment is surgical resection (parathyroidectomy).

Medical management (reserved for patients meeting the criteria): Modest intake of calcium (1000 mg/day) and vitamin D (400–600 IU/day). Theoretically, low calcium intake can stimulate PTH production, and therefore, it is not recommended; 25% of medically observed patients develop indications for surgery.

○ **What are the criteria for medical management of hyperparathyroidism?**

- Serum calcium level elevated only mildly.
- No previous episode of life-threatening hypercalcemia.
- Normal renal status (i.e., creatinine clearance of >70% without nephrolithiasis or nephrocalcinosis).
- T score above –2.5 at lumbar spine, hip, and forearm.
- Asymptomatic.

○ **What are the recommendations for the management and monitoring of a patient status post-parathyroidectomy?**

Immediate postoperative management focuses on establishing the success of the surgery and monitoring the patient for complications such as symptomatic hypocalcemia, bleeding, vocal cord paralysis, and laryngospasm. The serum calcium concentration typically reaches a nadir within 24 to 36 hours after surgery. The serum PTH level is in the normal range within 30 hours. The patient should maintain a low-calcium diet until the serum calcium concentration is normal.

● ● ● DISEASES OF THE ADRENAL GLAND ● ● ●

○ **What are the zones of the adrenal cortex?**

The adrenal cortex makes up 80% to 90% of the adrenal gland. The three zones from outer to inner include zona glomerulosa, zona fasciculate, and zona reticularis.

○ **What products are produced by the adrenal medulla?**

The adrenal medulla consists of 10% to 20% of the adrenal gland. It is derived from neuroectodermal cells of the sympathetic ganglia and is the source of catecholamine hormones (epinephrine and norepinephrine).

○ **What hormones are produced by the adrenal cortex?**

Mineralocorticoids, glucocorticoids, and androgenic sex steroids.

○ **What is the major glucocorticoid produced by the adrenal cortex? How is it regulated?**

Cortisol. It is regulated by the signals from the pituitary gland (specifically adrenocorticotropic hormone [ACTH]).

○ **What is the major mineralocorticoid? How is it regulated?**

Aldosterone. It is regulated by ACTH from the pituitary and by the renin angiotensin system.

○ **What is the major sex androgen produced by the adrenal cortex?**

Dehydroepiandrosterone (DHEA). It is regulated by ACTH from the pituitary and circulating levels of testosterone and estrogens.

○ **What controls the release of adrenocorticotropic hormone (ACTH) from the pituitary?**

Directly: Corticotropin-releasing hormone (CRH) from the hypothalamus, circulating cortisol levels, and antidiuretic hormone (ADH) otherwise known as vasopressin.
Indirectly: Circulating ACTH levels.

○ **What are the actions of cortisol (glucocorticoids)?**

Majorly affects protein, glucose, and fat metabolism. It strongly inhibits the entire process of inflammation and immune response. It inhibits muscle proteolysis and increases hepatic conversion of liberated amino acids into glucose (for storage as glycogen). It inhibits collagen synthesis, thereby reducing bone formation, connective tissue, and muscle mass. It increases arteriolar tone (through decreased endothelial permeability).

○ **What are the actions of aldosterone (mineralocorticoids)?**

Major regulator of sodium, potassium, and fluid balance. It acts on the renal tubule to increase sodium reabsorption and concomitant expansion of extracellular fluid, which results in maintenance of blood pressure. In turn, renal excretion of H+ and K+ occur, resulting in lowered plasma potassium concentrations.

○ **What are the actions of dehydroepiandrosterone (DHEA)?**

DHEA is a precursor steroid to testosterone and estradiol. In women, it supplies 50% of androgenic hormone requirement (while the remainder comes from the ovaries). After menopause, the adrenal cortex is the sole source of estrogens in women. In men, DHEA is negligible since the majority of the testosterone is produced from the testes.

○ **What is the definition of adrenal insufficiency?**

Inadequate function of the adrenal gland due to disease, destruction, or surgical removal of the adrenal cortices.

○ **What are the etiologies of primary adrenal insufficiency?**
- Acute, abrupt onset:
  ○ Adrenal hemorrhage (i.e., anticoagulation therapy)
  ○ Thrombosis (as seen in meningococcal disease)
  ○ Disseminated infection (i.e., sepsis)
  ○ Antiphosphoid syndrome
- Slow, insidious progression:
  ○ Autoimmune disease (Addison disease)
  ○ Infection (i.e., TB, coccidiomycosis, blastomycosis, histoplasmosis)
  ○ Metastatic carcinoma (most common lung, breast, kidney)
  ○ Lymphoma
  ○ AIDS (CMV, Kaposi sarcoma, etc.)

○ **What is the most common cause of primary adrenal insufficiency?**

Failure of the adrenal cortex due to autoimmune process (also known as Addison disease).

○ **What are the causes of secondary adrenal insufficiency?**
- Sheehan syndrome (postpartum pituitary necrosis)
- Bleeding into a pituitary macroadenoma
- Head trauma

○ **What are the common clinical manifestations of adrenal insufficiency?**

Fatigue, lethargy, anorexia, weight loss, hyperpigmentation, hyponatremia, and hyperkalemia are common.

Depression, dizziness, orthostatic hypotension, nausea and vomiting, diarrhea, generalized abdominal pain, WBC changes (i.e., lymphocytosis, eosinophilia), and normocytic, normochromic anemia are also significant manifestations.

○ **What are the clinical features of Addison disease (explain using the name as a mnemonic)?**

Anorexia

Diarrhea

Dehydration

Increased K+

Skin pigmentation

Orthostatic hypotension

Na level is abnormal

○ **What characteristic electrolyte imbalances are associated with primary adrenal insufficiency?**

Hyperkalemia, hyponatremia, hypoglycemia, azotemia (if volume depletion is present), and a mild metabolic acidosis.

○ **Are orthostatic hypotension and electrolyte abnormalities more common in primary or secondary adrenal insufficiency?**

Primary, because of the aldosterone deficiency and hypovolemia.

○ **What are the most specific signs of primary adrenal insufficiency?**

Hyperpigmentation of the skin and mucosal membranes due to high ACTH levels as a consequence of cortisol feedback and salt craving.

○ **What is the most common cause of secondary adrenal insufficiency and adrenal crisis?**

Iatrogenic adrenal suppression from prolonged steroid use. Rapid withdrawal of steroids may lead to collapse and death.

○ **Which hormone secretion is NOT impaired by secondary adrenal insufficiency?**

Aldosterone. Aldosterone secretion is more dependent upon angiotensin II than corticotrophin-releasing hormone signals from the pituitary gland. Aldosterone deficiency is not a problem in hypopituitarism.

○ **Besides serum cortisol levels and plasma ACTH, what are the three tests used to evaluate adrenal insufficiency?**

1. Corticotropin stimulation test

2. Insulin-induced hypoglycemia

3. Metyrapone test

○ **How is a corticotropin (ACTH) stimulation test performed to rule out adrenal insufficiency?**

After a baseline ACTH and cortisol level are obtained, 250 μg of Cosyntropin is given IV (or IM). Cortisol levels are obtained at 30 and 60 minutes postinjection. Adrenal function is thought to be normal if the cortisol level drawn at 30 or 60 minutes is ≥18 μg/dL and there are raises of minimum of >7 mg/dL above baseline.

○ **Are imaging studies of the adrenal glands necessary in primary adrenal insufficiency?**

Yes. In cases other than autoimmune or adrenal myeloneuropathy, a CT scan of the adrenal should be performed to aid in the differential diagnosis. Enlarged glands with/without calcifications in patients with TB are a sign of active disease and warrant anti-infective therapy. Enlargement also occurs in other fungal infections, lymphoma, cancer, and AIDS. A biopsy by CT guidance may also be helpful.

○ **What is the daily replacement of hydrocortisone for a stabilized patient with adrenal insufficiency?**

Hydrocortisone 15 mg in the morning and 10 mg in the afternoon. This matches the two-third a.m., one-third p.m. normal circadian release of cortisol physiologically. The dose should be the smallest possible to alleviate clinical symptoms yet prevent weight gain and osteoporosis. Measurements of urinary cortisol may help determine the appropriate dosing.

○ **What accounts for the almost immediate effect of cortisol on blood pressure in patients with adrenal insufficiency?**

Cortisol exerts a permissive effect on catecholamine vascular responsitivity and a vital role in the maintenance of vascular tone, vascular permeability, and distribution of body water within the vascular compartment.

○ **What added precautions should be taken by all patients with adrenal insufficiency?**

They should wear a medic alert bracelet, carry a card detailing their medications, and double or triple their dose of hydrocortisone when they have surgery or sustain injury/illness. They should secure ampules of glucocorticoids for self-injection or suppositories when vomiting or unable to take oral steroids.

○ **What is the amount of increased cortisol production that accompanies surgery?**

It depends upon the surgery; 85% above baseline for up to 2 days postlaparotomy and 35% above baseline for more minor procedures involving joints, breasts, or neck.

○ **Which drugs can increase the metabolism of cortisol?**

Phenytoin, phenobarbital, and Rifampin.

○ **What symptoms should increase the suspicion of adrenal insufficiency in the critically ill?**

Unexplained circulatory instability, high fever without cause, unresponsive to antibiotics, hypoglycemia, hyponatremia, hyperkalemia, neutropenia, eosinophilia, unexplained mental status changes, disparate anticipated severity of disease, and the actual state of the patient.

○ **What are the adverse effects of using excessive dosing when replacing cortisol production during times of stress?**

Catabolic effects on muscle, impaired wound healing, antagonizing insulin, and the effects on glucose metabolism as well as the anti-inflammatory effect on any active infection.

○ **What are the current dosing recommendations for stress doses in patients with suspected adrenal insufficiency?**

- Minor stress: 25 mg/day
- Moderate stress: 50 to 75 mg/day
- Major stress: 100 to 150 mg/day

○ **Two weeks after a myocardial infarction, a patient takes warfarin and has sudden onset of hypotension, right flank pain, right CVA pain, epigastric pain, fever, nausea, and vomiting. What is the most likely etiology?**

Adrenal gland hemorrhage (adrenal apoplexy).

○ **What is the Waterhouse-Fredrickson syndrome?**

Septicemia secondary to meningococcemia with associated bilateral adrenal gland hemorrhage. The patient will have a petechial rash, purpura, shaking, chills, a severe headache, and other signs of acute adrenal insufficiency.

○ **What are the causes of acute adrenal crisis?**

Major stress such as surgery, severe injury, myocardial infarction, or any other acute illness in a patient with primary or secondary adrenal insufficiency.

○ **What are the principal signs and symptoms of adrenal crisis? The most common cause is withdrawal of steroids:**

Abdominal pain, hypotension, and shock.

○ **What is the protocol for emergent steroid replacement in adrenal crisis?**

Treat by administering hydrocortisone; 100 mg IV bolus and 100 mg added to the first liter of D5 0.9 NS. Additional 50 to 100 mg IV q8h until stable.

○ **What are the two main causes of death during an adrenal crisis?**

Circulatory collapse and hyperkalemia-induced arrhythmias.

○ **Name four conditions that can be attributed to adrenocortical overstimulation:**

Cushing syndrome, hyperaldosteronism, adrenogenital syndrome, and feminization.

○ **What is Cushing disease?**

Pituitary adenoma leading to increased ACTH secretion with resultant bilateral adrenal hyperplasia and elevated cortisol levels.

○ **How is Cushing disease different from Cushing syndrome?**

Cushing syndrome is elevated cortisol levels from various causes, including paraneoplastic syndromes, primary adrenal tumors, and exogenous use of cortisol, whereas Cushing disease is specifically the elevation in cortisol levels due to ACTH-secreting pituitary adenomas (it is a subset of Cushing syndrome).

○ **What clinical manifestations are common to all patients with Cushing syndrome?**

Moon facies, buffalo hump, obesity, hypertrichosis, hypertension, growth retardation, easy bruising, purple striae on the hips and abdomen, and amenorrhea in women.

○ **What is the differential diagnosis for hypercortisolism state?**
- Pseudo-Cushing syndrome: major depressive disorder, alcohol excess.
- Hypercortisolism without Cushing syndrome: obesity, stress, trauma, acute illness, pregnancy, hyperthyroidism, drug induced (i.e., psychotropic medications).
- Metabolic syndrome and/or polycystic ovary syndrome may mimic Cushing syndrome with similar signs and symptoms.

○ **What is the recommended SCREENING test for suspected Cushing syndrome?**

Dexamethasone suppression test: abnormal is plasma cortisol >5 μg/dL at 8 a.m. after 1 mg dexamethasone ingested 11 p.m. day before.

○ **What is the recommended CONFIRMATORY test for hyperfunctioning adrenal status?**

24-hour urine cortisol levels:abnormal level in adult man is >10 mg/24 hours, in adult woman is >8 mg/24 hours, in elderly people slightly lower, and in pediatric patients depends on age but significantly lower.

○ **What is considered the definitive treatment for Cushing syndrome?**

Surgical resection, or if nonoperable etiology, then treat the underlying cause.

○ **What are the clinical manifestations of primary hyperaldosteronism (Conn syndrome)?**

Hyperplasia of the zona glomerulosa leading to hypertension, sodium and water retention, hypokalemia, and decreased serum renin levels.

○ **What are the hallmarks of polyglandular autoimmune disease type I?**

Autoimmune hypoparathyroidism, autoimmune adrenalitis (Addison disease), and chronic mucocutaneous candidiasis.

○ **What is a pheochromocytoma?**

Catecholamine-producing tumor of the neurochromaffin cells. Most arise from the adrenal medulla but extra-adrenal masses may occur at anatomical regions containing sympathetic ganglia.

○ **What are the classic signs and symptoms of pheochromocytomas?**

Paroxysmal episodes of hypertension, autonomic hyperactivity, and headaches lasting for 20 to 30 minutes. Concomitant underlying hypertension between episodes may be present. Abdominal mass present on examination or imaging.

○ **When is the peak incidence of pheochromocytoma?**

Third or fourth decade. However, it can occur from infancy to old age. Familial pheochromocytomas typically occur earlier in life and are bilateral.

○ **What laboratory tests help make the diagnosis of pheochromocytoma?**

An increased total 24-hour urinary catecholamines and their metabolites (i.e., epinephrine, norepinephrine, metanephrine, and VMA). Clonidine suppression test can also be administered in an inpatient setting.

○ **Which class of antihypertensive drugs are recommended for the temporary treatment of pheochromocytoma-associated hypertension?**

Alpha-adrenergic blocking agents such as phenoxybenzamine and prazosin.

○ **How do you manage a hypertensive crisis in a patient with a pheochromocytoma?**

1 mg of IV phentolamine or 0.5 to 0.8 mg/kg/min of sodium nitroprusside.

○ **What is the treatment of choice for pheochromocytoma (intra-adrenal or extra-adrenal)?**

Surgical resection.

• • • DISEASES OF THE PITUITARY GLAND • • •

○ **What is the radiologic study of choice to assess the pituitary or hypothalamic gland when hormonal abnormalities have been established?**

MRI with analysis of the sagittal and coronal sections. A CT scan can be helpful if bony invasion is suspected.

○ **What is the most common type of pituitary tumor?**

Prolactinomas.

○ **What are the common presenting signs of a prolactinoma?**

Headache, visual field impairment (typically bitemporal hemianopsia), amenorrhea, and galactorrhea.

○ **What is the most common presenting symptom of a prolactinoma in a woman?**

Secondary amenorrhea.

○ **What is the differential diagnosis for hyperprolactinemia?**

Hyperprolactinemia can be caused by pituitary adenomas, hypothyroidism, or drugs, such as reserpine, methyldopa, phenothiazine, or oral contraceptives.

○ **What is the serum prolacting level in hyperprolactinemia?**

50 ng/mL (typically >200 ng/mL in prolactinoma).

○ **What two options exist for the treatment of prolactinomas?**

Bromocriptine and surgery via a transsphenoidal approach.

○ **What is diabetes insipidus?**

A lack of ADH secretion, which results in an inability to concentrate the urine despite functioning kidneys.

○   **Compare and contrast CENTRAL diabetes insipidus from NEPHROGENIC diabetes insipidus:**

Central	Nephrogenic
Source: Posterior pituitary	Source: Distal tubules of kidney
Polyuria, Polydipsia	Polyuria, Polydipsia
Signs of dehydration	Signs of dehydration
Hypernatremia	Hypernatremia
Low urine osmolality	Low urine osmolality
High serum osmolality	High serum osmolality
Low vasopressin (ADH)	High circulating vasopressin (ADH)
Response to exogenous ADH	No response to exogenous ADH

○   **What is the danger of rigorously hydrating a patient who has hypernatremia due to diabetes insipidus?**
Cerebral edema, seizures, and death.

○   **What is the typically response to the administration of ADH in a patient with central diabetes insipidus?**
Response to exogenous ADH is typically a 50% increase in urine osmolality.

○   **What should the clinician consider if the patient with diabetes insipidus continues to diurese despite repeated doses of DDAVP (ADH)?**
The patient most probably has nephrogenic diabetes insipidus owing to unresponsive kidney receptors for ADH, irrespective of whether the ADH is endogenous or exogenous.

○   **If nephrogenic diabetes insipidus is assumed, what further pharmacological treatment may be helpful?**
Thiazide diuretics have a paradoxical effect and may work in decreasing fluid losses.

○   **What is the definition for SIADH?**
Syndrome of inappropriate antidiuretic hormone. There is an excessive release of ADH, resulting in a dilutional hyponatremia and hyposmolar state.

○   **What key laboratory results are expected with SIADH?**
Low serum sodium levels and high urine sodium levels in the setting of normovolemia and normal renal, thyroid, and adrenal function. It is the most common cause of normovolemic hyponatremia.

○ **What is the treatment for SIADH?**

Treatment of severe symptomatic hyponatremia includes a loop diuretic, such as furosemide, and the simultaneous infusion of small boluses of 3% saline over 4 hours or normal saline. If hyponatremia is corrected too rapidly, neurologic sequelae may result.

○ **What is the hormone abnormality in acromegaly?**

Excessive growth hormone.

○ **What are the clinical manifestations of acromegaly?**

Coarse facial features, enlarged tongue, enlargement of the distal extremities, and hypogonadism.

○ **What are the clinical manifestations of primary hypogonadism?**

Failure of development of the secondary sexual characteristics with abnormally small penis and testes.

○ **What is hypogonadotropic hypogonadism?**

Decreased levels of gonadotropins (FSH and LH) from the pituitary, which results in inadequate estrogen, progesterone, and/or testosterone production despite functioning ovaries or testes.

○ **How is the diagnosis of primary hypogonadism made?**

The levels of FSH and LH are abnormally elevated for the corresponding age. Testosterone levels remain low and show little response to the administration of hCG.

● ● ● **DIABETES MELLITUS** ● ● ●

○ **What is the most common cause of hypoglycemia seen in the emergency department?**

An insulin reaction in a diabetic patient.

○ **What are the key predisposing factors to hypoglycemia in diabetic patients on insulin?**

Exercise, poor oral intake, worsening renal function, and medications are the key predisposing factors to consider.

○ **What principal hormone protects the human body from hypoglycemia?**

Glucagon.

○ **What are the neurologic signs and symptoms associated with hypoglycemia?**

Hypoglycemia may produce mental and neurologic dysfunction. Neurologic manifestations can include paresthesias, cranial nerve palsies, transient hemiplegia, diplopia, decerebrate posturing, and clonus.

○ **Which is the most common type of hypoglycemia in children?**

Ketotic hypoglycemia. This condition usually develops in boys between 18 months and 5 years of age. Attacks typically arise from caloric deprivation. These attacks may be episodic and are more frequent in the morning and during periods of illness.

○ **In the first 2 years of life, what is the most common cause of *drug-induced* hypoglycemia?**

Salicylates.

Between ages 2 and 8 years, alcohol is the most likely cause.

Between ages 11 and 30 years, insulin and sulfonylureas are the primary causes.

○ **What drugs potentiate the hypoglycemic effects of sulfonylurea?**

Salicylates, alcohol, sulfonamides, phenylbutazone, and bishydroxycoumarin.

○ **How is sulfonylurea-induced hypoglycemia treated?**

IV glucose alone may be insufficient. It may require diazoxide, 300 mg slow IV over 30 minutes, repeated q4h.

○ **What are the classifications of impaired glucose regulation from normal to diabetes?**

Classification	Test	Result
Normal	Fasting glucose	<100 mg/dL
	2-h OGTT	<140 mg/dL
Impaired fasting glucose (IFG)	Fasting glucose	100–125 mg/dL
Impaired glucose tolerance	Fasting glucose	100–125 mg/dL
	2-h OGTT	140–199 mg/dL
Diabetes	Fasting glucose	≥126 mg/dL
	2-h OGTT	≥200 mg/dL

A1C is not yet recommended for diagnosis (although it may be in the future).

○ **How is the etiology of type 1 DM different from type 2 DM?**

Type 1 DM is associated with human leukocyte antigens (HLA), autoimmunity, and or islet cell antibodies.

Type 2 DM usually involves a genetic mutation resulting in inactive pancreatic and liver enzymes as well as insulin receptor defects leading to resistance.

○ **What etiologies are responsible for *secondary* DM?**

Exocrine pancreatic diseases such as cystic fibrosis, pancreatic cancer, and Cushing disease.

○ **What are the main signs and symptoms of diabetes mellitus?**

Patient presents with classic symptoms of polyuria (increased urination), polydipsia (increased thirst), and polydysplasia (increased appetite despite increased caloric intake). Other symptoms include fatigue, blurry vision, menstrual irregularities, delayed wound healing, or recurrent infections. In type 1 DM, typically, weight loss is seen. In type 2 DM, typically, weight gain is seen (obesity). Many cases of type 2 DM are asymptomatic.

○ **What are the diagnostic criteria for diabetes mellitus according to the World Health Organization?**

1. Symptoms of DM and a casual plasma glucose 200 mg/dL or higher. (Symptoms include polyuria, polydipsia, and unexplained weight loss.)

OR

2. Fasting plasma glucose 126 mg/dL or higher on two separate occasions.

OR

3. 2-hour plasma glucose is 200 mg/dL or greater during an oral glucose tolerance test (performed with glucose load of 75 g glucose).

○ **What is the significance of the HgbA1C?**

It represents the fraction of hemoglobin that has been nonenzymatically glycosylated. It provides an accurate estimation of the relative blood glucose level over the preceding 8 to 12 weeks.

○ **What are the two main side effects of uncontrolled diabetes mellitus on the retina?**

Diabetic retinopathy and neovascularization.

○ **What are the main side effects of uncontrolled diabetes mellitus on the nervous system?**

Peripheral polyneuropathy, gastrointestinal autonomic neuropathy (i.e., gastroparesis and diabetic enteropathy), genitourinary autonomic neuropathy (i.e., erectile dysfunction and bladder incontinence), and cardiovascular autonomic neuropathy (i.e., resting tachycardia, exercise intolerance, and orthostatic hypotension).

○ **Describe the classic presentation of diabetic peripheral polyneuropathy:**

Progressive peripheral nerve damage resulting in "stocking and glove" distribution of pain, numbness, tingling, and decreased sensation.

○ **What is the main side effect of uncontrolled diabetes mellitus on the renal system? How is it prevented?**

Diabetic nephropathy. Prevention includes glycemic control and angiotensin inhibition with antihypertensive agents (either angiotension converting enzyme inhibitor [ACE-I] or angiotensin receptor blocker [ARB]).

○ **What is the earliest manifestation of diabetic nephropathy?**

An increase in albumin excretion (microalbuminuria).

○ **What are the key factors predisposing diabetics to soft tissue infections?**

Microvascular disease, poor wound healing, and trauma often masked by neuropathy.

○ **What is the Somogyi effect?**

A hyperglycemic event that results from an overzealous response by counter regulatory hormones during a period of hypoglycemia.

○ **What is the Dawn phenomenon?**

A term used to describe an abnormal early-morning (usually between 4 and 8 a.m.) increase in blood sugar in patients with diabetes. The dawn phenomenon is more common in people with type 1 diabetes than with type 2 diabetes.

○ **Which ethnic groups are most at risk for diabetes mellitus?**

Hispanics: Prevalence is 1.7 to 2.4 times higher than in non-Hispanics and the death rate is twice as high.

Native Americans: Prevalence is 2.6 to 4.0 times higher than in nonnative Americans and the death rate is also twice as high.

Reasons for the high rate of disease in these groups is attributed to increased incidence of obesity and hyperinsulinemia.

○ **What is the recommended first-line oral hyperglycemic agent in type 2 diabetes (as long as not contraindicated)?**

Metformin.

○ **What is the formula for calculating the *initial* total daily amount of insulin necessary for type 1 diabetic patient?**

$0.5 \text{ U} \times \text{wt (kg)}$.

○ **What is the optimal formula used for dosing insulin in a type 1 diabetic patient?**

50% basal insulin and 50% bolus insulin.

○ **What are the onset time, peak, and duration of regular insulin?**

Onset: 0.5 to 1 hour
Peak: 2 to 3 hours
Total duration: 3 to 6 hours

○ **What are the onset time, peak, and duration of NPH insulin?**

Onset: 2 to 4 hours
Peak: 6 to 12 hours
Total duration: 10 to 16 hours

○ **What are the onset time, peak, and duration of glargine insulin?**

Onset: 1 to 2 hours
Peak: plateau release, no peak
Duration: 20 to 24 hours

○ **What is the appropriate mixture of regular and intermediate acting insulin in a twice daily insulin injection regimen?**

Two-third of the dose should be given 30 minutes prior to breakfast; the remaining one-third given 30 minutes prior to dinner. Both injections should be two-third intermediate acting and one-third regular (short acting) insulin.

○ **What are the ideal blood glucose and HgbA1C levels for a diabetic patient?**

Premeal glucose: 80 to 120 mg/dL
2 hours postprandial: 100 to 160 mg/dL
Bedtime glucose: 100 to 140 mg/dL
HbA1c: <7% (some experts are recommending <6.5%)

○   **Which common medications are likely to worsen glucose control in a diabetic patient?**

Thiazide diuretics, beta-blockers, steroids, estrogens, dilantin, cyclosporin, and diazoxide.

○   **What are the common causes of abdominal pain, nausea, and vomiting in a diabetic patient?**

Diabetic gastroparesis, gallbladder disease, pancreatitis, and, perhaps, ischemia bowel.

○   **What are some agents used to treat severe diabetic gastroparesis?**

Cisapride and metoclopramide are the key agents. Erythromycin has also been tried in very severe cases.

○   **What medications are likely to lead to acute hyperkalemia in a diabetic patient?**

NSAIDs, ACE inhibitors, beta-blockers, potassium-sparing diuretics, and salt substitutes (these are usually potassium salts).

○   **Which gastrointestinal condition should be considered in a diabetic patient with diffuse abdominal pain, bloody stools, and a high serum lactate?**

One should strongly consider ischemic or necrotic bowel.

○   **What is the most desirable agent used to treat severe hyperglycemia in pregnancy?**

Multiple injections of insulin.

○   **What are the major adverse effects of intravenous radiocontrast dye given to diabetic patients?**

Acute tubular necrosis is well known. One should also watch for worsening of CHF, precipitation of angina pectoris, and hemodynamic compromise.

○   **What side effect of propranolol may of be of concern to a diabetic patient?**

Hypoglycemia. Beta-blockers can also retard recovery from insulin-induced hypoglycemia. This latter effect is presumably due to diminished or absent early warning signs. Studies showed that the effects on glucose metabolism may be less prominent with beta-1 selective drugs.

○   **What are the signs and symptoms of diabetic ketoacidosis (DKA)?**
- Nausea/vomiting with abdominal pain
- Hyperventilation (Kussmaul respirations)
- Hypotension/shock
- Polyuria, polydipsia, and weight loss

○   **What do profound polyuria and dehydration in DKA reflect?**

Severe osmotic diuresis caused by glycosuria.

○   **What laboratory findings are expected with DKA?**

- Elevated serum glucose (typically >250 mg/dL but less than 800 mg/dL in DKA).
- Elevated serum ketoacids (β-hydroxybutyrate, acetoacetate) and natural ketone (acetone).
- Ketonuria and glucosuria are present.
- Serum osmolality is greater than 320 to 330 mOsm/kg.
- Serum bicarbonate levels, pCO_2, and pH are decreased, leading to a metabolic acidosis with increased anion gap.
- Hyponatremia and variable potassium levels (may be elevated but can be normal).
- Elevated white blood cell (WBC) count.

○   **What is the major mechanism of hyponatremia in DKA patients?**

Dilution of sodium due to shifting of water out of the cells into the vascular space.

○   **What is the most important initial step in treating DKA?**

Volume replacement, with the first liter administered over about 60 minutes.

○   **Outline the basic treatment including fluid replacement for DKA:**

- Start with normal saline (the total deficit may be 5–10 L), followed by potassium (100–200 mEq) in the first 12 to 24 hours.
- Prescribe insulin: 5 to 10 U bolus followed by 5 to 10 U/h. Change replacement fluids to D5W when the glucose falls below 200 mg/dL and keep at rate of 150 to 200 mL/h.
- Administer sodium bicarbonate (100 mmol diluted) if pH <6.9.

○   **Why should caution be used in administering bicarbonate therapy during DKA?**

Because of risk of paradoxical CSF acidosis, cardiac arrhythmias, decreased oxygen delivery to tissue, and fluid and sodium overload.

○   **What major insults are likely to lead to DKA in an otherwise controlled diabetic patient?**

Always look for infection (even a minor one), cardiac ischemia, medications, and lack of compliance with insulin and diet.

○   **What is the possible adverse effect seen during very rapid correction of severe hyperglycemia?**

Cerebral edema.

○   **What are the key features of nonketotic hyperosmolar coma?**

Hyperosmolality, hyperglycemia, and dehydration. Blood sugar levels should be >800 mg/dL, serum osmolality should be >350 mOsm/kg, and serum ketones should be negative.

○   **What are the key factors leading to hypernatremia in a patient with nonketogenic hyperosmolar coma?**

Profound dehydration with greater losses of water than of salts as well as impaired thirst.

○   **Besides the typical presentation seen with hyperglycemia emergency, what unique focal neurologic signs may be present in a patient with nonketotic hyperosmolar coma?**

Hemisensory deficits or perhaps hemiparesis. 10% to 15% of these patients will have a seizure.

○ **Outline the recommended treatment for nonketotic hyperosmolar coma:**

- Administer fluids (patients can be as much as 12-L deficient). Give normal saline until adequate blood pressure and urinary output established.
- Administer potassium (10–15 mEq/h).
- Administer insulin (only about 5–10 U).
- Add D5W replacement fluids when blood glucose level drops below 200 mg/dL.

○ **What is the drug of choice for a patient with nonketotic hyperosmolar coma and who experiences a seizure?**

The drugs of choice for this seizure disorder are lorazepam (Ativan) or diazepam (Valium). Phenobarbital is also appropriate. Phenytoin is contraindicated in patients with hyperglycemic, hyperosmolar, nonketotic coma.

○ **What is the overall mortality rate of nonketotic hyperosmolar coma?**

Approximately 50%.

● ● ● **REFERENCES** ● ● ●

Baron WF, Boulpaep EL. *Medical Physiology.* Elsevier Science; 2003.

Bickley LS. *Bates' Guide to Physical Examination and History Taking.* 9th ed. Baltimore, MD: Lippincott Williams and Wilkins. 2007.

DeGowin RL, LeBlond RF, Brown DD. *DeGowin's Diagnostic Evaluation. The Complete Guide to Assessment, Examination, and Differential Diagnosis.* 8th ed. New York, NY: McGraw-Hill; 2004.

Henderson KE, Baranski TJ, Bickel PE, et al. *The Washington Manual, Subspecialty Consult Series. Endocrinology Subspecialty Consult.* Lippincott Williams & Wilkins. 2005.

Levy MN, Koeppen BM, Stanton BA. *Berne and Levy Principles of Physiology.* 4th ed. Elsevier Science; 2005.

McPhee SJ, Papadakis MA, Tierney LM Jr. *Current Diagnosis and Treatment 2008.* New York, NY: McGraw-Hill; 2008.

Taniegra E. Hyperparathyroidism. Am Fam Phys. 2004;69(2):333–339.

Tintinalli JE, Kelen GD, Stapczynski JS. *Emergency Medicine: A Comprehensive Study Guide.* 6th ed. New York, NY: McGraw-Hill; 2004.

UpToDate (Online 17.1). www.uptodateonline.com. Accessed December 2008, February 2009, May 2009, June 2009.

Weiner CM, Fauci A, Braunwald E, et al. *Harrison's Principles of Internal Medicine, Self-Assessment and Board Review.* 17th ed. New York, NY: McGraw-Hill; 2008.

CHAPTER 5

Eyes, Ears, Nose, Throat (EENT)

David J. Klocko, MPAS, PA-C

● ● ● EYE ● ● ●

○ **What are cotton wool spots?**

Cotton wool spots are white patches on the retina that are observed upon funduscopic examination. These patches are due to the ischemia of the superficial nerve layer of the retina. They are most commonly associated with hypertension but also occur in patients with diabetes, anemia, collagen vascular disease, leukemia, endocarditis, and AIDS.

○ **Do visual changes in chronic open-angle glaucoma patients begin centrally or peripherally?**

Peripherally. Patients with chronic glaucoma experience a gradual and painless loss of vision. Those with acute- or subacute-angle closure glaucoma will have either dull or severe pain, blurry vision, lacrimation, and even nausea and vomiting. The pain may be more severe in the dark.

○ **Which is more common, chronic open-angle glaucoma or acute closed-angle glaucoma?**

Chronic open-angle glaucoma (90%). Four percent of the population older than 40 years have glaucoma.

○ **What is the most common cause of chronic open-angle glaucoma?**

Outflow obstruction through the trabecular meshwork. Other causes are obstruction of Schlemm canal and excess secretion of aqueous fluid.

○ **What is the normal range of intraocular pressure?**

10 to 23 mm Hg. Patients with acute angle-closure glaucoma generally have pressures elevated to 40 to 80 mm Hg.

○ **In what cases are topical steroids for the eyes absolutely contraindicated?**

If the patient has a herpetic infection. Herpetic lesions of the cornea are noted to have dendritic patterns of fluorescein uptake upon slit lamp examination.

○ **What is the most common finding upon funduscopic examination of a patient with AIDS?**

Cotton wool spots due to microvascular disease. Other findings are hemorrhage, exudate, or retinal necrosis.

○ **A patient presents with an itching, tearing, in both eyes. Upon examination, large cobblestone papillae are found under the upper lid. What is the probable diagnosis?**

Allergic conjunctivitis.

○ **A patient is seen with herpetic lesions on the tip of the nose. Why is this a problem?**

The tip of the nose and the cornea are both supplied by the nasociliary nerve. Thus, the cornea may also be involved. This is an ophthalmological emergency.

○ **A patient presents with conjunctiva and lid margin inflammation. Slit lamp examination reveals a "greasy" appearance of the lid margins with scaling, especially around the base of the lashes. What is the diagnosis?**

Blepharitis. This is often caused by a staphylococcal infection of the oil glands and skin next to the lash follicles. Treatment includes scrubbing with baby shampoo and, after consultation with an ophthalmologist, use of sulfacetamide drops and steroids.

○ **A patient presents with a painful red eye. Slit lamp examination reveals a localized, white, flocculent infiltrate in the anterior chamber. What is this?**

Hypopyon. This is an accumulation of white inflammatory exudate in the anterior chamber.

○ **A welder presents with severe eye pain. What is the expected finding upon slit lamp examination?**

Diffuse punctate keratopathy (welder's flash), which presents as a multiple pinpoint area of fluorescein uptake representing ruptured corneal epithelial cells.

○ **A patient presents with a painful pustular vesicle at the lid margin. What is the diagnosis and treatment?**

A hordeolum (sty) is a painful, red, swelling occurring on the upper or lower eyelids. An internal hordeolum is an abscess of the meibomian gland and "points" toward the conjunctival side of the eyelid. An external hordeolum is a painful swelling at the eyelid margin and "points" outward.

○ **A patient presents with a chronic, nontender, uninflamed nodule of the upper lid. What is the diagnosis?**

Chalazion. For persistent chalazion, surgical removal may be indicated.

○ **A patient presents with the sensation of a foreign body in the eye. Slit lamp examination reveals a dendritic (branchlike) lesion on the cornea. What is the treatment?**

Antiviral agents and cycloplegics. This is most probably a herpes simplex keratitis. Steroids are contraindicated because they allow for viral replication. Emergent ophthalmology consultation is indicated.

○ **A patient presents with sudden onset of vision loss in one eye that quickly returns. This should be diagnosed as what?**

Amaurosis fugax. This is usually caused by central retinal artery emboli from extracranial atherosclerosis.

○ **A patient presents with painless vision loss in one eye and describes it as a curtain slowly appearing in the visual field. What finding do you expect upon examination?**

A gray, detached retina. The patient may also complain of flashing lights in the peripheral visual field or spider webs in the visual field. Treatment consists of surgical repair.

○ **A patient was hit in the eye during a fight. He presents 8 hours after the incident, with proptosis and visual loss. Examination reveals an intact globe and an afferent pupillary defect. What is the problem?**

Retro-orbital hematoma with ischemia of the optic nerve or retina. The pressure in the orbit exceeds the perfusion pressure of the optic nerve and ocular globe, resulting in a lack of blood flow and loss of function. Treatment is to release the pressure by lateral canthotomy. A similar situation can occur with orbital emphysema.

○ **What are the complications of a hyphema?**

The 4 Ss:

1. **Staining** of the cornea due to hemosiderin deposits.

2. **Synechiae,** which interfere with iris function.

3. **Secondary rebleeds,** which usually occur between the second and fifth day after the injury (since this is the time of clot retraction) and tend to be worse than the initial bleed.

4. **Significantly increased intraocular pressure,** which can lead to acute glaucoma, chronic late glaucoma, and optic atrophy.

○ **Why do patients with sickle cell anemia and a hyphema require special consideration when presenting with ophthalmologic concerns?**

Increased intraocular pressure can occur if the cells sickle in the trabecular network, preventing aqueous humor from leaving the anterior chamber. Some medications, such as hyperosmotics and Diamox, increase the likelihood of sickling.

○ **A patient presents with a history of trauma to the orbit and dull ocular pain, decreased visual acuity, and photophobia. The examination reveals a constricted pupil and ciliary flush. What will be found on a slit lamp examination?**

Cells and flare in the anterior chamber are likely present with a traumatic iritis.

○ **What are the causes of a subluxed or dislocated lens?**

Trauma, Marfan syndrome, homocystinuria, and Weill-Marchesani syndrome.

○ **Physiologically, what causes flare?**

Flare is caused by inflammatory proteins resulting in the "dust in the movie projector lights" or "fog in the headlights" phenomena during slit lamp examination.

○ **Which is worse, acid or alkaline burns of the cornea?**

Alkaline burns, because these cause deeper penetration compared to acid burns. A barrier is formed from precipitated proteins with acid burns. The exceptions are hydrofluoric acid and heavy metal containing acids, which can penetrate the cornea.

○ **When do preexisting conditions contraindicate pharmacologic papillary dilation?**

Narrow-angle glaucoma and with an iris-supported intraocular lens.

○ **Why shouldn't topical ophthalmologic anesthetics be prescribed?**

These anesthetics inhibit healing and decrease a patient's ability to protect the affected eyes because of the loss of sensation.

○ **What is the most common organism in contact lens–associated corneal ulcers?**

Pseudomonas.

○ **How can Krazy-Glue (cyanoacrylate) be removed if a patient has stuck the eyelids together?**

Begin copious irrigation immediately and then apply mineral oil. Acetone and ethanol are unacceptable in the eyes. Surgical separation must be done with extreme care to prevent laceration of the lids or globe. Often the patient will have a corneal abrasion, which should be treated in the usual manner.

○ **Three hours ago, a patient experienced sudden, painless visual loss in her right eye. Central retinal artery occlusion (CRAO) is suspected. What findings are expected upon eye examination? What is the prognosis?**

Afferent pupillary defect, pale gray retina, and a small cherry red dot near the fovea. This dot is the choroidal vasculature seen at the macula where the retina is the thinnest. After 2 hours the prognosis is extremely poor for visual recovery. Digital massage or anterior chamber paracentesis may dislodge the clot. Immediate ophthalmic consultation is necessary.

○ **What conditions have been associated with central retinal vein occlusion?**

Hyperviscosity syndromes, diabetes, and hypertension. Funduscopic examination shows a chaotically streaked retina with congested dilated veins. There are superficial and deep retinal hemorrhages, cotton wool spots, and macular edema.

○ **A patient presents with a traumatic pain behind the left eye, an afferent papillary defect, central visual loss, and papilledema. What is the diagnosis? What are the potential etiologies?**

Optic neuritis. This may be idiopathic or may be associated with multiple sclerosis, Lyme disease, neurosyphilis, lupus, sarcoid, alcoholism, toxins, or drug abuse.

○ **A patient developed eye pain, nausea, vomiting, blurred vision, and sees halos around lights. Why would this patient be given mannitol, pilocarpine, and acetazolamide?**

This patient has acute angle closure glaucoma. The goal of treatment is to decrease intraocular pressure.
- Decrease the production of aqueous humor with carbonic anhydrase inhibitor.
- Decrease intraocular volume by making the plasma hypertonic to the aqueous humor with glycerol or mannitol.
- Constrict the pupil with pilocarpine, allowing increased flow of the aqueous humor out through the previously blocked canals of Schlemm.

○ **A patient presents with multiple vertical linear corneal abrasions. What should be suspected?**

A foreign body under the upper lid. This pattern is sometimes called an "ice rink" sign.

○ **What technique can be used to identify and narrow anterior chamber?**

Tangential light (from a penlight) is shone perpendicular to the line of vision across the anterior chamber. If the entire iris is in the light, then the chamber is most likely a normal depth. If part of the iris is in a shadow, then the chamber is narrow. This can occur with angle closure glaucoma and with perforating corneal injuries.

○ **What is the difference between a sympathomimetic and a cycloplegic medication when dilating the eye?**

A sympathomimetic simulates the iris's dilator muscle. The cycloplegic inhibits the parasympathetic stimulation, which constricts the iris and inhibits the ciliary muscle. Thus, cycloplegics will cause blurred near vision.

○ **While mowing the lawn, a patient felt something fly into his eye. On examination, there is a brown foreign body on the cornea and a tear drop iris pointing toward the foreign body. What is the diagnosis?**

Perforated cornea with extruded iris. A similar foreign body may appear black on the sclera with scleral perforation.

○ **A patient's cornea fluoresces prior to instillation of fluorescein. What should be considered?**

Pseudomonal infection. Several species are fluorescent.

○ **Which anesthetic is faster acting: proparacaine or tetracaine?**

Proparacaine has a rapid onset and a duration of 20 minutes. Tetracaine has a delayed onset and a duration of 1 hour.

○ **Place the following mydriatic-cycloplegic medications in the order of duration of activity: tropicamide, homatropine, atropine, and cyclopentolate:**

- Tropicamide (onset 15–20 minutes, brief duration)
- Cyclopentolate (onset 30–60 minutes, duration <24 hours)
- Homatropine (long lasting, 2–3 days)
- Atropine (very long lasting, 2 weeks)

○ **What organisms are typically responsible for causing bacterial conjunctivitis?**

Staphylococcus aureus, *Streptococcus pneumoniae*, and *Hemophilus influenzae*.

○ **A patient presents with a painful eye, blurred vision, and conjunctivitis. Upon slit lamp examination, you detect a dendritic ulcer. What is the most likely cause of this patient's symptoms?**

Herpes simplex keratitis. Treat with topical antivirals. Immediate ophthalmology consult is warranted. Corticosteroids are not to be used unless under direction of an ophthalmologist. If the eye has a bacterial superinfection, prescribe topical antibiotics.

○ **What are the most common causes of periorbital and orbital infections?**

Staphylococcus aureus, *Streptococcus pneumonia*, and *Hemophilus influenzae*.

○ **What condition should be suspected in a patient with vision loss and a pale fundus?**

Central retinal artery occlusion (CRAO). Vision loss is usually acute and painless.

○ **Describe the symptoms of optic neuritis:**

Variable loss of central visual acuity with a central scotoma and change in color perception. The disk margins are blurred from hemorrhage, the blind spot is increased, and the eye is painful, especially with movement.

○ **Describe a patient with acute angle-closure glaucoma:**

Symptoms include nausea, vomiting, and abdominal pain. Visual acuity is markedly diminished. The pupil is semidilated and nonreactive. There is usually a glassy haze over the cornea, and the eye is red and very painful. Intraocular pressure may be as high as 50 to 60 mm Hg.

○ **Describe the treatment of acute angle-closure glaucoma:**

Intravenous acetazolamide (a carbonic anhydrase inhibitor to minimize aqueous humor production), miotics (such as pilocarpine) to open the angle, topical beta-blocker, alpha-adrenergic receptor agonist, and, if necessary, intravenous hyperosmotic agent such as mannitol to reduce intraocular pressure. After the ocular pressure is stabilized, an iridectomy is eventually performed to provide aqueous outflow.

○ **What is the appropriate treatment of hyphema?**

Rest, elevation of the head, and topical steroids. Avoid aspirin and NSAIDS. Re-bleeding can occur in up to 20% at 3 days. Complications include glaucoma and corneal staining.

○ **What is the differential diagnosis of a red eye with decreased visual acuity?**

Conjunctivitis, keratitis, iritis, glaucoma, and central corneal lesions.

○ **What disease is associated with retrobulbar optic neuritis?**

Multiple sclerosis.

○ **Define strabismus, esotropia, and exotropia:**

- Strabismus: Lack of parallelism of the visual axis of vision.
- Esotropia: Medial deviation of the axis of vision.
- Exotropia: Lateral deviation of the axis of vision.

○ **An elderly patient presents with the complaint of seeing halos around lights. What diagnosis is suspected?**

Glaucoma. Another presenting complaint of glaucoma is blurred vision. Also, consider digitalis toxicity.

○ **What diseases are commonly associated with central retinal vein occlusion?**

Hypertension and glaucoma.

○ **What are the common eye findings in patients with AIDS?**

Cotton wool spots and hemorrhages are most commonly caused by cytomegalovirus (CMV) retinitis.

○ **What is a hordeolum?**

A Meibomian gland infection, usually of the upper lid.

○ **What is a pinguecula?**

It is a yellowish nodule, particularly on the nasal portion of the bulbar conjunctiva near the palpebral fissure. In some cases, they can also be located laterally.

○ **What is a pterygium?**

It is a chronic growth more commonly over the medial aspect of the conjunctive and part of the cornea approaching the pupil. It is often caused by chronic exposure to wind and dust.

○ **On funduscopic examination, microaneurysms and soft exudates are typical of what?**

Hypertension.

○ **On funduscopic examination, macular microaneurysms and hard exudates are typical of what?**

Diabetes.

○ **What medications are likely to exacerbate angle-closure glaucoma?**

Anticholinergics, antihistamines, antidepressants, benzodiazepine, carbonic anhydrase inhibitors, CNS stimulants, phenothiazine, sympathomimetics, theophylline, and vasodilators.

○ **An elderly patient presents with bilateral eye irritation and states that this persists despite using eye-lubricating drops. On physical examination, you notice that lower eyelid margins are rolled in and eyelashes appear to be rubbing against the conjunctiva and cornea. What is this condition called?**

Entropion. This is an inward turning of the eyelid margin from a degeneration of the eyelid fascia. For cases that involve continual irritation of the cornea from the eyelashes, surgery is indicated. Ectropion also occurs at an advanced age, and creates an outward turning or drooping of the lower eyelid. Complications from this are excessive tearing, exposure keratitis, and bad cosmetic appearance.

○ **What is the clinical history and physical examination findings of a central retinal vein occlusion?**

Sudden painless vision loss. Physical findings can range from a few hemorrhages and cotton wool spots to a massive superficial and deep hemorrhage with vitreous involvement. Diffuse hemorrhages in a quadrants of the fundus referred to as a "blood and thunder fundus."

○ **A patient presents with a painful reddened area over the tear duct at the nasal side of the right eye. A small amount of pus is draining from the tear duct. What is this condition called?**

Dacryocystitis. The most common pathogens for acute dacryocystitis are *S. aureus*, and beta-hemolytic streptococci. In chronic dacryocystitis, *Candida albicans*, anaerobic streptococci, and *Staphylococcus epidermidis* can be the causative pathogens. Treatment is with systemic antibiotics.

○ **An elderly patient complains of decreasing central vision clarity. He has long smoking history. Upon physical examination, you notice Drusen formations, and on direct ophthalmoscopic examination you see retinal atrophy. What condition is likely?**

Age-related macular degeneration.

• • • EAR • • •

○ **What is the most common type of hearing loss in the elderly?**

Presbycusis. This is an idiopathic, insidious, symmetrical decline in hearing that is associated with aging.

○ **What systemic sexually transmitted disease is associated with sensorineural hearing loss?**

Syphilis. Seven percent of patients with idiopathic hearing loss test positive for treponemal antibodies.

○ **Acute tinnitus is associated with toxicity of what medications?**

Salicylates, loop diuretics, and aminoglycosides. Other causes of tinnitus are vascular abnormalities, mechanical abnormalities, and damaged cochlear hair cells. Unilateral tinnitus is associated with chronic suppurative otitis, Meniere disease, and trauma.

○ **A patient experiences vertigo and disequilibrium after a Valsalva maneuver, coughing, or sneezing. What is the most likely diagnosis?**

Perilymphatic fistula.

○ **A patient presents with ear pain and fluid-filled blisters on the tympanic membrane. What is the diagnosis?**

Bullous myringitis, which is commonly caused by mycoplasma or a virus. Treat with erythromycin or azithromycin.

○ **A 16-year-old boxer presents with a hematoma of the external right ear after receiving a blow to the ear. What is the treatment?**

The hematoma should be aseptically drained by incision or aspiration and a mastoid conforming dressing should be applied. ENT follow-up is mandatory. If the ear is not treated appropriately, a cauliflower deformity may result.

○ **A patient presents with a swollen, tender, red left auricle. What is the diagnosis?**

Perichondritis. This is most often caused by *Pseudomonas*.

○ **What is the most common cause of hearing loss?**

Cerumen impaction.

○ **Describe the physical finding of unilateral sensorineural hearing loss:**

The patient will have air conduction greater than bone conduction (i.e., normal Rinne test) indicating no conductive loss. The Weber test will lateralize to the normal ear.

○ **Which medications should be suspected in a patient with bilateral sensorineural hearing loss?**

Ototoxins such as aminoglycosides, loop diuretics, antineoplastics, or salicylates.

○ **What is the most common neuropathy associated with acoustic neuroma?**

The corneal reflex may be lost due to trigeminal nucleus involvement.

○ **Name some causes of tympanic membrane perforation:**

Air or water blast injuries, foreign bodies in the ear (particularly cotton tip swabs), lightning strikes, otitis media, and associated temporal bone fractures.

○ **A young man who was involved in a barroom brawl complains of ear pain, significantly decreased hearing, and vertigo. A tympanic membrane rupture is determined by examination. What is the concern?**

Injury to the ossicles, temporal bone, or labyrinth. An urgent ENT consult is necessary.

○   **A diver on vacation decided to go scuba diving despite having an upper respiratory infection. While descending, she had acute ear pain followed by vertiginous symptoms and vomiting. What happened?**

Middle ear squeeze (barotitis media). Pressure from the middle ear could not be equalized because of abnormal eustachian tube function resulting from the illness. The middle ear volume decreased until the tympanic membrane retracted to the point of rupture. The inrush of cold water caused vestibular stimulation. This is the most common form of barotrauma in amateur scuba divers. Similar problems may occur while flying on aircraft.

○   **What organism usually causes pediatric acute otitis media?**

Streptococcus pneumoniae, followed by *Haemophilus influenzae* and *Moraxella catarrhalis*.

○   **Why are preschool children more susceptible to acute otitis media?**

Children have shorter, more horizontal eustachian tubes, which may prevent adequate drainage and allow aspiration of nasopharyngeal bacteria into the middle ear, particularly with URIs.

○   **What is the most common cause of sialadenitis?**

Stasis of the flow of saliva. The most common bacterial pathogens are *S. aureus, S. pneumonia, E. coli, H. influenzae*, and viruses. Signs and symptoms include fever, pain, swelling of the salivary glands, which may include the parotid gland.

○   **A patient presents with trismus, fever, and an erythematous, tender parotid gland. Pus is expressed from Stensen duct. What conditions predispose the patient to bacterial parotitis?**

Any situation that decreases salivary flow, including irradiation, phenothiazines, antihistamines, parasympathetic inhibitors, dehydration, and debilitation. Up to 30% of cases occur postoperatively.

○   **What are the incidences of salivary gland malignancies?**

Parotid 40%, submandibular 10%, and sublingual 1%.

○   **A 44-year-old man has lost sensorineural hearing in his left ear. What ear will the Weber test lateralize to?**

The right or normal ear. The damaged ear is less prone to detect sound waves via vibration.

○   **What is the most common complication of acute otitis media?**

Tympanic membrane perforation. Other complications include mastoiditis, cholesteatoma, and intracranial infections.

○   **A patient presents with hearing loss, nystagmus, facial weakness, and diplopia. Vertigo is provoked with sudden movement. A lumbar puncture reveals elevated CNS protein. What diagnosis is suspected?**

Acoustic neuroma.

○   **What is the most common causative organism of otitis externa?**

Pseudomonas species.

○   **Which medications put patients at risk for hearing loss?**

Aminoglycoside, antineoplastic agents, loop diuretics, and salicylates.

○ **A 17-year-old female patient presents with a history of ear discharge and pain, fever and swelling, and redness over the mastoid bone. She was treated for an otitis media 2 weeks ago. What is your clinical suspicion?**

Mastoiditis is a complication of otitis media and is caused by bacterial invasion into the mastoid air cells. The most common causative pathogens are *S. pneumonia, H. influenzae,* and *S. aureus.* If a subperiosteal abscess develops, surgical drainage is indicated.

○ **Describe the clinical presentation and treatment for Meniere disease:**

A patient will complain of aural pressure, episodic vertigo that lasts for hours, tinnitus, and hearing loss. The treatment includes a sodium-restricted diet, limiting caffeine and alcohol, and prescribing diuretics like hydrochlorothiazide. Acute episodes can be managed with vestibular suppressant benzodiazepines and antiemetics.

○ **Describe the signs and symptoms in a patient with vestibular neuronitis (labyrinthitis):**

The patient will have a rapid onset of severe vertigo (but some may have a gradual prodromal period) accompanied by nausea, vomiting, and imbalance. This is usually preceded by an upper respiratory infection. Rapid phase nystagmus and the feeling of body motion is toward the opposite ear with falling and past pointing toward the affected ear.

○ **What is a vestibular schwannoma?**

An acoustic neuroma or a tumor of the eighth cranial nerve. In addition to hearing loss and vertigo, patients also present with tinnitus. Surgical removal is the treatment of choice because this tumor may spread to the cerebellum and the brainstem.

○ **What are the most common initial symptoms of an acoustic neuroma?**

Tinnitus, hearing loss, and unsteadiness.

○ **Describe the signs and symptoms of acoustic neuroma:**

Unilateral high tone sensorineural hearing loss and tinnitus. Decreased corneal sensitivity, diplopia, headache, facial weakness, and positive radiographic findings may also be displayed. Vertigo usually appears late, is more often exhibited as a progressive feeling of imbalance, and can be provoked by changes in head movement. Nystagmus is frequently present and is usually spontaneous. The CSF may have elevated protein.

○ **A child with blurry vision has an abnormal pupillary reflex and a white reflex upon funduscopic examination. What is the likely diagnosis?**

Retinoblastoma. These can grow to other sites in the brain or body. Surgical removal is indicated. This condition is inheritable and thus the parents should be counseled about the risks.

○ **The Weber test is performed on a patient complaining of hearing loss. The patient hears sounds more loudly in his right ear. Which types of hearing loss may this patient have?**

Conductive hearing loss on the right or sensory neural hearing loss on the left.

○ **Describe Rinne test and explain the normal findings:**

Rinne test is performed by placing the tip of the tuning fork on the mastoid process until the patient can no longer hear the tone. The fork is then relocated to just in front of the pinna until the patient can no longer hear the tone. In normal patients, the air conduction to bone conduction ratio is 2:1.

○ **A 35-year-old woman with a history of flulike symptoms (URI) 1 week ago presents with vertigo, nausea, and vomiting. No auditory impairment or focal deficits are noted. What is the likely diagnosis?**

Labyrinthitis or vestibular neuronitis.

○ **Describe the key features of Meniere disease, also known as endolymphatic hydrops:**

Vertigo, hearing loss, and tinnitus. Meniere disease typically presents with the rapid onset of vertigo, nausea, and vomiting that lasts for hours to 1 day. Nystagmus may be spontaneous during the critical stage. Tinnitus may be present and is louder during attacks, and sensorineural hearing loss may occur. There also may be an aura with a sensation of fullness in the ear during an attack. Symptoms are unilateral in more than 90% of patients and recurring attacks are typical.

○ **What are the distinguishing characteristics of benign positional vertigo?**

Positional vertigo is usually provoked by certain head positions or movement. Nystagmus is always positional, of brief duration, and with fatigability.

○ **What are the key features of viral labyrinthitis or vestibular neuritis?**

Severe vertigo (usually lasting 3–5 days), with nausea and vomiting. Symptoms generally regress over 3 to 6 weeks. Nystagmus may be spontaneous during the severe stage.

○ **A 50-year-old female patient with acute vertigo, nausea, and vomiting reports similar episodes over the last 20 years that are sometimes associated with hearing change, hearing loss, and tinnitus. She has permanent right > left sensorineural hearing loss. What is the diagnosis?**

Meniere disease.

○ **For the following clinical presentations, identify which are associated with peripheral vertigo or with central vertigo:**

1. **Intense spinning, nausea, hearing loss, diaphoresis.**
2. **Swaying or impulsion, worse with movement, tinnitus, acute onset.**
3. **Unidirectional nystagmus inhibited by ocular fixation, fatigable.**
4. **Mild vertigo, diplopia, and ataxia.**
5. **Multidirectional nystagmus not inhibited by ocular fixation, nonfatigable.**

Peripheral vertigo: (1), (2), and (3); central vertigo: (4) and (5).

○ **What are the common features of central vertigo?**

Symptoms are gradual and continuous. They include focal signs, nausea, and vomiting. Hearing loss is rare.

○ **What are the signs and symptoms of peripheral vertigo?**

Symptoms are usually acute and intermittent. Hearing loss is common; nausea and vomiting are severe.

○ **What is the significance of bilateral nystagmus with cold caloric testing?**

It signifies that an intact cortex, midbrain, and brainstem are present.

○ **What is a mnemonic for remembering the drugs that cause nystagmus?**

MALES TIP:

Methanol   **T**hiamine depletion and **T**egretol (carbamazepine)

Alcohol   **I**sopropanol

Lithium   **P**CP and **p**henytoin

Ethylene glycol

Sedative hypnotics and **S**olvents

● ● ● **NOSE/SINUS** ● ● ●

○ **A 3-year-old child presents with a unilateral purulent rhinorrhea. What is the probable diagnosis?**

Nasal foreign body.

○ **What potential complications of nasal fracture should always be considered on physical examination?**

Septal hematoma and cribriform plate fractures. A septal hematoma appears as a bluish mass on the nasal septum. If not drained, aseptic necrosis of the septal cartilage and septal abnormalities may occur. A cribriform plate fracture should be considered in a patient who has a clear rhinorrhea after trauma.

○ **What four physical examination findings would make posterior epistaxis more likely than anterior epistaxis?**

1. Inability to see the site of bleeding. Anterior nosebleeds usually originate at Kiesselbach plexus and are easily visualized on the nasal septum.

2. Blood from both sides of the nose. In a posterior nosebleed, the blood can more easily pass to the other side because of the proximity of the choanae.

3. Blood trickling down the oropharynx.

4. Inability to control bleeding by direct pressure.

○ **Where is the most common site of bleeding in posterior nosebleeds?**

The sphenopalatine artery's lateral nasal branch.

○ **A patient returns to the emergency department with fever, nausea, vomiting, and hypotension 2 days after having nasal packing placed for an anterior nosebleed. What potential complication of nasal packing should be considered?**

Toxic shock syndrome. This syndrome is caused by toxin-releasing *Staphylococcus aureus*.

○ **A child with a sinus infection presents with proptosis, a red, swollen eyelid, and an inferolaterally displaced globe. What is the diagnosis?**

Orbital cellulitis and abscess associated with ethmoid sinusitis.

○ **A patient with frontal sinusitis presents with a large forehead abscess. What is the diagnosis?**

Pott puffy tumor. This is a complication of frontal sinusitis in which the anterior table of the skull is destroyed, allowing the formation of the abscess.

○ **An ill-appearing patient presents with a fever of 103°F, bilateral chemosis, extra ocular motion palsy, with a history of untreated sinusitis. What is the diagnosis?**

Cavernous sinus thrombosis. This life-threatening complication occurs from direct extension through the valveless veins. Complications of sinusitis may be local (osteomyelitis), orbital (cellulitis), or within the central nervous system (meningitis or brain abscess).

○ **Symptoms of itchy eyes, nasal congestion, sneezing, rhinorrhea with physical findings of bluish inflamed turbinates, and mucoid nasal discharge are consistent with what condition?**

Allergic rhinitis.

○ **What is the differential diagnosis for persistent nasal congestion?**

Allergic rhinitis, infection, perennial nonallergic rhinitis (vasomotor rhinitis), pollutants and irritants, medication-induced topical rhinitis (rhinitis medicamentosa), anatomic deformities like nasal polyps or deviated septum, and tumors and foreign bodies.

○ **What are the classifications of allergic rhinitis?**

Seasonal allergic rhinitis occurs when symptoms predictably appear seasonally in response to plant and tree pollination. Symptoms are exacerbated during windy periods. **Perennial allergic rhinitis** occurs all year long but can vary in intensity. Allergens responsible for this condition are usually indoor irritants like dust mites, smoke, chemicals, cockroaches, and animal dander.

○ **What are the two common pathogens in adult acute sinusitis?**

Streptococcus pneumoniae and *Haemophilus influenzae*.

○ **What is a frequent complication of ethmoid sinusitis?**

Orbital cellulitis.

● ● ●   MOUTH/THROAT   ● ● ●

○ **Hairy leukoplakia is characteristic of which two viruses?**

HIV and Epstein-Barr virus. Hairy leukoplakia is usually found on the lateral aspect of the tongue. Oral thrush may also be associated with HIV infection.

○ **How can Ellis class II and III dental fractures be differentiated?**

Class II fractures involve the dentin and enamel. The exposed dentin will be pinkish. Class III fractures involve the enamel, dentin, and pulp. A drop of blood is frequently noted in the center of the pink dentin.

○ **A patient presents 3 days after tooth extraction with severe pain and a foul mouth odor and taste. What is the appropriate diagnosis and treatment?**

Alveolar osteitis (dry socket) results from loss of the blood clot and local osteomyelitis. Treat by irrigation of the socket and application of a medicated dental packing or iodoform gauze moistened with Campho-Phenique or eugenol.

O   **What is the most common oral manifestation of AIDS?**

Oropharyngeal thrush. Other AIDS-related oropharyngeal diseases are Kaposi sarcoma, hairy leukoplakia, and non-Hodgkin lymphoma. Thrush can be differentiated from leukoplakia if it can be scraped from the mucosa with a tongue blade. Hairy leukoplakia cannot be removed.

O   **Retropharyngeal abscesses are most common in what age group? Why?**

Retropharyngeal abscesses occur from 6 months to 3 years of age. Retropharyngeal lymph nodes regress in size after age 3.

O   **Describe the overall appearance of a child with a retropharyngeal abscess:**

These children are often ill-appearing, febrile, stridorous, drooling, and in an opisthotonic position. They may complain of difficulty swallowing or may refuse to eat.

O   **What radiographic sign indicates a retropharyngeal abscess?**

Widening of the retropharyngeal space, which is normally 3 to 4 mm or less than half the width of the vertebral bodies. False widening may occur if the X-ray is not taken during inspiration and with the patient's neck extended. Occasionally, an air–fluid level may be noted in the retropharyngeal space.

O   **Retropharyngeal abscesses are most commonly caused by which organisms?**

β-Hemolytic streptococci and *Staphylococcus aureus*.

O   **What is the most common type of laryngeal cancer?**

Squamous cell carcinoma accounts for greater than 90% and is linked to tobacco and excessive alcohol use.

O   **A 48-year-old male patient presents with high fever, trismus, dysphagia, and swelling inferior to the mandible in the lateral neck. What is the diagnosis?**

Parapharyngeal abscess.

O   **Where is the most common origin of "Ludwig angina"?**

The lower second and third molar. Ludwig angina is a swelling in the region of the submandibular, sublingual, and submental spaces, which may cause upward and posterior displacement of the tongue. It is most commonly caused by hemolytic streptococci, staphylococci, and mixed anaerobic/aerobic bacteria.

O   **Herpangina is caused by what virus?**

Coxsackie virus group A. Sore throat, fever, malaise, and vesicular lesions on the posterior pharynx or the soft palate are prevalent with this disease.

O   **What is the IM treatment for adult streptococcal pharyngitis?**

1.2 million units of benzathine penicillin G. Use 0.6 million units of benzathine penicillin G for children weighing less than 27 kg.

○ **What viral agent most commonly induces laryngotracheitis?**

Parainfluenza virus type I, II, & III are most common, but can be Influenza A & B or RSV (respiratory syncytial virus). *Staphylococcus aureus* and *Streptococcus pneumoniae* are the most common bacterial pathogens.

○ **What is the initial antibiotic treatment for a child with epiglottitis?**

Treat with a second- or third-generation cephalosporin. The most likely cause of this condition is *H. influenzae* type b. This pathogen is seen in patients who lack Hib vaccination or have had vaccination failure. Other pathogens are group A streptococci and *Streptococcus pneumonia*.

○ **What are the signs and symptoms of a peritonsillar abscess?**

Sore throat, dysarthria ("hot potato" voice), odynophagia, ipsilateral otalgia, low-grade fever, trismus, and uvular displacement.

○ **What is the presentation of a patient with diphtheria?**

Sore throat, dysphagia, fever, and tachycardia. A dirty, tough gray fibrinous membrane so firmly adherent that removal causes bleeding may be present in the oropharynx. Corynebacterium diphtheriae exotoxin acts directly on cardiac, renal, and nervous systems. It can cause ocular bulbar paralysis that may suggest botulism or myasthenia gravis. The exotoxin may also cause flaccid limb weakness. Such weakness may also include decreased or absent DTRs—a finding suggestive of Guillain-Barré or tick paralysis.

○ **How does a patient present with a retropharyngeal abscess?**

Retropharyngeal abscesses are common among those younger than 3 years of age. On examination, the uvula and tonsil are displaced away from the abscess. The neck is held in hyperextension. Soft tissue swelling and forward displacement of the larynx are present. Soft tissue X-ray films of the neck may show the retropharyngeal space to be wider that the vertebral body of C4.

○ **How does an adult with epiglottitis present?**

Sore throat and severe dysphagia, drooling, muffled voice are prominent symptoms. Adults have an indolent course preceded by a viral URI. Pain is out of proportion to objective findings.

○ **Name the most likely pathogens to cause acute parotitis:**

The most likely causes of acute parotitis are paramyxovirus (mumps), influenza A virus, Coxsackievirus group A, cytomegalovirus, and echovirus.

○ **List the criteria that would be helpful to diagnose group A hemolytic streptococci:**

Tonsillar exudate, tender anterior cervical adenopathy, absence of cough, and a history of fever.

○ **What is the first-line drug of choice for treating streptococcus pyogenes?**

The first-line treatment for group A beta-hemolytic streptococci is penicillin. Clindamycin or erythromycin is recommended for patients with a penicillin allergy.

○ **A patient presents with a history of sore throat, fever, hot potato voice, and difficulty swallowing. What must you be clinically suspicious of?**

Peritonsillar abscess.

O   **A patient presents with a history of sudden pain and swelling over the submandibular gland. He states this occurred while eating lunch. What is your diagnosis?**

Sialolithiasis. Eighty percent of the time, salivary duct stones develop in the submandibular gland, with 10% to 20% occurring in the parotid gland. If the stone doesn't pass spontaneously, ENT referral for endoscopic extraction is indicated.

O   **A patient presents to you with a dental abscess. What antibiotic is indicated for this condition?**

Clindamycin or amoxicillin and clavulanic acid will provide good coverage for the oral flora and anaerobes such as *Bacteroides fragilis.*

O   **A patient presents with a painful cluster of vesicles on the lower lip. What is your diagnosis?**

Herpes simplex type 1 causes lesions to develop on the lips and mouth. HSV-1 can also cause genital lesions transmitted by oral–genital contact. Herpes simplex type 2 causes genital herpes. Approximately 25% of the population has serologic evidence of HSV-2.

O   **What anatomic abnormalities exist when a patient presents with stridor?**

Swelling or obstruction in the larynx or trachea. Inspiratory stridor indicates obstruction at glottis or supraglottis. Expiratory stridor is created in the trachea. Biphasic stridor is created at the subglottis.

O   **What are the incidences of salivary gland malignancies?**

Parotid 40%, submandibular 10%, and sublingual 1%.

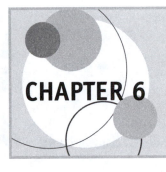

CHAPTER 6

Gastrointestinal/Nutritional

Travis Kirby, MPAS, PA-C

○ **A patient presents with chronic, progressive dysphagia of solids and liquids. A barium study shows a dilated esophagus with a distal "bird beak" appearance. What is the likely diagnosis?**

Achalasia.

○ **What study is the gold standard for diagnosing achalasia?**

Esophageal manometry.

○ **What infectious disease closely mimics idiopathic achalasia?**

Chagas disease. It is caused by *Trypanosoma cruzi*, a parasite that damages the myenteric plexus.

○ **What is the most common symptom of esophageal disease?**

Heartburn (pyrosis).

○ **What is the single, best diagnostic study for evaluating a patient with GERD?**

EGD (esophagogastroduodenoscopy).

○ **Is odynophagia (painful swallowing) a common symptom of GERD?**

No, odynophagia rarely results from GERD. It is normally associated with infectious or eosinophilic esophagitis, malignancy, or ingestion of corrosive agents.

○ **Name four common symptoms of Gastroesophageal reflux disease:**

1. Heartburn
2. Regurgitation of gastric juices
3. Dysphagia (difficulty swallowing)
4. Water brash (overproduction of saliva as a response to acid reflux)

○ **List four atypical symptoms associated with GERD:**

1. Cough
2. Hiccups
3. Throat clearing
4. Wheezing

○ **A hypotensive lower esophageal sphincter (LES) pressure is just one pathophysiological cause of GERD. Provide four dietary examples that can lower LES pressure:**

1. Fatty foods
2. Alcohol
3. Caffeine (coffee, tea, chocolate)
4. Peppermint

○ **List five medicines that can lower LES pressures, thus leading to GERD:**

1. Calcium channel blockers
2. Theophylline
3. Diazepam (Valium)
4. Meperidine (Demerol)
5. Morphine

○ **Do all patients with GERD need esophageal function testing?**

No, any additional testing beyond an EGD should be reserved for patients who either fail medical therapy and lifestyle modification or in whom the correlation of reflux symptoms are in doubt.

○ **Provide five extraesophageal manifestations of GERD:**

1. Asthma
2. Laryngitis/pharyngitis
3. Dental decay
4. Recurrent sinusitis
5. Recurrent otitis media

○ **What are the most serious complications from chronic GERD (gastroesophageal reflux disease)?**

Esophageal stricture and Barrett esophagitis.

○ **Barrett esophagitis is associated with which type of cancer?**

Esophageal adenocarcinoma.

○ **How often should patients with Barrett esophagitis have routine endoscopic surveillance?**

Every 2 to 3 years.

○   **Name four risk factors for the development of esophageal cancer:**

1. Smoking
2. Alcohol
3. Uncontrolled, chronic GERD
4. Obesity

○   **What is the most predominant type of cancer of the <u>proximal</u> esophagus?**

Squamous cell carcinoma usually involves the proximal esophagus, whereas adenocarcinoma is predominantly of distal esophageal origin.

○   **What percentage of patients with esophageal cancer is also afflicted with distant metastasis?**

80%. The 5-year survival rate is 5%.

○   **What is the most common benign esophageal neoplasm?**

Leiomyoma.

○   **What is the most common cause of infectious esophagitis?**

Candida albicans.

○   **Name three medications that may predispose a patient to fungal esophagitis:**

1. Antibiotics
2. Steroids (both systemic and inhaled)
3. H2 blockers/PPIs (acid suppression therapy)

○   **List four medical conditions that are strongly associated with fungal esophagitis:**

1. HIV
2. Diabetes mellitus
3. Cushing disease
4. Alcoholism

○   **A <u>globus sensation</u> is a feeling of a "lump in the throat." Name three potential causes of this symptom:**

1. GERD
2. Anxiety disorder
3. Goiter (causing external compression on the hypopharyngeal area)

○   **What is the most common viral cause of infectious esophagitis?**

Herpes simplex virus (HSV).

○   **The most common cause of oropharyngeal dysphagia in the elderly is of neuromuscular etiology. Give three examples:**

1. Cerebrovascular accident (CVA)
2. Parkinson disease
3. Motor neuron disorders

○ **What is a Zenker diverticulum?**

It is a diverticular outpouching usually located posteriorly in the hypopharynx.

○ **List the common symptoms associated with a Zenker diverticulum:**
- Halitosis
- Regurgitation of undigested foods
- Lower neck dysphagia

○ **A 24-year-old female patient with dysphagia is found to have an esophageal web on barium studies. What blood disorder should be considered?**

Iron deficiency anemia (related to Plummer-Vinson syndrome).

○ **Repeated violent bouts of vomiting can result in both Mallory-Weiss tears and Boerhaave syndrome. Differentiate between the two:**

Mallory-Weiss tears involve the submucosa and mucosa, typically in the right posterolateral wall of the gastroesophageal junction.

Boerhaave syndrome is a full thickness tear, usually in the unsupported left posterolateral wall of the distal esophagus.

○ **What are the signs and symptoms of Boerhaave syndrome?**

Substernal and left-sided chest pain with a history of forceful vomiting, leading to spontaneous esophageal rupture. The abdomen can become rigid and shock may follow.

○ **What is the test of choice to confirm the diagnosis of Boerhaave syndrome?**

An esophagram. A water-soluble contrast medium should be used in place of barium to confirm the diagnosis.

○ **What is Hamman sign?**

It is air in the mediastinum following an esophageal perforation. This condition produces a "crunching" sound over the heart during systole.

○ **What is the best way to remove a meat bolus causing esophageal obstruction?**

Upper endoscopy.

○ **What test must be performed after a food bolus is cleared or passes through spontaneously?**

Either a barium study or preferably an endoscopy to check for underlying pathology (e.g., strictures, masses).

○ **What are the most common symptoms of gastritis?**
- Dyspepsia (epigastric discomfort or burning)
- Postprandial fullness or bloating
- Nausea
- Vomiting

○ **List three common causes of <u>acute gastritis</u>:**

1. NSAIDs

2. Alcohol

3. Biphosphonates

○ **What etiologies are more commonly associated with <u>chronic gastritis</u>?**

- *H. pylori* infection
- Alcohol
- NSAIDs
- Bile acid reflux

○ **What are potential risk factors for exposure to *Helicobacter pylori* infection?**

Crowded living conditions, suboptimal sanitation, and low socioeconomic status.

○ **List the various methods in which *H. pylori* can be diagnosed:**

- <u>Invasively</u> via endoscopic gastroduodenal biopsies
- <u>Noninvasively</u> via:
  - serology (*H. pylori* antibody)
  - urea breath test
  - stool antigen test

○ **Does *H. pylori* play a role in either gastric or duodenal ulcers?**

Yes, most gastric ulcers occur in the setting of *H. pylori* gastritis (~60%–80%). The association is quite strong with duodenal ulcers as well.

○ **Can *H. pylori* be considered a "potential suspect" in causing gastric cancer?**

Yes, gastric cancer is the second most common cancer in the world and is classified as a group I carcinogen by the World Health Organization (WHO). Patients with *H. pylori* have a fivefold higher incidence of gastric cancer.

○ **What continents and countries have the highest prevalence of gastric cancer?**

Asia and South America have the highest rate of gastric cancer. Japan, Chile, and Costa Rica have the greatest risk.

○ **What lifestyle or dietary factors are suspected to be linked to gastric cancer?**

- Highly salted meats or fish
- Smoked meats
- Tobacco smoking

○ **What is the most common type of gastric carcinoma? What percent of these are ulcerative, polypoid, or linitis plastica?**

Adenocarcinomas account for 90% of gastric cancers. Of these, 75% are ulcerative, 10% are polypoid, and 15% are diffuse infiltrative (linitis plastica).

○ **What percentage of gastric carcinomas produces a positive hemoccult test?**

50%.

○ **What percentage of gastric carcinomas is associated with a palpable mass?**
25%.

○ **What is a Krukenberg tumor?**
It is a gastric carcinoma that has metastasized to the ovary.

○ **Stomach cancer is associated with the enlargement of what lymph nodes?**
Supraclavicular nodes (sentinel nodes).

○ **Is peptic ulcer disease (PUD) more common in men or women?**
Men (a 3:1 male-to-female ratio).

○ **Are patients with duodenal PUD usually younger or older?**
Younger. Duodenal PUD is more often associated with *H. pylori*. Older people tend to develop gastric ulcers as a result of NSAID use.

○ **Do gastric or duodenal ulcers heal faster?**
Duodenal.

○ **What medical conditions are associated with an increased incidence of peptic ulcer disease?**
• COPD
• Cirrhosis
• Chronic renal failure

○ **Are gastric and duodenal <u>perforations</u> more commonly associated with malignant or benign ulcerations?**
Benign ulcers.

○ **Is gastrointestinal bleeding common with a perforated ulcer?**
No.

○ **After the fluid and blood resuscitation of a bleeding ulcer, what is the most useful diagnostic test?**
Upper endoscopy is the most useful test because it can also be therapeutic via cryo- or electrocautery of an arterial bleeder.

○ **What are some indications for surgery in a bleeding ulcer?**
• A visible vessel in the ulcer bed
• More than 6 units of blood transfused in 24 hours
• More than 3 to 4 units transfused per day for 3 days

○ **Name two endocrine problems that can cause PUD:**
Zollinger-Ellison syndrome and hyperparathyroidism (hypercalcemia).

○ **A 48-year-old female diabetic patient presents with a multimonth history of chronic nausea, early satiety, and postprandial bloating. What is the most likely diagnosis?**

Diabetic gastroparesis.

○ **Define gastroparesis:**

It is a motility disorder of the stomach that results in impairment of the normal gastric emptying mechanism. "Delayed gastric emptying."

○ **What is the most common etiology of gastroparesis?**

Idiopathic. Other associated factors may include diabetes, gastric cancer, prior gastric bypass surgery, chronic gastritis, or exposure to viral gastroenteritis.

○ **How prevalent are gallstones in the Western population?**

Approximately 10% to 15% of adults have gallstones, with women being twice as likely. Approximately 20% of those adults will develop symptoms.

○ **List the ultrasound findings that are suggestive of acute cholecystitis:**
- Formation of gallstones or sludge
- Thickening of the gallbladder wall by more than 5 mm
- Presence of pericholecystic fluid
- A dilated common bile duct (>10 mm may suggest common bile duct obstruction).

○ **A patient with a history of gallstones presents with acute, postprandial RUQ pain. What is the KUB likely to show?**

Nothing specific. Only about 10% to 15% of gallstones are radiopaque.

○ **Gallbladder stones are made predominantly of what two materials?**

Cholesterol (80%) and bile pigments (20%).

○ **What is the diagnostic test of choice to evaluate a patient suspected to have gallstones?**

Abdominal ultrasound has a 95% detection rate for gallstones.

○ **If the abdominal ultrasound is nondiagnostic for gallstones, could the patient still have gallbladder disease? If so, what additional tests can be ordered?**

Yes, although structurally things may look normal, a patient may still exhibit symptoms from a functional disorder of the gallbladder. Biliary dyskinesia and acalculous cholecystitis are two examples. The test of choice would be a HIDA scan (radionuclide biliary scan) with cholecystokinin to calculate a gallbladder ejection fraction and to gauge if CCK administration reproduces the patient's episodic symptoms.

○ **A 54-year-old man, 2 days postop for a right knee replacement, presents with RUQ abdominal pain, nausea, and low-grade fevers. His ultrasound fails to reveal any gallstones or other obvious GB abnormality. What is the probable diagnosis?**

Acalculous cholecystitis: This is a condition most often seen in postoperative, posttraumatic, and burn patients secondary to dehydration.

○ **Which types of patients are at greatest risk for gallbladder perforation?**

The elderly patients, diabetic patients, and those with recurrent cholecystitis.

○ **What dietary history would be suspicious for underlying biliary disease?**

The ingestion of fried, fatty, greasy, oily or rich foods within 20 minutes to 2 hours prior to symptom onset. Patients may describe any of the following: epigastric or RUQ abdominal pain accompanied by nausea and/or vomiting, bloating, belching, and heartburn.

○ **What clinical sign can assist in the diagnosis of cholecystitis?**

Murphy sign is pain on inspiration with palpation of the RUQ. As the patient breathes in, the gallbladder is lowered in the abdomen and comes in contact with the peritoneum just below the examiner's hand. This will aggravate an inflamed gallbladder, causing the patient to abruptly discontinue breathing deeply.

○ **Which ethnic group has the largest proportion of people with symptomatic gallstones?**

Native Americans. By the age of 60 years, 80% of native Americans with previously asymptomatic gallstones will develop symptoms as compared to only 30% of Caucasian Americans and 20% of African Americans.

○ **Eight years after cholecystectomy, a woman develops RUQ pain and jaundice. What is the chance of recurrent biliary tract stones developing?**

At least 10%; the recurrence may be due to either retained stones or in situ formation by the biliary epithelium.

○ **What is the significance of a porcelain gallbladder?**

Defined as intramural calcification of the gallbladder wall that is normally seen on CT or plain radiographs. It has a 20% association with gallbladder carcinoma, and if discovered, cholecystectomy is recommended.

○ **Should the presence of gallbladder polyps necessitate cholecystectomy?**

Yes, all lesions >1 cm in size should be removed to rule out malignancy. Smaller lesions should be followed closely with ultrasound every 6 months.

○ **An 11-year-old child with sickle cell anemia presents with fever, RUQ abdominal pain, and jaundice. What is the most likely diagnosis?**

Charcot triad suggests ascending cholangitis. The precipitating cause in this case is probably pigment stones resulting from chronic hemolysis.

○ **What is the difference between cholelithiasis, cholangitis, cholecystitis, and choledocholithiasis?**

Cholelithiasis: Gallstones within the gallbladder sac.
Cholangitis: Inflammation of the common bile duct, often caused by infection or choledocholithiasis.
Cholecystitis: Inflammation of the gallbladder.
Choledocholithiasis: Gallstones that have migrated from the gallbladder sac into the common bile duct.

○ **What is the most frequent complication of choledocholithiasis?**

Cholangitis (60%). Other complications include bile duct obstruction, pancreatitis, biliary enteric fistula, and hemobilia. Cholangitis is a medical emergency when fever exceeds 101°F or is associated with sepsis, hypotension, peritoneal signs, or a bilirubin level >10 mg/dL. CT or abdominal ultrasonography is supportive of the diagnosis.

○ **What is the most likely diagnosis for a patient who presents with epigastric pain that radiates to the back and is partially relieved by sitting up?**

Pancreatitis.

○ **What are the major causes of acute pancreatitis?**

Alcoholism (40%) and gallstone disease (40%). The other causes of acute pancreatitis are familial inheritance, hyperparathyroidism, infection, hypertriglyceridemia, drugs, trauma, and protein deficiency.

○ **Name two metabolic causes of acute pancreatitis:**

Hypertriglyceridemia and hypercalcemia

○ **What are some of the drugs known to cause pancreatitis?**

Sulfonamides, estrogens, tetracyclines, thiazides, furosemide, and valproic acid.

○ **What are some of the infectious causes of pancreatitis?**

Mumps, viral hepatitis, Coxsackie virus group B, and mycoplasma.

○ **What is the most common cause of <u>chronic</u> pancreatitis in Western society?**

Chronic alcohol abuse.

○ **Does acute pancreatitis <u>commonly</u> progress to chronic pancreatitis?**

No, only rarely.

○ **What are the laboratory abnormalities associated with pancreatitis?**

Leukocytosis, hyperglycemia, elevated amylase, elevated lipase, hepatic enzyme elevation, hypoxemia, and prerenal azotemia.

○ **What are some abdominal X-ray findings associated with acute pancreatitis?**

- A sentinel loop (either of the jejunum, transverse colon, or duodenum)
- A colon cutoff sign (an abrupt cessation of gas in the mid or left transverse colon)
- Calcification of the pancreas

○ **Serum amylase is frequently elevated in acute pancreatitis. What other conditions can cause a similar rise in amylase?**

Salivary stones, renal failure, mumps, cholecystitis, bowel infarction, perforated ulcer, ovarian disorders, pancreatic cancer, and macroamylasemia.

○ **When is surgery indicated in pancreatitis?**

When a patient has an infected pancreatic necrosis or an abscess that cannot be adequately drained and treated.

○ **Should immediate surgery be performed in gallstone-induced pancreatitis?**

NO, it should be performed after the pancreatitis has subsided.

○ **What is <u>Cullen sign</u>?**

Periumbilical ecchymosis indicative of <u>pancreatitis</u>, severe upper GI bleeding, or ruptured ectopic pregnancy.

○ **What is <u>Courvoisier sign</u>?**

It is a palpable, distended gallbladder in the RUQ of patients with jaundice. It is usually the result of a malignant bile duct.

○ **Where is the most common site of pancreatic cancer?**

The pancreatic duct system (~80%) found in the <u>head of the pancreas</u>.

○ **With regards to pancreatic cancer, distinguish between periampullary lesions and lesions of the body and tail.**

Periampullary lesions most commonly develop at the head of the pancreas. These lesions are usually adenocarcinomas and are associated with jaundice, weight loss, and abdominal pain.

Lesions in the body and tail tend to be much larger at presentation because of their retroperitoneal location and their distance from the common bile duct. Weight loss and pain are typical.

○ **What are the risk factors for pancreatic cancer?**

- Smoking
- High-fat diet
- Chronic pancreatitis

○ **What are the associated symptoms of pancreatic cancer?**

- Weight loss
- Abdominal pain
- Nausea and anorexia
- Easy fatigability
- Painless jaundice

○ **What is the tumor marker that can assist in diagnosing pancreatic cancer?**

CA 19-9.

○ **What is the survival rate for pancreatic cancer?**

<20% survive beyond 1 year from their initial diagnosis and <30% survive longer than 5 years.

○ **What are the two most common causes of ascites?**

- Chronic liver disease
- Peritoneal carcinomatosis

○ **What are the two main mechanisms of liver injury?**

Hepatocellular injury indicates damage or destruction of the liver cells; most often due to viral hepatitis, autoimmune hepatitis, and drugs/toxins.

Cholestatic injury indicates impaired transport of bile. This may be caused by

- Extrahepatic obstruction (gallstones)
- Intrahepatic duct narrowing (primary sclerosing cholangitis)
- Bile duct damage (primary biliary cirrhosis)

○ **How is cholestatic injury best detected?**

By an elevated alkaline phosphatase (AP) level. However, keep in mind that alkaline phosphatase can be derived from other body tissue (e.g., bone, intestine), so a concurrent elevation of GGT or 5′-nucleosidase helps to support a cholestatic mechanism.

○ **What is the test of choice to assess for hepatocellular injury?**

ALT level. The AST level may also be elevated but is not as specific.

○ **Name the two most common causes of drug-induced liver disease:**

Alcohol and acetaminophen.

○ **What recreational drugs are associated with hepatotoxicity?**

Cocaine and ecstasy.

○ **How are hepatitis viruses transmitted?**

- A and E = fecal, oral route
- B, C, D = blood borne

○ **Name four other viruses, other than Hepatitis A through E, which can affect the liver:**

1. Cytomegalovirus
2. Herpes simplex virus
3. Epstein-Barr virus
4. Arthropod-borne flaviviruses (e.g., dengue, yellow fever)

○ **What are the predominant characteristics of <u>autoimmune hepatitis</u>?**

This condition affects mostly women (∼70%) and is typically diagnosed in the fourth to fifth decade of life. It is essentially an idiopathic, unresolving inflammation of the liver, which can lead to cirrhosis, portal hypertension, liver failure, or even death.

○ **Differentiate primary biliary cirrhosis (PBC) with primary sclerosing cholangitis (PSC):**

- Primary biliary cirrhosis mainly affects women in their fifties and is characterized by destruction of the septal bile ducts.
- Primary sclerosing cholangitis mainly affects men in their forties and involves diffuse inflammation and fibrosis of the entire biliary tree.

Both are chronic cholestatic liver diseases of unknown etiology that can eventually progress to end-stage liver disease.

○ **What other gastrointestinal condition is strongly associated with primary sclerosing cholangitis?**

Inflammatory bowel disease.

○ **What is hemochromatosis?**

It is a disease of <u>iron overload</u> in the liver and other organs with the most likely defect occurring in a regulatory mechanism for iron absorption in the small intestine.

○ **What is the most common screening test for hemochromatosis?**

Serum ferritin—an elevated level >400 mg/dL suggests the possibility of iron overload, but unfortunately serum ferritin can be an acute phase reactant. Thus, supportive testing (e.g., iron saturation, genetic testing, or liver biopsy) is needed to confirm the diagnosis.

○ **What is the treatment for genetic hemochromatosis?**

Phlebotomy, with removal of 1 to 2 units per week.

○ **A 52-year-old patient presents with tremor, ataxia, dementia, cirrhosis, and grey-green rings around the edge of the cornea. What is the diagnosis?**

Wilson disease—this is a disorder of <u>copper storage</u> and is associated with deficiency of an enzyme derived from hepatic cells. Deposition of copper may be seen in the eye (*Kayser-Fleischer rings*) and in parts of the brain.

○ **How is Wilson disease accurately diagnosed?**

A <u>diminished serum ceruloplasmin level</u> is strongly suggestive of Wilson disease. A quantitative copper level in liver tissue from liver biopsy should provide a definitive diagnosis.

○ **List six extra hepatic manifestations of alcoholic liver disease:**

1. Ascites
2. Spider angiomata
3. Asterixis
4. Palmar erythema
5. Korsakoff syndrome
6. Wernicke encephalopathy

○ **What are the most common vascular tumors of the liver?**

Hemangiomas.

○ **What is the most common cause of jaundice in pregnancy?**

Viral hepatitis.

○ **What is the most common liver disorder <u>related to pregnancy</u>?**

Intrahepatic cholestasis.

○   **What is the most common clinical symptom of intrahepatic cholestasis of pregnancy?**

Severe pruritus in the third trimester.

○   **Nonalcoholic steatohepatitis (NASH) is becoming a growing concern in the United States. What other clinical conditions are associated with primary NASH?**

- Morbid obesity
- Non-insulin–dependent diabetes
- Hyperlipidemia

○   **What is the most common laboratory abnormality in patients with NASH?**

A two- to threefold increase in the serum AST and ALT.

○   **What is the most specific imaging technique used to evaluate NASH?**

Hepatic ultrasound.

○   **Patients with cirrhosis or chronic active hepatitis should have what routine testing performed to screen for hepatomas?**

Alpha-fetoprotein levels and a hepatic ultrasound should be performed every 6 months. These patients have a higher risk for developing hepatic cancer.

○   **A 43-year-old patient presents with a 6-week history of frequent, malodorous diarrhea that leaves an oily sheen to the surface of the toilet water. You suspect a malabsorption disorder. What is the best study to screen for fat malabsorption?**

A microscopic stool examination using Sudan stain; it has 100% sensitivity and 96% specificity.

○   **What is the best test to differentiate malabsorption caused by small bowel versus pancreatic etiology?**

d-Xylose test.

○   **What is the most sensitive and specific serum marker for celiac disease?**

Tissue transglutaminase (tTG).

○   **What condition should be considered in a celiac patient who had previously responded well to a gluten-free diet, but now has developed refractory symptoms?**

Small bowel lymphoma.

○   **What are the signs and symptoms of Whipple disease?**

- Weight loss
- Diarrhea
- Arthralgias
- Cardiac involvement

○   **What gastrointestinal disease is most commonly associated with *Dermatitis Herpetiformis*?**

Celiac disease (gluten enteropathy).

○ **List the signs and symptoms of Crohn disease:**

- Abdominal pain (especially RLQ)
- Weight loss
- Diarrhea
- Fever
- Perianal fistulas
- Arthritis
- Hematochezia

○ **What other diseases can mimic Crohn disease?**

- Ischemic colitis
- Diverticulitis
- Colorectal cancer
- Infection with *Yersinia* species

○ **Name five potential treatment options for Crohn disease:**

1. 5-Aminosalicylic acid (5ASA) agents
2. Immunosuppressant therapy (azathioprine, 6-mercaptopurine)
3. Steroids (prednisone)
4. Biologic therapy
5. Surgery

○ **What effect does smoking have on Crohn disease and ulcerative colitis?**

- Crohn disease: <u>detrimental effect;</u> cigarette smokers are more likely to develop Crohn, have a worse prognosis, and have an increased number of recurrent flares.
- Ulcerative colitis: <u>protective effect;</u> the incidence of ulcerative colitis is higher in non- and ex-smokers than in current smokers.

○ **What is the greatest risk factor for ulcerative colitis?**

Family history. Approximately 15% of patients with ulcerative colitis have a first-degree relative with the disease.

○ **What are the signs and symptoms of ulcerative colitis?**

- Diarrhea
- Rectal bleeding (hematochezia)
- Tenesmus
- Passage of mucus

○ **Name five extraintestinal manifestations of ulcerative colitis:**

1. Arthritis
2. Erythema nodosum
3. Uveitis
4. Ankylosing spondylitis
5. Primary Sclerosing cholangitis

○ **What is the least common site of primary gastrointestinal cancer?**

Small bowel. Although it contains 75% of the length and 90% of the mucosal surface area, the small bowel only accounts for 1% to 2% of GI cancers. Adenocarcinoma remains the most prevalent type followed by lymphoma.

○   **Define carcinoid syndrome:**

Carcinoid syndrome refers to systemic symptoms resulting from the secretion of humoral factors by the Carcinoid (neuroendocrine) tumor. These symptoms may include:

- Episodic flushing of the face and upper trunk
- Watery diarrhea
- Bronchospasm

○   **What is the most likely distribution of carcinoid tumors?**

Carcinoid tumors are slow growing and can occur anywhere along the GI tract. Most are found incidentally, thus at the time of discovery, most patients are asymptomatic. Only 5% of patients with carcinoid tumors have carcinoid syndrome (see above). Common sites for carcinoid growth include the <u>appendix</u> (most common), followed by the <u>ileum</u>, then <u>stomach</u>, <u>rectum</u>, <u>colon</u>, and <u>pancreas</u>.

○   **If carcinoid syndrome is strongly suspected, what is the best initial diagnostic study to pursue?**

A <u>urine analysis for 5-HIAA</u> (hydroxyindoleacetic acid) will be increased. If the urine for 5-HIAA is increased then a <u>CT of the abdomen and pelvis</u> or an <u>Octreoscan</u> (Octreotide scintigraphy) should identify the primary site of the tumor in 80% of cases.

○   **What is the most common cancer arising in the colon?**

Adenocarcinoma.

○   **How does colorectal cancer rank in mortality for the population of the United States?**

Second, behind lung cancer.

○   **Considering those within the U.S. population who do not have a significant family history of colorectal cancer, at what age should general screening begin?**

Caucasians and other races = age 50 years
African Americans = age 45 years

○   **What two clinical conditions should raise the suspicion for the presence of colon cancer?**

1. An unexplained iron deficiency anemia
2. Sepsis with *Streptococcus bovis*

○   **What percentage of colon cancer is related to genetic inheritance?**

15%.

○   **What is the "gold standard" for identifying colorectal cancer?**

Colonoscopy.

○   **Name two metabolic disorders that can cause constipation:**

1. Hypothyroidism
2. Diabetes mellitus

○   **A 72-year-old female patient presents with a 2-day history of progressively worsening LLQ abdominal pain associated with constipation and "chills." What is the most likely diagnosis?**

Diverticulitis.

○   **What are potential complications of diverticulitis?**

- Abscess formation
- Perforation leading to peritonitis
- Diverticular bleeding
- Obstruction from diverticular strictures or luminal narrowing

○   **List three risk factors for diverticulosis:**

1. Increasing age
2. Chronic constipation that leads to increased luminal pressures
3. Westernized diet—low in fiber and high in refined carbohydrates

○   **What groups are most at risk for perforation of appendicitis?**

- Children younger than 5 years of age
- Elderly patients
- Diabetic patients
- Immunosuppressed patients

○   **What is the most common tumor of the appendix?**

Carcinoid tumor.

○   **What antibiotics are commonly associated with *Clostridium difficile* colitis?**

C. difficile colitis can occur with any antibiotic, even a single dose preop. But the most likely suspects remain clindamycin, ampicillin, and third-generation cephalosporins.

○   **What is the first-line treatment of *C. difficile* colitis?**

Metronidazole (Flagyl). Improvement should begin with 2 to 4 days and resolution of diarrhea by 2 weeks. If the patient does not respond to metronidazole, then vancomycin should be considered.

○   **List the most common sources of upper gastrointestinal bleeding:**

- Duodenal ulcers
- Gastric erosions
- Gastric ulcers
- Esophagitis

○   **What is the most likely source of acute hematemesis in a 43-year-old male patient with a history of cirrhosis?**

Esophageal varices (50%).

○   **What is the most common cause of hematochezia (bright red rectal bleeding) or lower GI bleeding in <u>adults</u>?**

Internal hemorrhoids.

○ **List four other causes of lower GI bleeding:**

1. Diverticulitis
2. Vascular ectasias
3. Neoplasms
4. Ischemic colitis

○ **What is the most common cause of lower GI bleeding in <u>children</u>?**

Meckel diverticulum—located in the ileum, it is the most common congenital abnormality of the gut.

○ **What is the most common complication of a Meckel diverticulum?**

Bleeding. It presents with painless melena or hematochezia described as "currant jelly" like stools. Diagnosis is established via a Meckel scan (technetium-99m scintiscan).

○ **An 82-year-old male patient presents with an acute onset of crampy LLQ abdominal pain with the urge to defecate and expulsion of bloody diarrhea. Associated symptoms include nausea, fever, and tachycardia. Plain film abdominal X-rays reveal "thumbprinting" changes. What is the most likely diagnosis?**

Ischemic colitis.

○ **A differential diagnosis for <u>bloody diarrhea</u> would include:**

- Ischemic colitis
- Infectious colitis
- Radiation proctitis
- Inflammatory bowel disease (UC or Crohn disease)
- Meckel diverticulum

○ **How much blood is needed to produce a positive hemoccult (fecal occult blood test)?**

As little as 2 mL.

○ **What is the test of choice to accurately diagnose celiac sprue (gluten enteropathy)?**

Upper endoscopy with biopsies obtained from the duodenum that demonstrates <u>flattened small bowel villi in association with increased epithelial lymphocytes.</u>

○ **Name two methods used to diagnose lactose intolerance:**

1. Dietary history and response to empiric therapy
2. Hydrogen breath test

○ **What are the four types of stimuli for abdominal pain?**

1. Stretching or tension
2. Inflammation
3. Ischemia
4. Neoplasms

○ **What is the single best test to evaluate HIV-infected patients who present with abdominal pain?**

CT of the abdomen and pelvis.

○ **What gastrointestinal symptoms may occur in patients with pheochromocytoma?**

- Weight loss
- Anorexia
- Abdominal pain due to cholelithiasis

○ **What is the significance of <u>Sister Mary Joseph node</u>?**

It is an umbilical metastasis manifesting as periumbilical lymphadenopathy from an internal malignancy. It usually indicates advanced disease with an average survival time of up to 10 months.

○ **What other type of <u>node</u> may represent an intra-abdominal malignancy?**

Virchow node, presenting as a supraclavicular mass, may indicate a bowel carcinoma.

○ **What is a common cause of acute abdominal pain in illicit drug users?**

<u>Acute mesenteric ischemia</u> ("crack belly") can be seen in cocaine abusers.

○ **What is the differential diagnosis of yellowish discoloration of the skin?**

- Jaundice
- Hypercarotemia (overingestion of carotene, e.g., carrots, squash)
- Lycopenoderma (overingestion of lycopenes, e.g., red veggies, tomatoes)
- Profound hypothyroidism

○ **What type of gastroenteritis is closely associated with the consumption of seafood?**

Vibrio parahaemolyticus.

○ **What is the most common cause of gastroenteritis in the United States?**

Viruses.

○ **What is the most common cause of childhood diarrhea?**

Rotavirus.

○ **Ordering stool cultures is appropriate in patients presenting with what characteristics?**

- Bloody diarrhea
- High fever
- Presence of fecal leukocytes
- Immunocompromised patients
- Diarrhea persisting longer than 72 hours

○ **Name the most common bacterial causes of infectious diarrhea in the United States:**

Remember C, C, S, S, Y, and sometimes E:

Campylobacter
Clostridium
Salmonella
Shigella
Yersinia
E. coli O157:H7

○ **What is the most common bacterial source to infectious diarrhea in the United States?**

Campylobacter jejuni.

○ **What is the most common parasitic diarrhea infection in the United States? In the world?**

<u>Giardia lamblia</u> is the most common in the United States
<u>Amebiasis</u> (*Entamoeba histolytica*) is the most common in the world.

○ **Deficiency of what two vitamins can cause a macrocytic anemia?**

Folate and B12.

○ **What is the leading cause of death in bulimia nervosa?**

Cardiac arrhythmia.

○ **What proportion of adults in the United States is obese?**

Approximately one-third.

○ **What vitamin deficiency does the Schilling test evaluate?**

Vitamin B12.

○ <u>**Pellagra**</u> **is caused primarily by a deficiency of what nutrient?**

Niacin.

○ **What are the three D's of pellagra?**

Dermatitis
Diarrhea
Dementia

○ **What is the most common dermatologic finding in patients with hemochromatosis?**

Bronze pigmentation of the skin.

○ **What two dermatologic signs may assist in the diagnosis of acute pancreatitis?**

1. Cullen sign (periumbilical bruising)
2. Grey Turner sign (flank bruising)

○   **What is a possible finding on an upper GI series from a woman with telangiectasias, tight knuckles, and acid indigestion?**

Aperistalsis. The defective peristalsis can be associated with connective tissue disorders such as <u>scleroderma,</u> or in this clinical scenario, a <u>CREST syndrome</u>:

Calcinosis cutis

Raynaud phenomenon

Esophageal dysfunction

Sclerodactyly

Telangiectasias

○   <u>**Rickets**</u> **is associated with a deficiency of what vitamin?**

Vitamin D.

○   **A 38-year-old male patient presents with anorexia, lethargy, arthralgias, and swollen gums. What vitamin deficiency may be present?**

Vitamin C (scurvy).

○   **Deficiencies in either of these two micronutrients may cause paresthesias, tetany, seizures, or arrhythmia:**

Calcium or magnesium.

○   <u>**Night blindness**</u> **may be associated with what vitamin deficiency?**

Vitamin A.

○   **What is the most common risk factor for hepatitis C?**

<u>Intravenous drug abuse</u> accounts for 43% of cases.

○   **List four factors that increase the risk for colorectal cancer:**

1. Increasing age

2. Family history of polyps or CRC

3. Inflammatory bowel disease

4. Diets high in fat and low in fiber

○   **What are three basic mechanisms of weight loss?**

1. Decreased food intake (e.g., esophageal stricture)

2. Increased metabolism (e.g., hyperthyroidism)

3. Increased loss of energy (e.g., intestinal malabsorption with steatorrhea)

○   **What are the leading causes of** <u>**unexplained weight loss in the elderly?**</u>

- Psychiatric
- Malignancy
- Gastrointestinal disorders

○ **What is the most common digestive complaint in the United States?**

Constipation.

○ **List four common causes of acute abdominal pain in the elderly from <u>most to least prevalent</u>:**

1. Biliary tract disease

2. Bowel obstruction

3. Incarcerated hernias

4. Appendicitis

○ **Identify six causes of chronic hiccups:**

1. Abdominal distention

2. Brain stem lesion

3. Gastric malignancy

4. Pleural irritation

5. Pancreatitis

6. Chronic renal failure

● ● ● **REFERENCES** ● ● ●

Edmundowicz, SA. *20 Common Problems in Gastroenterology.* New York, NY: McGraw-Hill; 2002.

Feldman M, Friedman LS, Sleisenger MH. *Sleisenger & Fordtran's Gastrointestinal and Liver Disease.* 7th ed. Philadelphia, PA: W.B. Saunders; 2002.

Hauser, S. *Mayo Clinic Gastroenterology and Hepatology Board Review.* 3rd ed. Florence, KY: Mayo Clinic Scientific Press and Informa Healthcare; 2008.

McNally PR. *GI/Liver Secrets.* 2nd ed. Philadelphia, PA: Hanley & Belfus; 2001.

Schilling-McCann. *Professional Guide to Signs and Symptoms.* 4th ed. Philadelphia, PA: Lippincott, Williams & Wilkins; 2004.

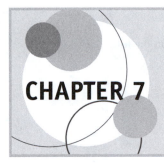

CHAPTER 7 Genitourinary

Daniel Thibodeau, MHP, PA-C

● ● ● BENIGN CONDITIONS OF THE GU TRACT ● ● ●

○ **What is the most common tumor found in men?**

Benign prostatic hyperplasia (BPH).

○ **A 56-year-old man who reports that his urinary stream has weakened. He also complains of nocturia, decreased force of stream, and hesitancy. He also states he is having postvoid dribbling. On the basis of patient's history, what do you expect to find on his physical examination?**

In most cases of suspected BPH, the prostate will have a smooth symmetric and firm elastic consistency. If you detect an irregular, harder nodule or lesion, cancer must be suspected.

○ **What percentage of men with BPH are afflicted with occult prostate cancer?**

10% to 30%.

○ **How well does the size of the prostate in BPH correlate with the symptoms?**

Not well. Symptoms can arise because of a small fibrous prostate as well as a large one. Additional symptoms can also develop as a result of median bar hypertrophy of the posterior vesicle neck, detrusor muscle decompensation, or instability.

○ **Name three tests that can be used to determine the presence of BPH:**

1. Intravenous urography (IVU)
2. CT scan
3. Ultrasound.

○ **What class of drugs is used as a first-line treatment of BPH?**

α-Blockers.

○ **Name the most common surgical procedure for the treatment of BPH:**

Transurethral resection of the prostate (TURP).

○   **Why is surgical correction of cryptorchism important?**

Surgical correction is required to preserve fertility, but the procedure has no bearing on the future development of testicular cancer. Surgery must be performed before age 5 to preserve fertility.

○   **Which children are at higher risk for having cryptorchism?**

Premature births have up to 20% prevalence.

○   **What is the most common systemic cause of erectile dysfunction?**

Diabetes.

○   **Name some systemic conditions that can cause erectile dysfunction:**

Diabetes, hypercholesterolemia, heart disease, depression, renal failure, adrenal and thyroid dysfunction.

○   **Name treatments for improving erectile dysfunction:**

Hormonal replacement, vacuum constriction device, vascular surgery, vasoactive therapy, and penile prosthesis.

○   **A 4-year-old boy presents with a painless mass in his scrotum that fluctuates in size with palpation. The mass transilluminates. What is the probable diagnosis?**

A communicating hydrocele. An inguinal scrotal ultrasound should distinguish hydrocele from bowel and a testicular nuclear scan should rule out testicular torsion.

○   **When do communicating hydroceles need repair?**

If after 1 year to 18 months they do not reduce in size or become larger, surgery is indicated.

○   **Varicoceles are most common in which side of the scrotum?**

The left. Varicoceles are a collection of veins in the scrotum. These patients have a higher incidence of infertility, presumably because of the increased temperature of the testes surrounded by the warm blood of the varicocele. Incidentally, the left testis is the first to descend and also hangs lower than the right in the majority of men. Hernias are also more common on the left side, too.

○   **Are varicoceles commonly treated surgically?**

No, most are left alone. Treatment is reserved for cases of suspicion of infertility.

○   **Name the two common types of causes of urinary incontinence:**

Stress and urge incontinence.

○   **What is a third type?**

Overflow incontinence.

○ **What is the mnemonic that refers to the correctable causes of urinary incontinence?**

DIAPPERS

Delirium

Infection

Atrophic urethritis and atrophic vaginitis

Pharmaceuticals: sedatives, hypnotics, alcohol, diuretics, and anticholinergics

Psychologic disorders: depression, psychosis

Endocrine disorders: hyperglycemia, hypercalcemia

Restricted mobility

Stool impaction

○ **What is the most common form of urge incontinence?**

Detrusor instability.

○ **What is the most common form of stress incontinence?**

Urethral incompetence.

○ **What are some examples of stress incontinence?**

Incontinence after laughing, coughing, sneezing, or lifting heavy objects.

○ **What are Kegel exercises?**

Kegel exercises are pelvic floor muscle exercises. If properly performed, they can help improve the symptoms of urinary incontinence.

○ **What is the most effective treatment for stress incontinence?**

Surgery, which has a 75% to 80% cure rate. This is used as a last resort.

○ **A 33-year-old male patient presents with a history of sudden onset of right flank pain that was sharp and doubled the patient over. This was also associated with nausea and vomiting and radiation of pain around the flank to the lower quadrant of the abdomen and scrotum. Based on this history, what is the likely diagnosis?**

Kidney stone.

○ **Which gender has more kidney stones?**

Men (a 3:1 male-to female ratio).

○ **Which t is the test of choice for ruling out a kidney stone?**

Spiral CT scan.

○ **What is the one greatest factor in the prevention of kidney stones?**

The amount of fluid intake by the patient. The more a patient is able to take in fluid, the less likely he or she will develop a stone. If a patient has a history of a stone, the recommendation is to try to double the amount of fluids.

○ **What percentage of urinary calculi are radiopaque?**

85%.

○ **What are the admission criteria for patients with renal calculi?**

Infection with concurrent obstruction, a solitary kidney and complete obstruction, uncontrolled pain, intractable emesis, or large stones. Only 10% of stones >6 mm pass spontaneously. Other indications include renal insufficiency and complete obstruction or urinary extravasation, as demonstrated by the IVP.

○ **What percentage of patients with urinary calculi do not have hematuria?**

10%.

○ **A urinary pH of 7.3 is conducive to the formation of what kind of stones?**

Struvite and phosphate stones. Alkalotic urine actually inhibits the formation of uric acid and cystine stones. Conversely, struvite and phosphate stones are inhibited by a more acidic urine.

○ **Which type of stone formation is caused by a genetic error?**

Cysteine stones. These stones are produced because there is an error in the transport of amino acids that results in cystinuria.

○ **Where is kidney stone formation most likely to occur?**

In the proximal portion of the collecting system.

○ **Differentiate between radiolucent and radiopaque renal calculi:**

90% of all stones are radiopaque and are composed of calcium oxalate, cysteine, calcium phosphate, or magnesium ammonium phosphate. Radiolucent obstruction consists of uric acid stones and blood clots.

○ **What is the 5-year recurrence rate for kidney stones?**

50%. The 10-year recurrence rate is 70%.

○ **What percentage of patients spontaneously pass kidney stones?**

80%. This is largely dependent on size. 75% of stones <4 mm pass spontaneously, while only 10% of those >6 mm pass spontaneously. Analgesics and increased fluid intake aid in outpatient management of kidney stones.

○ **Which bacterium is associated with magnesium ammonium phosphate uretero lithiasis?**

Proteus, a bacterium that produces urease. These are infected stones and need to be removed. Antibiotics will help treat the UTI and will generally cease stone formation and urinary acidification. A urease inhibitor like acetohydroxamic acid will also prevent stone growth.

○ **Name the three most common anatomical sites where kidney stones are likely to get stuck:**

1. Ureterovesicular junction (UVJ)
2. Crossing over the iliac vascular structures
3. Opening of the urethrovesicular junction

○ **What is phimosis?**

A condition in which the foreskin cannot be retracted posterior to the glans. The preliminary treatment is a dorsal slit.

○ **What is paraphimosis?**

A condition in which the foreskin is retracted posterior to the glands and cannot be advanced over the glans.

○ **What is a nonsurgical method to attempt to reduce a paraphimosis?**

Firmly squeeze the inflamed tissue for 5 to 10 minutes to reduce the size, then retract the paraphimosis distally while pushing the glans penis proximally.

○ **How is testicular torsion distinguished from epididymitis?**

By the rate of the pain onset. Torsional pain typically begins instantaneously at maximum intensity, whereas epididymal pain grows steadily over hours or days. In torsion, you classically have a loss of the cremasteric reflex and a swollen firm high riding testicle. Clinically, elevation of the scrotum may relieve pain related to epididymitis but is not effective with torsional pain (Prehn sign). This test is not, however, considered diagnostic.

○ **How is testicular torsion diagnosed?**

By emergency surgical exploration. A Doppler examination is also very sensitive but should not delay treatment.

○ **What is the testicular viability after 6, 10, and 24 hours of ischemia?**

After 6 hours: 6% to 80%
After 10 hours: 10% to 20%
After 24 hours: 24% to near 0%

○ **What does a blue dot sign suggest?**

Torsion of the epididymis or appendix testis. With transillumination of the testis, a blue reflection occurs. When detected early, a patient with torsion of the appendix testis will experience intense pain near the head of the epididymis or testis, which is frequently associated with a palpable tender nodule. If normal flow to the affected testis can be confirmed by a testicular ultrasound, immediate surgery can be avoided. Most appendages will calcify or degenerate within 10 to 14 days without harm to the patient.

○ **What is the postvoid residual volume that suggests urinary retention?**

A volume greater than 60 mL.

○ **Testicular torsion is most common in which age group?**

14-year-olds. Two-thirds of the cases occur in the second decade. The next most common group is newborns.

○ **A baby is brought to the emergency department because of vomiting and persistent crying. On examination, a testicle is tender and enlarged. What is the diagnosis?**

Testicular torsion.

○   **True/False: Testicular torsion frequently follows a history of strenuous physical activity or occurs during sleep:**

True.

○   **True/False: 40% of patients with testicular torsion have a history of similar pain in the past that resolved spontaneously:**

True.

○   **How do you manually attempt to reduce a testicular torsion?**

Standing in front of the patient, you manually twist simultaneously the right testicle counterclockwise and the left testicle clockwise. Remember; open the book to reduce the testicles.

○   **What is the definitive treatment for testicular torsion?**

Bilateral orchiopexy in which the testes are surgically attached to the scrotum.

• • • INFECTIOUS/INFLAMMATORY CONDITIONS • • •

○   **What is the most common pathogen of urinary tract infections (UTIs)?**

Escherichia coli (80%). *E. coli* is also the most common cause of pyelonephritis and pyelitis because of its ascension from the lower urinary tract. *Staphylococcus saprophyticus* accounts for 5% to 15% of UTIs.

○   **What are some clinical complaints of patients with cystitis?**

Urinary frequency, dysuria, urgency, suprapubic pain, and hematuria.

○   **Name three commonly used antibiotics for the treatment of uncomplicated cystitis:**

1. Trimethoprim-sulfamethoxazole
2. Cephalexin
3. Nitrofurantoin

○   **What is the drug of choice for treating urinary tract infection due to *Proteus mirabilis* ?**

Ampicillin. This condition is common in young boys.

○   **What is the most common cause of epididymitis in the following age groups: prepubertal boys, men younger than 35 years, and men older than 35 years?**

Prepubertal boys: *Coliform* bacteria

Men younger than 35: *Chlamydia* or *Neisseria gonorrhoeae*

Men older than 35: *Coliform* bacteria

Epididymitis is also frequently caused by urinary reflux, prostatitis, or urethral instrumentation.

○   **What does epididymitis in childhood suggest?**

Obstructive or fistulous urinary defects. Epididymitis is rare in children.

○ **How does the pain associated with epididymitis differ from that produced by prostatitis?**

Epididymitis: Pain begins in the scrotum or groin and radiates along the spermatic cord. It intensifies rapidly, is associated with dysuria, and is relieved with scrotal elevation (Prehn sign).

Prostatitis: Patients have frequency, dysuria, urgency, bladder outlet obstruction, and retention. They may have low back pain and perineal pain associated with fever, chills, arthralgias, and myalgias.

○ **What percentage of patients with epididymitis will also have pyuria?**

25%.

○ **What is the most common cause of epididymitis?**

Chlamydia trachomatis in men younger than 35 years. *E. coli* in prepubertal and older patients.

○ **Acute testicular pain and relief of pain with elevation of the scrotum (Prehn sign) is classically associated with:**

Epididymitis.

○ **Aside from antibiotics, what other instructions do you give a patient with acute epididymitis?**

Rest with scrotal elevation. For a sexually transmitted bacterium, the sexual partner must also be treated.

○ **Name etiologies for acute orchitis:**

Infectious etiologies (viral, bacterial, mycobacterial), mumps, and epididymitis.

○ **What is the basic treatment for uncomplicated orchitis?**

Supportive care, rest, analgesia, and a recumbency position.

○ **A 35-year-old male patient has a 4-day history of dysuria, with perineal pain, and subjective fevers. On examination, you note a tender, boggy prostate. What is the likely diagnosis?**

Acute prostatitis.

○ **What are the causative organisms of prostatitis?**

E. coli (80%), *Klebsiella*, *Enterobacter*, *Proteus*, and *Pseudomonas*.

○ **What is the outpatient treatment for prostatitis?**

TMP-SMX, double strength po bid for 30 days; or ciprofloxacin, 500 mg po bid for 30 days; or norfloxacin, 400 mg po bid for 30 days.

○ **A 23-year-old female patient presents with 5 days of fever, right flank pain, along with dysuria and nausea with vomiting. On examination, there is right-sided CVA tenderness and the abdomen and pelvic examinations are benign. What is the likely diagnosis?**

Acute pyelonephritis.

○   **What are the likely pathogens for an acute, uncomplicated pyelonephritis?**

Gram-negative rods such as *E. coli, Proteus, Klebsiella, Enterobacter,* and *Pseudomonas. S. aureus* can also cause, but this is usually spread hematogenously.

○   **In making a correct diagnosis of pyelonephritis, what are some differentials to consider?**

Acute cholecystitis, appendicitis, diverticulitis, and pancreatitis. Also consider a patient with a history of kidney stones to have an infected stone in the renal pelvis.

○   **What is the treatment for an uncomplicated case of pyelonephritis?**

Intravenous ampicillin or an aminoglycoside prior to obtaining culture results. As an outpatient treatment, quinolones or nitrofurantoin are used. Aggressive fluid intake is also done along with analgesia for pain.

○   **What is the course for a pregnant patient with pyelonephritis?**

This requires inpatient care with aggressive fluids and IV antibiotics. In some early cases of pregnancy, outpatient therapy can be done with very close follow-up.

○   **Outpatient management of pyelonephritis should be reserved for what patients?**

Young, otherwise healthy patients who are not vomiting, are hemodynamically stable, are defervescing with antipyretics, and are able to drink fluids. These patients should be treated with IV fluids, antipyretics, and a dose of IV antibiotics, such as gentamicin, a third-generation cephalosporin, or TMP-SMX.

○   **What are the risk factors for subclinical pyelonephritis?**

Multiple prior UTIs, longer duration of symptoms, recent pyelonephritis, diabetes, anatomic abnormalities, immunocompromised patients, and indigents.

○   **What is the most common cause of urethritis in men?**

Neisseria gonorrheae (gonococcal urethritis) or *Chlamydia trachomatis* (nongonococcal urethritis). Gonorrhea presents with a purulent discharge from the urethra, whereas chlamydia is generally associated with a thinner, white mucous discharge. Treatment should cover both gonorrhea and chlamydia because there is a high incidence of coinfection. Ceftriaxone for gonorrhea and doxycycline or tetracycline for chlamydia are the drugs of choice.

○   **What are the most common causes of nongonococcal urethritis?**

Chlamydia trachomatis. Ureaplasma urealyticum is another common cause.

○   **What is the most common clinical manifestation of disseminated gonococcal infection?**

Gonococcal arthritis–dermatitis syndrome. Arthritis, a pustular or papular rash, and tenosynovitis are exhibited with this syndrome.

○ **A 75-year-old diabetic man presents with a fever, appearing toxic, complaining of acute onset of pain and swelling in his scrotum. He denies urinary symptoms and has a painful, erythematous, edematous scrotum with crepitus. What is the diagnosis and treatment?**

Fournier gangrene. This usually presents in immunocompromised elderly patients and is due to infection or trauma of the perianal area. *Bacteroides fragilis* and *E. coli* predominate. Treatment is supportive plus broad-spectrum parenteral antibiotics against anaerobes and gram-negative enteric organisms. Urological consult for surgical debridement is necessary.

○ **What is the inflammation of the foreskin called?**

Balanitis or balanoposthitis.

• • • NEOPLASTIC DISEASES • • •

○ **A 66-year-old male patient presents with a 3-day history of painless hematuria. There are no other complaints and his examination is normal with exception of mild bloody discharge from the urethral meatus. There is no history of trauma. What is the most likely etiology?**

Bladder cancer.

○ **What is the number one risk factor for bladder cancer?**

Smoking, which accounts for 60% of all cases.

○ **How is bladder cancer confirmed as a diagnosis?**

By cystoscope and biopsy.

○ **Which is the most common type of bladder cancer?**

Transitional cell carcinoma. Schistosomiasis infection, aniline dyes, smoking, and the male gender are all risk factors.

○ **What is the most common physical examination finding in men with prostate cancer?**

They will have a normal examination with a normal palpated prostate.

○ **Do prostate cancers present with voiding problems?**

No, they normally are asymptomatic and are found by the PSA. Larger growths can cause voiding issues, but these are usually later stage cancers.

○ **What percentage of men with PSAs greater than 10 ng/mL will have prostate cancer?**

Between 50% and 70%.

○ **What is the standard method for diagnosing prostate cancer?**

Transrectal ultrasound guided biopsy.

○ **Which is the most common type of prostate cancer?**

Acinar adenocarcinoma (95%).

○ **Where is prostate cancer most commonly found?**

In the peripheral regions of the prostate.

○ **What is the biggest risk factor for prostate cancer?**

Age. The median age for diagnosis of prostate cancer is 72 years.

○ **Where is the most common site for prostate cancer to metastasize?**

Bone. Most typical area is the axial skeleton.

○ **What are the six Whitmore-Jewett stages of prostatic cancer?**

1. A1–A2: No palpable tumor confined to capsule with a positive random biopsy.

2. B2–B3: Palpable tumor confined to 1 gland or a nodule confined to 1 lobe. Both are contained within the capsule.

3. C1: Extension beyond the capsule.

4. C2: Involvement of the seminal vesicles.

5. D1: Metastasis to regional lymph nodes.

6. D2: Metastasis beyond regional lymph nodes.

○ **What is the best screening method for prostate cancer?**

A combination of a digital rectal examination (DRE) and PSA test.

○ **What is the definitive surgical treatment for prostate cancer?**

Radical prostatectomy. In some localized tumors, radiation therapy may be indicated as an alternative.

○ **What types of radiation therapy are available for treating prostate cancer?**

Directed beam radiation and transperineal radioactive seed implantation.

○ **A 64-year-old male patient presents to the emergency department with a 1-month history of mild hematuria, flank pain, weight loss, and subjective fever. On examination, you palpate a firm small mass on trapping the right kidney. What is the likely diagnosis in this patient?**

Renal cell carcinoma.

○ **What percentage of patients with renal cell carcinoma present with hematuria (gross or microscopic)?**

60%.

○ **What is the only significant risk factor for developing renal cell carcinoma?**

Smoking.

○ **What is the best method for detecting renal cell carcinoma?**

CT scan is the preferred test. Most tumors are found incidentally.

○ **While considering the work-up for a patient with a suspected renal cell carcinoma, what other tests should be ordered?**

The CT scan will also evaluate the contralateral kidney. In addition, chest X-ray to rule out pulmonary metastasis as well as a bone scan should be performed. Alkaline phosphatase may be elevated in these patients.

○ **What is the definitive treatment for a patient with renal cell carcinoma?**

Radical nephrectomy. In some cases where the tumor is isolated, a partial nephrectomy can be performed.

○ **Is chemotherapy an effective treatment option for renal cell carcinoma?**

No, there are no drugs that are effective in treating this disease.

○ **A 27-year-old male patient presents with a painless nodular growth on his right testicle that has been present for the last 3 months. There is no history of pain, urinary symptoms, or difficulty with ejaculate. What is the most likely problem that this patient has?**

Testicular cancer until proven otherwise.

○ **Which testicle is more likely to have a cancer, the right or the left?**

The right. This parallels with the higher amount of cryptorchidism on that side.

○ **What imaging technique is used to confirm a testicular mass?**

Testicular ultrasound.

○ **How is the diagnosis of testicular cancer made?**

By orchiectomy.

○ **What are the treatments for testicular cancer?**

Orchiectomy and retroperitoneal radiation.

○ **What is the most common cancer in young adult males?**

Testicular cancer is one of the leading cancers in incidence in young adult men with an average age of about 32 years. There is a significantly increased incidence of carcinoma developing in cryptorchid testes.

○ **What is the best tumor marker for testicular cancer?**

Placental alkaline phosphatase (PLAP). 70% to 90% of patients with testicular cancer have elevated PLAP. Other tumor markers are a-fetoprotein and β-hCG.

○ **What is an important difference between testicular teratomas in children and adults?**

In children, teratomas are benign lesions. In adults, they may metastasize.

○ **What is the most common neoplasm in men younger than 30 years?**

Seminomas. This is also the most common type of testicular neoplasm. Peak incidence is between ages 20 and 40 years, with a smaller peak occurring below age 10. 90% to 95% are germinal tumors. However, only 60% to 70% are germinal in children. Cryptorchidism is a significant risk factor for this cancer.

○ **A mother brings in her 3-year-old son because she has noticed that his abdomen has increased in size. In addition, the child has been having subjective fever. On examination, the child is found to be hypertensive and has a palpable mass on the left side of the abdomen. There is also microscopic hematuria and mild anemia on laboratory reports. Given this history, what is the likely diagnosis of the child?**

Wilms tumor

○ **What is the most common malignant renal tumor in children?**

Wilms tumor is a highly malignant tumor of mixed histology. A suspected hereditary form of Wilms tumor that is transmitted as an autosomal dominant disorder accounts for about 40% of all tumors. An abdominal mass is the presenting complaint in these children with peak ages at diagnosis of 1 to 3 years.

○ **One to two percent of the affected patients will have a recurrence of the Wilms tumor. Where is this recurrence most likely to be?**

The chest.

○ **What is the treatment for a patient with a Wilms tumor?**

Surgical exploration of the abdomen to view the contralateral kidney as well as the liver and lymph nodes. Surgical resection of the tumor is attempted with effort to not spill and seed the abdomen.

○ **What is the prognosis for a Wilms tumor?**

The overall cure rate is 90%.

● ● ● **RENAL DISEASES** ● ● ●

○ **What are some common physical examination findings in patients with chronic renal disease?**

In general, the patients appear ill and complain of fatigue, weakness, and malaise. They may have a fishy odor on breath. Hypertension is frequently seen. Skin may be yellow and easy to bruise. Cardiovascular examination may have cardiomegaly with a displaced PMI, rales, and edema.

○ **What is the most common cause of acute renal failure?**

Acute tubular necrosis. This occurs after toxic or ischemic renal injuries caused by shock, surgery, or rhabdomyolysis.

○ **What is the most common cause of chronic renal failure?**

NIDDM.

○ **When are renal insufficiency symptoms displayed?**

When 90% of the nephrons have been destroyed. Hypertension, diabetes mellitus, glomerulonephritis, polycystic kidney disease, tubulointerstitial disease, and obstructive uropathy are all causes of chronic renal failure.

○ **What is the most common cause of cardiac arrest in a uremic patient?**

Hyperkalemia.

○ **What is the most common cause of intrinsic renal failure?**

Acute tubular necrosis (80%–90%), resulting from an ischemic injury (the most common cause of ATN) or from a nephrotoxic agent. Less frequent causes of intrinsic renal failure (10%–20%) include vasculitis, malignant hypertension, acute GN, or allergic interstitial nephritis.

○ **What type of anemia is characteristic of chronic renal failure?**

Normochromic, normocytic.

○ **Name an abnormal ultrasound finding that suggests chronic renal failure:**

Kidneys <9 cm in length are abnormal. A difference of >1.5 cm in length between the two kidneys suggests unilateral kidney disease. Kidneys with a small or absent renal cortex are also indicative of chronic renal failure.

○ **What is the life expectancy of chronic renal patients after the disease has progressed to dialysis?**

Patients between the ages of 55 and 64 years have an average 22-year life expectancy. Patients older than 60 and with end-stage renal disease have a 5-year life expectancy.

○ **What is the most common cause of death in patients with renal failure?**

Cardiac dysfunction (45%), followed by infection (14%), and then cerebrovascular disease (6%).

○ **What are the causes of advanced chronic renal failure and large kidneys?**

Amyloidosis, polycystic kidney disease, diabetic nephropathy, HIV-ATN (AIDS nephropathy), and multiple myeloma.

○ **What does acute renal failure in a patient with alcoholic cirrhosis and a urine sodium of less than 10 suggest?**

Prerenal azotemia or hepatorenal syndrome.

○ **Acute renal failure caused by Wegener granulomatosis may respond best to what treatments?**

This is usually rapidly progressive GN and responds to high-dose steroids and cyclophosphamide.

○ **Total and persistent anuria with renal failure should prompt a work-up for what?**

These patients are presumed to be obstructed until proven otherwise.

○ **A renal biopsy in a patient with acute renal failure, hematuria, and red cell casts will most likely reveal what lesion?**

A proliferative glomerulonephritis, usually with crescents.

○ **What continuous modes of renal replacement therapy used in ARF?**

CVVH and peritoneal dialysis. Hemodialysis is an intermittent therapy.

○ **What are the first-line oral phosphate binders used in CRF?**

Calcium carbonate and calcium acetate. Aluminum-containing agents are best avoided.

○ **What are the causes of high levels of PTH in CRF?**

Hyperphosphatemia, hypocalcemia due to deficiency of vitamin D, and parathyroid receptor resistance.

○ **What is the etiology of CRF associated with cerebral berry aneurysms?**

Adult polycystic kidney disease is associated with cerebral berry aneurysms.

○ **What are the indications for emergent dialysis in ARF?**

Intractable acidosis, intractable hyperkalemia, intractable volume overload, BUN over 80 to 100, encephalopathy, pericarditis, uremic bleeding, and certain intoxications.

○ **At what GFR will patients with CRF due to diabetes need to start dialysis?**

Dialysis usually begun at GFR of 10 to 15 mL/min.

○ **Sudden ARF, seen after initiation of ACE inhibitors, should prompt a work-up for what diseases?**

ACE inhibitors are likely to cause ARF in patients with bilateral renal artery stenosis or renal artery stenosis in a solitary kidney.

○ **What type of ARF is usually seen with rhabdomyolysis?**

Acute tubular necrosis.

○ **What pathology is usually seen in patients with CRF, nephrotic syndrome, and AIDS?**

Usually focal segmental glomerulosclerosis is seen at biopsy.

○ **What type of acute renal failure is seen in a patient with systemic lupus erythematosus (SLE)?**

SLE with diffuse proliferative GN is likely to cause renal failure, nephrotic syndrome, hematuria, and cylindruria. This may be treated with steroids and pulse IV cyclophosphamide.

○ **What is the most common cause of intrinsic renal failure?**

Acute tubular necrosis.

○ **What four clinical findings are indicative of acute glomerulonephritis (GM)?**

1. Oliguria
2. Hypertension
3. Pulmonary edema
4. Urine sediment containing RBCs, WBCs, protein, and RBC casts

○ **What is the most common cause of postinfectious glomerulonephritis?**

Poststreptococcal group A β-hemolytic. However, other infections may also produce GN-related infections. GN is caused by an immune complex deposition in glomeruli. Most patients recover renal function spontaneously within a few weeks.

○ **What syndrome is characterized by a rapidly progressive, antiglomerular basement membrane antibody-induced GN that is preceded by pulmonary hemorrhage and hemoptysis?**

Goodpasture syndrome.

○ **A urinalysis reveals RBC casts and dysmorphic RBCs. What is the probable origin of hematuria?**

Glomerulus.

○ **What is the most common cause of proteinuria?**

Pathology of the glomerulus. Other causes include tubular pathology or overproduction of protein.

○ **What is the classic presentation of poststreptococcal glomerulonephritis (PSGN)?**

Sudden development of gross hematuria, hypertension, edema, and renal insufficiency following a throat or skin infection with group A β-hemolytic streptococcus. Patients frequently also have generalized complaints of fever, malaise, lethargy, abdominal pain, etc.

○ **What signs and symptoms are prevalent with poststreptococcal glomerulonephritis?**

Facial edema and decreased urinary output. Urine may be dark. Other laboratory results include normochromic anemia because of hemodilution, increased sedimentation rate, numerous RBCs and WBCs in the urine with casts, and hyperkalemia. Hospitalization is advised.

○ **How early in the development of "strep throat" will antibiotic therapy decrease the risk for PSGN?**

Antibiotics have not been found to decrease the risk for PSGN.

○ **What laboratory test best confirms PSGN as the diagnosis?**

Anti-DNAse B antibody titer.

○ **What is the most common form of lupus nephritis?**

Diffuse proliferative nephritis (WHO class IV). Unfortunately, this is also the most severe form.

○ **The biopsy of the kidney from a 24-year-old male patient with nephrotic syndrome shows increased mesangial cells and, on immunofluorescence, C3 deposits in the mesangium. What is the man's diagnosis and prognosis?**

This man has membranoproliferative glomerulonephritis (a type of chronic glomerulonephritis). Prognosis is poor, with many patients progressing to end-stage renal failure.

○ **What findings mark the presentation of a patient with rapidly progressive glomerulonephritis?**

Hematuria (most common), edema (periorbital), HTN, ascites, pleural effusion, rales, and anuria.

○ **The laboratory reports from a patient with hematuria show depressed levels of C3. What etiologies should you suspect?**

Chronic infection, lupus, poststreptococcal glomerulonephritis, or membranoproliferative glomerulonephritis.

○ **What is the most common cause of nephrotic syndrome in children? In adults?**

Children: Minimal change disease.
Adults: Idiopathic glomerulonephritis.

○ **What is the diagnostic triad of the nephrotic syndrome?**

Edema, hyperlipidemia, and proteinuria with hypoproteinemia.

○ **What is the main goal of treatment in nephrotic syndrome?**

Treat the underlying cause of the syndrome. In most cases, treating hypertension and fluid overload is paramount. Some patients may require strict sodium and fluid restrictions as well as diuretics, and some patients may require dialysis.

○ **Name some risk factors for developing polycystic kidney disease:**

Younger age of onset for kidney disease, black race, male gender, hypertension, and a presence of polycystin-1 gene.

○ **What is the best testing method to detect polycystic kidney disease?**

Renal ultrasound for patients older than 30 years, and CT or MRI for patients younger than 30 years.

○ **What are some extrarenal manifestations of polycystic renal disease?**

Cerebral hemorrhages, including subarachnoid, saccular aneurysms, aortic and root dilatation, as well as mitral valve prolapse and aortic regurgitation. These are mainly due to the abnormalities of collagen.

● ● ● ELECTROLYTE AND ACID/BASE DISORDERS ● ● ●

○ **What are the two main reasons for hyponatremia?**

Either an increase in intracellular volume and water gain, or due to a primary sodium loss.

○ **What is the most common drug that can induce hyponatremia?**

Thiazide diuretics.

○ **Name three medical conditions that can commonly cause hyponatremia to occur:**

1. Congestive heart failure
2. Cirrhosis of the liver
3. Nephrotic syndrome

○ **What disorder causes hyponatremia, normovolemia, and has a large release of arginine vasopressin (AVP) in the setting of increased water intake?**

Syndrome of inappropriate antidiuretic hormone (SIADH). Some of the causes for this are neuropsychiatric, malignant tumors, surgery, and some medications.

○ **What is *beer potomania*?**

These are patients who drink excessive amounts of beer and have poor protein intake in their diet, which results in an overload of volume, thus causing hyponatremia.

○ **What are the two main goals in the treatment of hyponatremia?**

1. Water restriction to lower the overall water volume.
2. Treatment of the underlying cause of the hyponatremia.

○ **A 93-year-old female patient is admitted for severe malnutrition and hyponatremia with a serum level of 121 mmol/L. She has mental status changes that are related to the hyponatremic state. What is the main therapy for this severely ill patient?**

Patients with severe hyponatremia and neurological symptoms on examination require hypertonic solution to be infused so that the serum concentration is raised to 1 to 2 mmol/L for the first 3 to 4 hours and then to 12 mmol/L for the first 24 hours total.

○ **What is the risk of treating hyponatremia too fast?**

You can create osmotic demyelination syndrome, which will cause paralysis, dysarthria, and dysphagia.

○ **What is the single biggest factor for a patient with hypernatremia?**

Loss of overall water in the body.

○ **What are some causes for hypernatremia?**

Varying degrees of hyperosmolality with a mild thirst response. In other situations, deprivation of water, infants, physically handicapped, and mentally impaired patients are at risk of not getting adequate water intake.

Nonrenal etiologies for hypernatremia include diarrhea, insensible losses through the skin and respiratory tract (fevers, burns, infections).

○ **What is the most common reason for hypernatremia?**

Drug-induced osmotic diuresis, or diabetes insipidus.

○ **Name physical examination features that can be present in a patient with hypernatremia:**

Contracted volume with hypotension, dry mucous membranes, and neurological symptoms of altered mental status, weakness, irritability, focal deficits, coma, and seizures.

○ **What is the main goal of treatment of hypernatremia?**

First determine the cause of the reason behind the electrolyte imbalance, and then prevent further damage.

○ **What is the safest and most effective corrective treatment of hypernatremia?**

Water by mouth or nasogastric (NG) tube placement.

○ **How would geophagia (eating clay) affect an individual's electrolyte?**

It will cause hypokalemia because the clay will bind the potassium. This was a common finding in the African American population in the south, and can still be seen in some populations.

○ **What effect does diabetic ketoacidosis have on potassium?**

It will cause a depletion of potassium by way of the Na^+ K^+-ATPase pump stimulation.

○ **What are some gastrointestinal problems, which can cause hypokalemia?**

Vomiting, diarrhea, excessive loss of laxatives, and volume depletion.

○ **What is the main cause in a patient who suffers from chronic potassium loss?**

Renal-induced potassium wasting.

○ **A 46-year-old female patient is evaluated for hypokalemia and a value of 2.9 mg/dL. She is given potassium supplements and is rechecked a week later only to find that she is still at a low level of 3.0 mg/dL despite taking 40 mEq daily. She is not on any medications. What could be this patient's disorder causing the hypokalemia?**

Primary hyperaldosteronism, which is sometimes caused by a primary tumor of the adrenal gland resulting in hypokalemia. Other possibilities include renal cell carcinoma, ovarian carcinoma, and Wilms tumors in children. These other possibilities are a result of hyperreninemia, which will draw off potassium.

○ **Can Cushing disease present with hypokalemia?**

Yes, and is a result of the elevated glucocorticoid levels, which cause an inactivation of cortisol.

○ **Name some physical examination features in patients with hypokalemia:**

Muscle fatigue, weakness, myalgias, and in more serious cases hypoventilation and paralysis can occur.

○ **What electrophysiological effects can be seen on an EKG in a patient with hypokalemia?**

Flattening of the T-wave, prominent U-wave, and in some cases a prolonged PR interval.

○ **Name some causes of hyperkalemia:**

Renal failure, decreased arterial volume circulation, decreased secretion of potassium by either hypoaldosteronism or enhanced chloride absorption, and drugs such as ACE inhibitors and NSAIDs.

○ **What are some physical symptoms of patients with hyperkalemia?**

Muscle weakness, which can progress to paralysis and respiratory depression (hypoventilation).

○   **What electrophysiological effects can be seen on an EKG in a patient with hyperkalemia?**

Peaked T-wave, prolonged PR interval, and QRS duration. This can eventually lead to ventricular fibrillation or asystole.

○   **A 66-year-old male patient presents to the emergency department with an arrhythmia, which is determined to be a widened QRS complex that has resulted in the patient going in and out of ventricular fibrillation. His potassium on initial evaluation is 7.6 mg/dL and the patient's renal function is intact. What would be the treatment of choice for this life-threatening illness?**

Calcium gluconate.

○   **What is the other treatment for hyperkalemia in a non–life-threatening illness?**

Regular insulin and glucose to draw the potassium into the cells. Another alternative is administration of a thiazide loop diuretic to waste potassium.

○   **What is the fastest and most reliable treatment for hyperkalemia?**

Hemodialysis.

○   **What are some presenting symptoms in patients with mild hypercalcemia? Severe cases?**

In general, most patients are asymptomatic. Some will experience trouble concentrating, depression, and personality changes. Some other symptoms will be nausea, constipation, pancreatitis, and anorexia.

In severe hypercalcemia, the symptoms will be lethargy, coma, and stupor.

○   **What are some primary disorders that can cause hypercalcemia?**

Parathyroid adenomas and hyperplasia of the parathyroid.

○   **What is one factor that could mislead you in a correct diagnosis of hyper- or hypocalcemia?**

Serum albumin levels, which bind to calcium. If this level is either high or low, it can impact the serum levels of calcium.

○   **What is the most common cause of hypercalcemia?**

Primary hyperparathyroidism followed by malignancy.

○   **What is the treatment of choice for hypercalcemia?**

Bisphosphonates.

○   **What are the most common reasons for hypocalcemia?**

Impaired vitamin D production and impaired parathyroid hormone production.

○   **Name some physical examination characteristics in patients with hypocalcemia:**

Paresthesias of the fingers and toes and circumoral regions are some symptoms. Chvostek sign as well as carpal spasm can be present. Severe hypocalcemia can present with seizures, bronchospasm, laryngospasm, and prolonged QT interval on EKG.

○ **What is the treatment for a patient with severe hypocalcemia?**

Calcium gluconate.

○ **For patients with chronic hypocalcemia, what is the long-term management treatment?**

Elemental calcium supplements, 1 to 1.5 g/day.

○ **What are some physical examination characteristics in patients with hypomagnesemia?**

Tetany, weakness, seizures, muscle weakness, ataxia, nystagmus, vertigo, depression, irritability, delirium, and psychosis.

○ **What are some EKG findings in patients with hypomagnesemia?**

Prolonged PR or QT intervals and flattening of T waves. Digitalis toxicity may be enhanced with low magnesium levels.

○ **What is the most common cause of hypermagnesemia in a patient with renal failure?**

Patient use of compounds high in magnesium, such as antacids. This can result in neuromuscular paralysis.

Consider IV calcium. Saline and furosemide-assisted diuresis may not help a patient with renal failure, so consider dialysis as well.

○ **What are some common causes of increased anion gap?**

Aspirin, methanol, uremia, diabetes, idiopathic (lactic), ethylene glycol, and alcohol are all reasonably common.

Numerous etiologies may produce the entity above-listed demurely as "lactic." Lactic acidosis may be the result of shock, seizures, acute hypoxemia, INH, cyanide, ritodrine, inhaled acetylene and carbon monoxide, and ethanol. Sodium nitroprusside, povidone-iodine ointment, sorbitol, and xylitol can induce an anion gap acidosis.

Other causes of anion gap acidosis include toluene intoxication, iron intoxication, sulfuric acidosis, short bowel syndrome (D-lactic acidosis), formaldehyde, nalidixic acid, methenamine, and rhubarb (oxalic acid). Inborn errors of metabolism, such as methylmalonic acidemia and isovaleric acidemia, may also elicit a gap acidosis response.

Recall some pearls for sorting out the differential diagnosis:

1. Methanol—Visual disturbances and headache are common. May produce wide gaps because each 2.6 mg/dL of methanol contributes 1 mOsm/L to gap. Compare this with alcohol: each 4.3 mg/dL adds 1 mOsm/L to gap.
2. Uremia—Must be quite advanced before it causes an anion gap.
3. Diabetic ketoacidosis—Both hyperglycemia and glucosuria typically occur. Alcoholic ketoacidosis (AKA) is often associated with low blood sugar and mild or absent glucosuria.
4. Salicylates—High levels contribute to gap.
5. Lactic acidosis—Check serum level. This condition also has broad differential, as cited above.
6. Ethylene glycol—Also causes calcium oxalate or hippurate crystals in urine. Each 5.0 mg/dL contributes 1 mOsm/L to gap.

○ **What are the major physiologic causes of metabolic acidosis?**

Increases in endogenous acids (lactate and ketoacids), loss of bicarbonate, and accumulation of endogenous acids (renal failure).

○   **What is the treatment of metabolic acidosis with a pH <7.20?**

Sodium bicarbonate IV.

○   **What are the three major conditions of metabolic acidosis?**

1. Lactic acidosis
2. Diabetic ketoacidosis (DKA)
3. Alcoholic ketoacidosis

○   **Name some drugs and toxins that can cause metabolic acidosis:**

- Salicylates
- Alcohols
- Ethylene glycol
- Methanol
- Isopropyl alcohol.

○   **Name some causes for a patient to have metabolic alkalosis:**

Exogenous bicarbonate loads such as alkali ingestion, extracellular volume contraction, and potassium deficiency such as GI (vomiting, aspiration), renal disorders (diuretics, lactic acidosis recovery), hypercalcemia, drugs (PCNs), magnesium deficiency, potassium deficiency, and high and low renin volume expansion disorders (renal artery stenosis, accelerated hypertension, licorice ingestion).

○   **What is the expected change in serum bicarbonate in chronic respiratory acidosis or alkalosis?**

Bicarbonate increases by approximately 3 mEq/L for each 10 mm Hg increase in $Paco_2$ in chronic respiratory acidosis. Bicarbonate decreases by 4 to 5 mEq/L for each 10 mm Hg decrease in $Paco_2$ in chronic respiratory alkalosis.

○   **A 45-year-old obese man presents with dyspnea, peripheral edema, snoring, and excessive daytime sleepiness. A room air arterial blood gas in drawn and the pH is 7.34, $Paco_2$ 60 mm Hg, the PaO_2 is 58 mm Hg, and the calculated HCO_3^- is 28 mEq/L. What is the acid–base disturbance?**

Chronic, compensated respiratory acidosis. If this was acute respiratory acidosis, the pH would be 7.24 with a normal HCO_3^-.

○   **What are some common causes of respiratory alkalosis?**

Respiratory alkalosis is defined as a pH above 7.45 and a Pco_2 less than 35. Common causes of respiratory alkalosis include any process that may induce hyperventilation: shock, sepsis, trauma, asthma, CVA, PE, anemia, hepatic failure, heat stroke, exhaustion, emotion, pregnancy, salicylate poisoning, hypoxemia, pregnancy, and inadequate mechanical ventilation.

○   **What is respiratory alkalosis?**

A pH above 7.45 and a Pco_2 less than 35. Alkalosis shifts the O_2 disassociation curve to the left. It also causes cerebrovascular constriction. The kidneys compensate for respiratory alkalosis by excreting HCO_3^-.

○ **What are some causes of respiratory acidosis?**

Respiratory acidosis is defined as a pH of 7.35 or less and a P_{CO_2} of 35. Common causes of respiratory acidosis include drugs, CVA, infection, asthma, lung disease such as emphysema, bronchitis, ARDS, neurologic disorders such as poliomyelitis, myasthenia, and muscular dystrophy. Obesity, kyphoscoliosis, and hypoventilation are other etiologies.

○ **What are some reasons for volume contraction?**

Vomiting, diarrhea, nasogastric suctioning, diuretics, hyperaldosteronism, and diabetes insipidus.

○ **Name some etiologies that have hypovolemia with normal extracellular or expanded volume:**

Decreased cardiac output by myocardial or valvular disease, low albumin (cirrhosis, nephrotic syndrome), acute pancreatitis, ischemic bowel, rhabdomyolysis, and sepsis.

○ **How is renal tubular acidosis (RTA) classified?**

RTA is classified into one of three types: type 1 (distal RTA), type II (proximal RTA), or type IV (mineralocorticoid deficiency). There is no type III.

○ **What are the mechanisms for the different types of RTA?**

In type I, there is a deficiency in the secretion of the hydrogen ion by the distal tubule and collecting duct. In type II, there is a decrease in the bicarbonate reabsorption in the proximal tubule. For type IV (most common type), there is aldosterone deficiency, which leads to impairment of sodium reabsorption as well as potassium and hydrogen excretion.

○ **Which isolated form of RTA will be most likely to lead to renal failure?**

Distal (type I), though most cases of type I RTA have an excellent prognosis.

○ **What type of RTA usually presents as an isolated condition?**

Type I (distal RTA).

○ **What are the characteristic acid–base electrolyte abnormalities associated with type I and type II RTA?**

Hypokalemic, hyperchloremic metabolic acidosis.

○ **What are the characteristic acid–base/electrolyte abnormalities associated with type IV RTA?**

Hyperkalemic, hyperchloremic metabolic acidosis.

○ **What is the underlying cause of type IV RTA?**

Decreased sodium reabsorption secondary to lack of aldosterone effect.

○ **What diseases are associated with type IV RTA?**

Diseases of the adrenal gland; most commonly Addison disease and congenital adrenal hyperplasia.

○ **What treatments are used to ameliorate bleeding in a uremic patient?**

Dialysis may lessen bleeding as may DDAVP, cryoprecipitate, or even platelet transfusions. Estrogens may lessen bleeding from angiodysplasia.

○ **What medications are likely to cause acute renal failure with interstitial nephritis?**

Beta-lactam antibiotics, cimetidine, NSAIDs, Dilantin, rifampin are but a few.

○ **What medications may be associated with hemolytic uremic syndrome?**

Mitomycin, estrogens, and cyclosporin are known culprits.

○ **What comorbid factors are likely to increase the risk of contrast-induced ATN?**

Azotemia, diabetic nephropathy, CHF, multiple myeloma, and dehydration.

○ **What are some common causes of prerenal acute renal failure?**

Volume depletion and decreased effective volume (CHF, sepsis, cirrhosis).

○ **What are the causes of postrenal failure?**

Ureteral and urethral obstruction.

○ **What arrhythmia is frequently encountered during renal dialysis?**

Hypokalemia-induced ventricular fibrillation.

○ **What are some causes of false-positive hematuria?**

Food coloring, beets, paprika, rifampin, phenothiazine, Dilantin, myoglobin, or menstruation.

○ **Name some common nephrotoxic agents:**

Aminoglycosides, NSAIDs, contrast dye, and myoglobin.

○ **What is the definition of oliguria? Of anuria?**

Oliguria: Urine output < 500 mL/day
Anuria: Urine output < 100 mL/day

○ **What is the initial treatment for priapism?**

Terbutaline, 0.25 to 0.5 mg subcutaneously.

○ **If a urine dipstick is positive for blood, but a urine analysis is negative for RBCs, what is the probable disease?**

Rhabdomyolysis. Severe muscle damage can result in free myoglobin in the blood. Very high levels can lead to acute renal failure.

○ **What is the most common manifestation of Goodpasture disease?**

Hemoptysis. These patients usually develop pulmonary hemorrhage before any signs of renal failure develop.

○ **What two common medications can induce nephrogenic diabetes insipidus?**

Lithium and amphotericin B.

○ **A patient with nephrogenic diabetes insipidus has a serum sodium level of 117 mEq/L. How do you determine how much NaCl to administer to keep the risk of cerebral edema at a minimum?**

Amount of NaCl to add in mEq/L = 0.6 × wt (in kg) × (140 − serum sodium).

○ **What percentage of kidney transplants donated from a relative (usually a parent) are still functional after 3 years?**

75% to 80%.

○ **Patients born with what disease are more likely to have horseshoe kidneys?**

Turner syndrome.

○ **What is the antihypertensive of choice in patient with chronic diabetic nephropathy?**

Angiotensin-converting enzyme inhibitors are preferred.

○ **What is the major therapy used to treat allergic interstitial nephritis not responding to discontinuation of the culprit medication?**

Corticosteroids.

○ **Chronic renal failure with hypertension, small shrunken kidneys, and gout at an early age should suggest what?**

Lead nephropathy should be considered.

○ **What is the most common anatomical abnormality associated with chronic urinary tract infections?**

Vesicoureteral reflux.

○ **What factors predispose one to acute papillary necrosis?**

Analgesic abuse, sickle cell disease, diabetes mellitus, and alcoholism are usual predisposing factors.

○ **What major renal toxicity is seen with amphotericin B?**

Tubulointerstitial disease with a distal hypokalemic renal tubular acidosis and hypomagnesemia.

○ **Acute renal failure seen after use of cocaine may be due to what?**

Rhabdomyolysis leading to ATN.

○ **What causes priapism?**

Prolonged sex, leukemia, sickle cell trait and disease, blood dyscrasias, pelvic hematoma or neoplasm, syphilis, urethritis, and drugs including phenothiazine, prazosin, tolbutamide, anticoagulants, and corticosteroids.

○ **What medication is the best treatment for preventing nephropathy in diabetic patients?**

ACE inhibitors. They are found to reduce endpoint renal disease, dialysis, and transplantation by 50%.

● ● ● REFERENCES ● ● ●

Brunicardi FC, Anderson DK, Billiar TR, et al. *Schwartz's Principles of Surgery.* 8th ed. New York, NY: McGraw-Hill; 2005.

Fauci Anthony S., B. E. (2008, 7 1). Harrisons Online. New York, NY.

McPhee SJ, Papadakis MA, eds. *Current Medical Diagnosis and Treatment 2009.* New York, NY: McGraw-Hill; 2009.

McPhee SJ, Ganong WF. *Pathophysiology of Disease: An Introduction to Clinical Medicine.* 5th ed. New York, NY: McGraw-Hill; 2006.

Tanagho E, McAninch JW *Smith's General Urology.* 17th ed. New York, NY: McGraw-Hill; 2008.

CHAPTER 8 **Reproductive**

Jacqueline Jordan Spiegel, MS, PA-C

● ● ● **REPRODUCTIVE PHYSIOLOGY** ● ● ●

○ **What are the three events that occur in the normal course of female puberty (in order of occurrence and with definition of each)?**

1. Thelarche—the development of breasts

2. Pubarche—the development of axillary and pubic hair

3. Menarche—the first menstrual cycle

○ **What is the classification system commonly used to define the progression of breast and pubic hair development in puberty, and How many stages does the system have?**

Tanner classification. There are five stages.

○ **Define the normal menstrual cycle:**

The normal menstrual cycle is 28 days, with a flow lasting 2 to 7 days. The variation in cycle length is set at 24 to 35 days.

○ **In a normal menstrual cycle, when does ovulation typically occur?**

Ovulation in a 28-day cycle typically occurs on day 14. The luteal (secretory) phase of the cycle is normally 14 days long. The estrogenic (proliferative) phase of the cycle can be variable (typically 14–16 days).

○ **What are the hormones, and their source, that are involved in maintaining a normal menstrual cycle?**

From the ovary: Estrogen and progesterone.

From the pituitary: Follicle-stimulating hormone (FSH) and luteinizing hormone (LH). In addition, prolactin- and thyroid-stimulating hormone are also vital in maintaining a normal menstrual cycle.

From the hypothalamus: Gonadotropin-releasing hormone (GnRH).

○ **Describe the effect of estrogen on the endometrium:**

Estrogen causes growth of the endometrium. The endometrial glands lengthen and the glandular epithelium becomes pseudostratified. Mitotic activity is present in both the glands and the stroma.

○ **When does implantation of the fertilized ovum typically occur?**

At approximately 9 days following ovulation (day 23).

○ **What is the lifespan of a normal corpus luteum in the absence of pregnancy?**

Approximately 14 days.

○ **What is the action of oxytocin?**

It stimulates uterine contractions during labor and elicits milk ejection by myoepithelial cells of the mammary ducts.

○ **What is the function of FSH?**

It stimulates maturation of the follicle(s) and the production of estradiol from the follicles.

○ **What is the function of LH?**

It causes follicular rupture, ovulation, and establishment of the corpus luteum.

○ **During the luteal phase of the ovary, describe the corresponding phase of the uterus:**

The secretory phase. After ovulation, the expelled follicle is called the corpus luteum. The corpus luteum secretes estradiol and progesterone, which cause secretory ducts to develop in the endometrial lining.

○ **What does a biphasic curve on a basal body temperature (BBT) chart of a 25-year-old woman indicate?**

Normal ovulation and the effect of progesterone. A monophasic BBT curve indicates an anovulatory cycle. A temperature that remained elevated following a normal biphasic curve would indicate pregnancy.

○ **What is the cause of midcycle spotting or light bleeding?**

The decline in estradiol that occurs immediately prior to the LH surge.

○ **Decline in which hormone heralds the onset of menses?**

Normal menses occurs because of progesterone withdrawal.

○ **What is the function of prolactin?**

It initiates and sustains lactation by the breast glands and it may influence synthesis and release of progesterone by the ovary and testosterone by the testis.

○ **What is the main physiological stimulus for prolactin release?**

Suckling of the breast.

○ **What is oxytocin?**

Oxytocin is a decapeptide synthesized by the posterior pituitary gland. It is a powerful uterotonic agent causing the uterus to contract. In nature, it is secreted in pulsatile fashion throughout labor. (The fetus also produces oxytocin and at least some traverses the placenta, escaping enzymatic breakdown.)

○ **What is the definition of Mittelschmerz?**

The cyclic abdominal pain located on either side of the abdomen, which can be felt during ovulation and may persist for approximately 2 days after.

○ **What is the squamocolumnar junction? Describe its importance and how it changes.**

It is the junction between the columnar epithelium and the squamous epithelium of the cervix. This is also known as the transformation zone. Throughout a woman's life, the squamous epithelium of the ectocervix (and vagina) invades the columnar epithelium of the endocervix. It is important because it is the squamous epithelium in this transformation zone that is most likely to become dysplastic.

○ **What pelvic type is the most common in women?**

Gynecoid. It is estimated that approximately 50% of women have gynecoid pelvis. (It should be noted that in reality most women have intermediate pelvic shapes rather than true gynecoid, anthropoid, android, or platypelloid).

• • • UTERUS • • •

○ **What percentage of the female population has endometriosis?**

More than 15%, and 7% of these women have it during their reproductive years.

○ **What is thought to be the most common etiology for endometriosis?**

Retrograde menstruation.

○ **What are chocolate cysts?**

Endometriomas (cystic forms of endometriosis on the ovary).

○ **What percentage of women with endometriosis also have infertility?**

25% to 50%.

○ **Where is the most common site of endometriosis?**

The ovaries (60%). Other sites include the cul-de-sac, uterosacral ligaments, broad ligaments, fallopian tubes, uterovesical fold, round ligaments, vermiform appendix, vagina, rectosigmoid colon, cecum, and ileum.

○ **What is considered the preferred means of establishing a diagnosis of endometriosis?**

Direct visualization during diagnostic laparoscopy or laparotomy. Clinical presentation, laboratory evaluation, and/or pelvic ultrasound are considered inadequate to make a definitive diagnosis.

○ **What are the pharmacotherapeutic options for treating endometriosis?**

Combined oral contraceptive agents, Progestin-only contraceptives, GnRH agonists, danazol (a 17-alpha-ethinyl testosterone derivative).

○ **What are common side effects of danazol (Danocrine)?**

Hirsutism, amenorrhea, deepening of the voice, acne, weight gain, hot flashes, labile emotions, and decreased vaginal lubrications.

○ **A 66-year-old postmenopausal woman presents with vaginal bleeding. What is the provisional diagnosis (top on list of differentials)?**

Endometrial cancer; 15% of women with postmenopausal bleeding have endometrial cancer.

○ **What are the most common etiologies of endometrial cancer?**

30% of these tumors are due to exogenous estrogens, 30% are due to atrophic endometriosis or vaginitis, 10% are due to cervical polyps, and 5% are due to endometrial hyperplasia.

○ **What are the risk factors for endometrial cancer?**

Nulliparity, early menarche, late menopause, significant amounts of unopposed estrogen, and prior ovarian, endometrial, or breast cancer.

○ **Describe the initial office evaluation of a woman whose history is suspicious for endometrial cancer:**

Pelvic examination, Pap smear, biopsy of any abnormal cervical or vaginal lesion, and endometrial biopsy.

○ **What percentage of women with endometrial cancer will have an abnormal Papanicolaou smear?**

Approximately 50%.

○ **What is the most common clinical condition associated with the development of endometrial hyperplasia?**

Polycystic ovary syndrome.

○ **What is Lynch syndrome type II?**

A hereditary predisposition to the development of colon, breast, ovarian, and endometrial cancer.

○ **What is the most common type of benign gynecologic pelvic neoplasm?**

Uterine leiomyomas (or uterine fibroids).

○ **What type of leiomyoma is symptomatic?**

Submucosal myomas, though small, can cause profuse bleeding, potentially requiring a hysterectomy. Most other myomas are asymptomatic until grown large enough to cause obstruction or significantly distort the endometrial cavity.

○ **What is the difference between leiomyoma and leiomyosarcoma?**

Uterine leiomyoma (aka uterine fibroids) are benign growths that arise from the uterine muscle and are seen in reproductive-aged patients typically presenting with menorrhagia and secondary dysmenorrhea. Leiomyosarcomas are a rare cancer of the uterine muscle wall and are seen in postmenopausal-aged patients typically presenting with postmenopausal vaginal bleeding and rapidly enlarging uterus.

○ **What are the indications for performing a dilation and curettage?**
- Removal of endometrial polyp or hydatid mole
- Termination of pregnancy/incomplete abortion
- Removal of retained placental tissue
- Relief of profuse uterine hemorrhage

○   **What major complication is associated with the performance of a dilation and curettage?**

Perforation of the uterus.

○   **A woman presenting with pelvic pain and pressure when standing, the feeling of something protruding from the vaginal opening, and possible urinary incontinence or constipation is likely to have what?**

Pelvic organ prolapse.

○   **Define the following: cystocele, rectocele, uterine prolapse, and vaginal prolapse:**

- Cystocele is the downward displacement of the bladder into the vagina along the anterior wall and is usually associated with childbirth (e.g., delivery of a large baby, multiple deliveries, prolonged labor).
- Rectocele represents the displacement of the rectum into the posterior wall of the vagina and is also typically associated with multiparous women with history of long end-stage labor. There also maybe a link to those women who undergo midline episiotomy.
- Uterine prolapse is the descent of the uterus and cervix down the vaginal canal toward the introitus secondary to broken uterosacral ligaments or relaxation of the musculature of the pelvic floor. This is more likely to occur in women with a retroverted uterus.
- Vaginal prolapse is the downward displacement of the vaginal apex also due to loss of muscle and ligamental support and it typically follows a hysterectomy.

○   **Define total vs. subtotal, vaginal vs. abdominal, and simple vs. radical hysterectomy:**

- "Total" or "subtotal" are used to denote whether the cervix is removed or retained. Total hysterectomy includes removal of the entire uterus and cervix. Subtotal hysterectomy includes uterus removal while the cervix remains intact.
- "Vaginal" or "abdominal" are used to specify the route of removal. Abdominal hysterectomy can be further clarified as either a laparoscopic or cesarean (open) approach.
- "Simple" or "radical" are used to denote whether vaginal tissue and pelvic lymph nodes are removed. Radical hysterectomy includes the removal of uterus, cervix, vaginal, and pelvic lymph nodes. Determining simple or radical depends on the condition being treated surgically.
- Oophorectomy denotes the removal of the ovaries and is separate from hysterectomy. Oophorectomy can be unilateral or bilateral.

○   **What are the indications for cesarean hysterectomy?**

Most common include severe, life-threatening intrauterine infection, an unrepairable uterine scar, laceration of major uterine vessels, uterine atony (which is unresponsive to medical or therapeutic intervention), large leiomyomata, severe cervical dysplasia or early cervical cancer, and placenta accreta.

Uterine rupture and uterine inversion may also require hysterectomy.

○   **What is the most frequent complication of hysterectomy?**

Infection. The most common organisms are those found in normal vaginal flora. Because the vagina is difficult to cleanse, most experts recommend antibiotic prophylaxis for all patients undergoing vaginal hysterectomy.

○   **What must be identified and located prior to clamping the infundibulopelvic ligament?**

The ureter.

● ● ● OVARY ● ● ●

○   **What is the most common cause of pelvic pain in an adolescent woman?**

Ovarian cysts.

○   **What is the most common type of ovarian cyst?**

Follicular. The other types are corpus luteum and theca lutein cysts.

○   **What is the recommended treatment for uncomplicated follicular cysts?**

Most resolve spontaneously within a few menstrual cycles (60 days) without treatment. Combined oral contraceptive agents can be used if recurrent.

○   **What is the most common complication of ovarian cysts?**

Torsion of the ovary. Torsion is more common in small- to medium-sized cysts and tumors. Emergency surgery is required.

○   **By how much is the incidence of functional cysts reduced by OCP use?**

80% to 90%. Oral contraceptives suppress FSH and LH ovarian stimulation.

○   **What is Halban syndrome?**

This is the persistence of a corpus luteum. Patients commonly present with delayed menses, pelvic mass, and negative pregnancy test. Clinically, this is often confused with an ectopic pregnancy

○   **What are the clinical manifestations of polycystic ovarian disease (PCO)? Explain using the mnemonic OVARIAN:**

Obesity

Virilization

Anovulation

Resistance to insulin (diabetes)

Increased hair

Androgen increase

No period/**Amenorrhea**

○   **Is the Stein-Leventhal syndrome a unilateral or bilateral phenomenon?**

Bilateral. Both ovaries are cystic and enlarged with a thickened and fibrosed tunica. Patients are often infertile, obese, and hirsute. This syndrome is a subtype of polycystic ovarian disease.

○   **What laboratory findings are seen in PCO?**

Most patients have increased LH-to-FSH ratio at 2:1 (or more), high fasting insulin and elevated serum glucose, and elevated sex androgens including DHEA-sulfate and/or testosterone.

○ **How are patients with PCO treated?**

Weight loss is the first-line treatment for PCO. In addition, combined oral contraceptive pills for menstrual regulation and ovarian suppression; Biguanides (metformin) for menstrual regulation, weight reduction, and to reestablish fertility; anti-androgen (spironolactone) for sex androgen suppression and hirsutism.

○ **What serum marker is associated with ovarian cancer?**

CA-125.

○ **If a woman has ascites, what is the most likely tumor to be found?**

An ovarian carcinoma.

○ **What is Meigs syndrome?**

Ascites and hydrothorax in the presence of an ovarian tumor.

○ **What is the treatment for stage 1A or 1B ovarian cancer?**

Surgical excision alone (abdominal hysterectomy and bilateral salpingo-oophorectomy).

○ **What is the treatment for all other stages of ovarian cancer besides stage 1A or 1B?**

Surgical resection followed by adjuvant chemotherapy or radiation.

○ **What are considered protective factors for the risk of ovarian cancer?**

Multiparity, combined oral contraceptive use, and breast-feeding.

● ● ● **CERVIX** ● ● ●

○ **What is a nabothian cyst?**

A mucous inclusion cyst of the cervix (usually asymptomatic and benign).

○ **What are the American College of Obstetrics and Gynecology (2003) recommendations for Pap smear screening?**

Pap smears should be initiated 3 years following the onset of sexual activity or age 21 (whichever comes first). Annually with conventional slide cytology or every 2 years with liquid-based cytology.

After the age of 30 years, women with three consecutively normal readings may be screened every 2 to 3 years. If the patient is at high risk despite age, continue annual screening.

No cytology screening after total hysterectomy if surgery for benign condition. If surgery for CIN I, II, or III, then annually three times before discontinuing.

○ **According to the American Cancer Society (2002) recommendations, at what age can routine Pap smears be discontinued in a woman with an intact cervix?**

Age 70, if the patient has had three consecutive normal readings.

○   **What is the recommendation for HPV testing in women?**

HPV testing should occur at the time of Pap screening in any high-risk patient or in reflex following an abnormal Pap smear.

○   **What do ASC-US, LSIL, HSIL on a Pap screening pathology report represent?**

ASC-US: atypical squamous cells of undetermined significance
LSIL: low-grade squamous intraepithelial lesion, i.e., mild dysplasia, CIN I
HSIL: high-grade squamous intraepithelial lesion, i.e., moderate to severe dysplasia, CIN II-III, carcinoma in situ

○   **What is the recommended further evaluation in a woman with ASC-US Pap result and HPV positive?**

Colposcopy.

○   **How many times more likely is a woman with condyloma acuminatum (genital warts) to develop cervical cancer than a woman without this lesion?**

4 times more likely. These women should have yearly Pap smear and be screened for other sexually transmitted infections.

○   **What are the known subtypes of HPV associated with cervical cancer?**

HPV types 16, 18, and 31 are risk factors for cervical dysplasia, which can lead to cervical cancer.

○   **What are the risk factors for carcinoma of the cervix?**

Multiple sexual partners, early age at first intercourse, early first pregnancy, and HPV positive.

○   **What is the most common type of cervical cancer?**

80% are squamous cell and arise from the squamocolumnar junction of the cervix.

○   **What is the most common presenting symptom for patients with cervical cancer?**

Up to 80% of patients present with abnormal vaginal bleeding, most commonly postmenopausal. Only 10% note postcoital bleeding. Less frequent symptoms include vaginal discharge and pain.

○   **What clinical triad is strongly indicative of cervical cancer extension to the pelvic wall?**

1. Unilateral leg edema
2. Sciatic pain
3. Ureteral obstruction

○   **A colposcopically directed cervical biopsy from a 25-year-old G0P0 reveals a small focus of invasive squamous cell carcinoma. What is the next step in this patient's management?**

Cervical cone biopsy to establish the full extent of invasion.

○   **When performing a radical hysterectomy for cervical cancer, is it required to perform an oophorectomy too?**

No. Early cervical cancer rarely spreads to the ovaries.

○ **What are the advantages of radical hysterectomy relative to radiation therapy for stage I cervical cancer?**

- Ovarian preservation is possible
- Unimpaired vaginal function
- Extent of disease can be established

• • • VAGINA/VULVA • • •

○ **What is the normal pH of the vagina?**

3.8 to 4.4 (a vaginal pH greater than 4.9 indicates a bacterial or protozoal infection).

○ **What is the predominant organism in a healthy woman's vaginal discharge?**

Lactobacilli (95%).

○ **What is the treatment of choice for a Bartholin gland abscess?**

Marsupialization with the placement of a Word catheter. This prevents recurrences.

○ **What is the most common cell type in vulvar and/or vaginal carcinoma?**

Squamous cell (90% in vulvar carcinoma; 85% in vaginal carcinoma).

○ **What is the most common location for vaginal carcinoma?**

Upper one-third of the posterior vaginal wall.

○ **What causes condylomata acuminata (genital warts)?**

Human papilloma virus types 6 and 11.

○ **What other sexually transmitted infection is commonly seen in combination with condylomata acuminata?**

Trichomonas vaginitis.

○ **What are the recommended treatment options for condylomata acuminata (genital warts)?**

Liquid nitrogen, podophyllin resin, Aldara (topical imiquimod); not necessarily curative but treatment is focused on destruction of warts.

○ **What is the most frequent gynecologic disease of children?**

Vulvovaginitis, the cause of which is poor perineal hygiene.

○ **What is the most common cause of vaginitis?**

Candida albicans.

○ **What predisposes a woman to vaginal candidiasis infections?**

Diabetes, oral contraceptives, and antibiotics.

○   **What are the recommended forms of treatment for vaginal candidiasis infections?**

Antifungal drugs commonly used to treat candidiasis are topical clotrimazole (Gyne-Lotrimin), topical tioconazole (Monistat), and oral fluconazole (Diflucan). It has been reported that a one-time dose of fluconazole (Diflucan) is 90% effective in treating a vaginal yeast infection.

In severe infections (generally in hospitalized patients), amphotericin B, caspofungin, or voriconazole may be used.

○   **What are the signs and symptoms typical for gardnerella vaginitis?**

On physical examination, a frothy, grayish white, fishy smelling vaginal discharge is noted.

○   **What would you expect on microscopic evaluation with saline and with 10% KOH on a patient with gardnerella vaginitis?**

"Clue cells," which are epithelial cells with bacilli attached to their surfaces. On saline wet mount adding 10% KOH to the discharge produces a fishy odor.

○   **What is the recommended treatment for gardnerella vaginitis?**

Metronidazole (Flagyl) either orally or vaginally.

○   **When should you avoid treating a woman with Flagyl (orally or vaginally)?**

If she is in her first trimester of pregnancy, metronidazole may have teratogenic effects. Clotrimazole (Gyne-Lotrimin) may be used instead.

○   **A 42-year-old woman complains of painful urination and "leaking a bit" after she urinates. On pelvic examination, you feel a small mass under the urethra that emits a purulent discharge from the urethral meatus if compressed. What is the likely diagnosis?**

Urethral diverticulum.

○   **What is the most common type of urinary fistula?**

Vesicovaginal fistulas. These most commonly occur after surgical procedures, but they can also occur with invasive cervical carcinoma or radiotherapy due to cervical cancer.

○   **A patient presents with pain in her eyes, canker sores in her mouth, and sores and scars in her genital area. What is the diagnosis?**

Behçet disease. This is a rare disease involving ocular inflammation, oral aphthous ulcers, and destructive genital ulcers (generally on the vulva). No cure is known, but remission may occur with high estrogen levels.

○   **What causes toxic shock syndrome (TSS)?**

An exotoxin composed of certain strains of *Staphylococcus aureus*. Other organisms that cause toxic shock syndrome are group A streptococci, *Pseudomonas aeruginosa*, and *Streptococcus pneumoniae*.

○   **What are the known risk factors for the development of toxic shock syndrome (TSS)?**

Tampons, IUDs, septic abortions, sponges, soft tissue abscesses, osteomyelitis, nasal packing, and postpartum infections can all house these organisms.

○ **What dermatological changes occur with TSS?**

Initially, the patient will have a blanching erythematous rash that lasts for 3 days, and 10 days after the start of the infection there will be a full thickness desquamation of the palms and soles.

○ **What criteria are necessary for the diagnosis of TSS?**

All of the following must be present: Temperature > 38.9°C (102°F), rash, systolic BP < 90 mm Hg with orthostasis, and involvement of three organ systems (GI, renal, musculoskeletal, mucosal, hepatic, hematologic, or CNS). The patient must also have negative serologic tests for diseases such as RMSF, hepatitis B, measles, leptospirosis, and VDRL.

○ **How should a patient with TSS be treated?**

Fluids, pressure support, fresh frozen plasma or transfusions, vaginal irrigation with iodine or saline, and antistaphylococcal penicillin or cephalosporin with anti-β-lactamase activity (nafcillin or oxacillin). Rifampin should be considered to eliminate the carrier state.

● ● ● SEXUALLY TRANSMITTED INFECTIONS/PELVIC INFLAMMATORY DISEASE ● ● ●

○ **A 22-year-old patient presents with a complaint of painful blisters on the vulva and vaginal introitus. She admits to a prodrome of burning, tingling, and/or pruritus prior to the appearance of lesions. Upon examination, you note vesicles on an erythematous base. What is the probable diagnosis?**

Herpes simplex virus.

○ **What is the causative bacterium in syphilis?**

Treponema pallidum.

○ **What is the hallmark presenting sign of primary syphilis?**

Painless ulcer (chancre).

○ **What are the presenting signs associated with secondary syphilis?**

Nonpruritus maculopapular rash that includes the palms and soles (Condyloma latum), lymphadenopathy, and constitutional symptoms (fatigue/malaise). These symptoms present 4 to 6 weeks after the hallmark syphilitic chancre and persist for 2 to 6 weeks before the infection enters the latent phase.

○ **What is the presenting feature of tertiary syphilis?**

Neurosyphilis (neuro deficits including difficulty with coordination, memory loss, paralysis, gradual blindness, or dementia).

○ **What is the treatment for syphilis?**

Benzathine PCN G, 2.4 million units IM × 1 dose. Additional doses if infection has been for >1 year or if the patient is pregnant. If the patient is penicillin-allergic, treat with doxycycline.

○   **What causes a greenish gray frothy vaginal discharge with mild itching?**

Trichomonas vaginitis.

○   **What is considered the hallmark pelvic examination finding in 20% of trichomonas infections?**

Petechiae on the cervix (also known as a "strawberry cervix").

○   **What microscopic findings are indicative of trichomonas infections?**

The presence of mobile and pear-shaped protozoa with flagella is indicative of trichomonas.

○   **A 30-year-old woman complains of a <u>painful</u> sore on her vulva that first resembled a pimple. On examination, you find an ulcer with vague borders, gray base, and foul-smelling discharge. What is the probable diagnosis? Causative agent?**

Chancroid. Gram stain, culture, and biopsy (used in combination because of the high false-negative rates) should show the causative agent *Haemophilus ducreyi*.

○   **What is considered the most appropriate treatment for chancroid?**

Ceftriaxone 250 mg IM × 1 dose **or** azithromycin 1g PO × 1 dose.

○   **What is the typical clinical presentation of lymphogranuloma venereum (LGV)? Causative agent?**

Vesicopustular eruption, unilateral inguinal bubo, possible anal discharge, and rectal bleeding. The causative organism is a serotype of *Chlamydia trachomatis*.

○   **What is the most common sexually transmitted infection in the United States and sometimes asymptomatic in women?**

Chlamydia trachomatis.

○   **What finding on Gram stain is indicative of *Neisseria gonorrhea***

Gram-negative diplococci.

○   **What is the treatment for *Neisseria gonorrhea***

Ceftriaxone 125 to 250 mg IM × 1 dose **or** cefixime 400 mg PO × 1 dose **or** cefpodoxime 400 mg PO × 1 dose.

Plus include either azithromycin 1 g × 1 dose **or** doxycycline 100 mg BID × 7 days since 50% of patients are also infected with *Chlamydia trachomatis*.

○   **Which two organisms cause most cases of PID?**

Neisseria gonorrhea and *Chlamydia trachomatis*.

○ **What are the risk factors for pelvic inflammatory disease?**

- Age < 25 years (cervix not fully matured)
- African American race
- Early onset of sexual activity
- Frequent sexual intercourse
- Multiple sexual partners
- Douching
- Presence of IUD
- Women with one episode are at increased risk for a second episode

○ **Why is a woman with pelvic inflammatory disease (PID) likely to have an exacerbation of symptoms when she menstruates?**

The breakdown in cervical mucus, which typically acts as an antibacterial barrier, allows bacteria to ascend from the lower tract to the upper tract. Pelvic examination, intercourse, and exercise can all exacerbate symptoms.

○ **What are the criteria for diagnosis of PID (pelvic inflammatory disease)?**

All of the following must be present:

- Adnexal tenderness
- Cervical and uterine tenderness
- Abdominal tenderness

In addition, one of the following must be present: (1) temperature > 38°C, (2) endocervix Gram stain positive for gram-negative intracellular diplococci, (3) leukocytosis > 10,000/mm^3, (4) inflammatory mass on ultrasound or pelvic examination, or (5) WBCs and bacteria in the peritoneal fluid.

○ **Which patients with PID should be admitted?**

Admit patients who are pregnant, have a temperature > 38°C (100.4°F), are nauseated or vomiting (which prohibits oral antibiotics), have pyosalpinx or tubo-ovarian abscess, have peritoneal signs, have an IUD, show no response to oral antibiotics, or for whom diagnosis is uncertain.

○ **What percent of patients with pelvic inflammatory disease become infertile?**

10%.

• • • **BREAST** • • •

○ **Breast hyperplasia is a normal physiologic phenomenon in the neonatal period. How many months does this typically last?**

Up to 6 months of age.

○ **What are the American Cancer Society's 2003 recommendations for screening mammography?**

Age ≥ 20 years—monthly breast self-examinations

Age 20 to 39 years—MD examination every 3 years

Age ≥ 40 years—annual MD examination and mammogram

For patients with (+) FH or risk factors, screening should begin earlier

○ **According to the American Cancer Society in 2007, what are the recommendations for the use of MRI in breast cancer screening?**

Screening MRI is recommended for women with an approximately 20% to 25% or greater lifetime risk of breast cancer, including women with a strong family history of breast or ovarian cancer (+BRCA mutations) and women who were treated for Hodgkin disease.

○ **After the establishment of fibrocystic breast disease, what is the recommended treatment?**

Breast pain associated with fibrocystic change is best treated by avoiding trauma and by wearing a bra with adequate support. Some find that combined oral contraceptive agents limit the severity of the cyclical changes in the breast tissue. The role of caffeine is controversial. Many patients report relief of symptoms after abstinence from coffee, tea, and chocolate.

○ **What is the most common type of benign breast tumor?**

Fibroadenomas. These are usually solitary, mobile masses with distinct borders. They are more prevalent in women younger than 30 years.

○ **What is the recommended work-up for suspected fibroadenoma?**

Diagnostic mammogram with ultrasound. If indeterminant, fine needle aspiration of the mass with pathology.

○ **What is the most common cause of unilateral bloody nipple discharge?**

Benign intraductal papilloma. Growths usually develop just before or during menopause and they are rarely palpable. They are typically mobile and painless.

○ **What pattern of nipple discharge would one expect with benign galactorrhea?**

Bilateral, induced, clear/white/yellow color.

○ **What diagnosis must be considered in a patient presenting with crusty, eczematous erosion of the nipple without nipple discharge?**

Paget disease. This rare cancer occurs in 3% of breast cancer patients. It involves the excretory ducts of the breast.

○ **What is Peau d'orange?**

French for skin of the orange. It describes the dimpling and thickening of the skin of the breast seen with breast cancer.

○ **A hard mass in the upper outer quadrant of the right breast of a 45-year-old woman is detected. What are the next steps?**

Mammogram followed by an excision biopsy. A negative needle aspiration alone cannot rule out malignancy. False negative rates for fine needle biopsy are 3% to 30%.

○ **What are the risk factors for breast cancer?**

Risk factors include family history, age over 40, high fat intake, nulliparity, early menarche, late menopause, cellular atypia in fibrocystic disease, radiation exposure to breast(s), and prior ovarian, endometrial, or breast cancer.

○ **Is there an increased risk of breast cancer associated with estrogen replacement therapy?**

There may be a slightly increased risk of breast cancer especially with long duration of use (10 or more years).

○ **What are the two genetic markers known to be linked to breast cancer?**

BRCA-1 and BRCA-2.

○ **Geographically, where is breast cancer most common?**

North America and northern Europe have an incidence and mortality rate five times that of most Asian and African countries.

Asians and Africans immigrants to North America or northern Europe maintain a lower rate of incidence; however, their offspring quickly assume a higher one. This points to environmental and dietary factors.

○ **Who have higher incidences of estrogen receptor–positive tumors, premenopausal or postmenopausal women?**

Postmenopausal (60%). If the tumors are both estrogen and progesterone sensitive, then the antiestrogen drug tamoxifen is 80% effective. Otherwise, it is 40% to 50% effective.

○ **What is the most common histologic type of breast cancer?**

Infiltrating ductal carcinoma (70%–80%). Subtypes are colloid, medullary, papillary, and tubular.

○ **What does a high cathepsin D level indicate in a woman with breast cancer?**

A high risk of metastasis.

○ **What is the surgical treatment of choice for breast cancer?**

Modified radical mastectomy: the removal of the breast tissue, pectoralis minor, and axilla. (A radical mastectomy includes the pectoralis major.) For small primary tumors, a partial mastectomy may be performed. This is a local lumpectomy with axillary node dissection and postoperative irradiation of the breast. It has not been shown whether radiation following a modified radical mastectomy affects survival.

○ **What is the most accurate prognostic indicator of breast cancer mortality?**

Axillary node involvement, which is related to the size of the tumor, not the location; 40% to 50% of patients have axillary node involvement when diagnosed.

○ **Are the majority of breast cancers in the ducts or in the lobes?**

Invasive ductal tumors account for 90% of all breast cancers. Only 10% are lobular.

○ **When does breast milk production typically begin?**

Colostrum secretion usually persists for 3 to 4 days after delivery. Day 5 the fluid begins to change in composition. Mature milk is usually present by 1 to 2 weeks postpartum.

○   **How does colostrum differ from breast milk?**

Colostrum is more cellular and has more minerals, but is lower in calories. True milk has more fat and carbohydrate (especially lactose), but less protein.

○   **How many extra calories above baseline does a woman need when breast-feeding?**

About 500 per day.

○   **How much daily dietary of calcium is recommended for lactating women?**

1200 to 1500 mg per day.

○   **Why does lactation not occur during pregnancy even though the prolactin levels are elevated?**

The receptor sites in the breast are competitively bound by estrogen and progesterone, preventing prolactin from activating lactation. When the placenta is delivered, these levels of estrogen and progesterone rapidly drop and the prolactin floods the receptors.

○   **What is the proper postpartum management of a mother who chooses not to breast-feed?**

A firmly fitting (but not binding) bra, ice packs as needed, and decreased stimulation to the nipples such as loose clothes rubbing across the breast or direct contact from a shower.

Pharmacologic suppression including bromocriptine is no longer an indication due to severe maternal side effects and should not be prescribed. The introduction of 35 µg or higher oral contraceptives within 2 weeks of delivery may inhibit lactation in some women and may be of use to decrease the production of milk.

○   **What is likely occurring in a 2-week-old infant who wants to have feed every 1 to 2 hours but nurses only for 5 minutes at a time before falling asleep? What can the mother do to improve this?**

Her infant is not nursing long enough with each episode. The infant is only receiving the "foremilk," which is high in proteins, carbohydrates, and water. The infant falls asleep before getting the "hindmilk," which is high in fat and satiates the appetite plus takes longer to digest.

The infant should be stimulated when he or she dozes off, changed to the opposite breast. If this fails, the mother can pump or express the hindmilk at that time and it can be given by another caregiver later so the mother can rest.

○   **Which vitamin is not found in human breast milk?**

Vitamin K. It is administered to newborns at birth. Formula is also deficient in vitamin K.

○   **How does human milk differ from cow's milk?**

While the two are similar in calories, human milk has more lactose, less protein (and very different protein constitution), and slightly more fat (especially more polyunsaturated fatty acids and cholesterol, which are needed for brain development.) There is significantly more calcium, phosphorous, and iron in bovine milk.

○   **A breast-feeding mother presents to your office complaining of fever, chills, and a swollen red breast. What is the most likely diagnosis and causative organism?**

Mastitis. *Staphylococcus aureus* is the most common cause of mastitis. Mastitis is seldom present in the first week postpartum. It is most often seen 3 to 4 weeks postpartum.

○ **What is the treatment for acute mastitis?**

Warm compresses to breast, analgesics, dicloxacillin, or a cephalosporin.

○ **Can a nursing mother with mastitis continue to nurse?**

Yes, as long as there is no abscess formation. Nursing facilitates the drainage of the infection and the infant will not be harmed because he/she is already colonized.

• • • MENSTRUAL DISORDERS • • •

○ **Define the following: menorrhagia, metrorrhagia, menometrorrhagia, polymenorrhea, and oligomenorrhea:**

Menorrhagia—excessive amount of vaginal bleeding or duration of bleeding during menses

Metrorrhagia—bleeding between menstrual periods

Menometrorrhagia—excessive amount of blood at irregular frequencies

Polymenorrhea—menstrual periods < 21 days apart

Oligomenorrhea—menstrual periods > 35 days apart

○ **What is secondary amenorrhea?**

No menstruation for 6 months or more in a woman who previously had regular menses.

○ **What is the most common cause of secondary amenorrhea?**

Pregnancy. The second most common cause is hypothalamic hypogonadism, which can be due to weight loss, anorexia nervosa, stress, excessive exercise, or hypothalamic disease.

○ **A 27-year-old woman presents with secondary amenorrhea for 6 months. What is the appropriate initial evaluation?**

Pelvic examination, Pap smear, pregnancy test, laboratory studies (prolactin, FSH, LH, TSH), and progestin challenge.

○ **A 26-year-old woman with secondary amenorrhea and an essentially normal work-up is given progestin 10 mg for 7 days (or an IM injection of progesterone 100 mg). She responds with a normal menstrual period. What does this tell you?**

She has a functional endometrium and a normal production of estrogen. Patients producing less than 40 pg/mL of estrogen will not bleed. This test is called the progesterone challenge.

○ **What are the two major differential diagnoses in a patient with secondary amenorrhea who fails a progestin challenge?**

Premature ovarian failure and hypothalamic dysfunction. Premature ovarian failure can be diagnosed if the serum FSH level is high; hypothalamic dysfunction can be diagnosed in setting of low FSH and LH.

○ **List the differential diagnosis of persistent vaginal bleeding in a preadolescent woman:**

Neoplasia, precocious puberty, ureteral prolapse, trauma (including sexual assault), vulvovaginitis, exposure to exogenous estrogen, Shigella infection, group A and β-hemolytic streptococcal infection, and foreign body in vagina.

Foreign body is the most common and presents with bloody, foul smelling discharge.

○   **What blood tests would be appropriate in the evaluation of a female child with precocious puberty?**

Serum levels of FSH, LH, prolactin, TSH, estradiol, testosterone, dehydroepiandrosterone sulfate (DHEAS), and HCG.

○   **In a woman of reproductive age, what is the first step in the evaluation of abnormal uterine bleeding following the history and physical examination?**

A pregnancy test.

○   **What is the recommended treatment for massive intractable dysfunctional uterine bleeding?**

25 mg IV conjugated estrogens.

○   **What are the recommended pharmacotherapeutic interventions for primary dysmenorrhea?**

NSAIDs or combined oral contraceptive agents.

If nonresponsive to the above interventions, tocolytic agents (salbutamol) or calcium channel blockers (nifedipine) or progestins (medroxyprogesterone) have been shown to be effective.

○   **What are the four main etiologies of secondary dysmenorrhea?**

1. Endometriosis
2. Pelvic inflammatory disease
3. Uterine fibroids
4. Pelvic congestion (typically occurs in multiparous women who have pelvic vein varicosities and congested pelvic organs)

○   **A 37-year-old woman, G2 P2 presents with a history of lengthening menses and acquired dysmenorrhea. This problem had been subtly going on for 2 years and now is a quality-of-life issue. Examination reveals a top normal size globular-shaped uterus. What is the most likely diagnosis?**

Adenomyosis.

● ● ● **MENOPAUSE** ● ● ●

○   **What are some causes of premature menopause?**

Smoking, radiation, chemotherapy, and anything else that limits the ovarian blood supply.

○   **What is the median age for menopause?**

51 years.

○   **What is the most common cause of postmenopausal bleeding?**

Atrophic endometrium and/or atrophic vaginitis.

○ **What are the common changes associated with estrogen depletion?**

Menstrual cycle changes, cardiovascular disease, osteoporosis, genitourinary atrophy, vasomotor, and psychological symptoms.

○ **What are the expected changes in gonadotropin levels after menopause?**

FSH increases 10- to 20-fold and LH increases three fold, reaching a maximum 1 to 3 years after menopause. With the lack of ovarian response to FSH and LH, there is less estrogen and progesterone being produced. In turn, no negative feedback is in place to inhibit the rise of FSH and LH.

○ **Which hormones decline as a result of menopause?**

Estrogen and androstenedione. Progesterone production also decreases.

○ **What hormone is secreted more by the postmenopausal ovary than the premenopausal ovary?**

Testosterone. Prior to menopause, the ovary contributes 25% of circulating testosterone, and in menopause the ovary contributes 40% of circulating testosterone.

○ **What is the cause of mild hirsutism in menopause?**

Increased free androgen to estrogen ratio as a result of decreased SHBG and estrogen.

○ **After menopause, what is the percent of bone loss per year?**

2.5% for the first 4 years, and then 1% to 1.5% annually.

○ **What risk factors are associated with bone loss and osteoporosis?**

White and Asian race, thin women, sedentary lifestyle, smoking, coexisting endocrine disease, long-term steroid use, and age of menopause.

○ **How does estrogen therapy help maintain bone mass?**

Estrogen has a direct effect on osteoblasts, improves intestinal absorption of calcium, and decreases renal excretion of calcium.

○ **Why does vaginitis and vaginal atrophy increase during the postmenopausal years?**

Because of estrogen deficiency, the vaginal pH increases from 3.5–4.5 to 6.0–8.0, predisposing it to colonization of bacterial pathogens.

○ **What effect does estrogen therapy have on colorectal cancer?**

It significantly decreases the risk of colon cancer (50%).

○ **What effect does estrogen have on Alzheimer disease?**

Alzheimer disease is less frequent among HRT users and cognitive function in affected individuals is improved.

○ **A 63-year-old woman asks you about the risk–benefit ratio for estrogen therapy. What do you tell her?**

Estrogen therapy is currently recommended for postmenopausal women who are NOT in a high-risk category for breast cancer; to improve cardiovascular health—research suggests that estrogen decreases the risk of CHD by 35%; to limit the risk of osteoporosis, including decreased risk of hip fractures by 25% and risk of vertebral fractures by 50%; for control of vaginal atrophy and vasomotor side effects of hypoestrogenic state. Hormone replacement therapy should be used with caution since unopposed estrogen increases the risk of endometrial cancer eight times (addition of progestins will eliminate this risk); it could potentially increase the risk of breast cancer in those with known risk factors; it can lead to hypercoagulable state (DVT).

○ **What are the contraindications to estrogen therapy?**

Estrogen-sensitive cancers, chronically impaired liver function, undiagnosed genital bleeding, acute vascular thrombosis, neurophthalmologic vascular disease, and known or suspected pregnancy.

○ **What is the mainstay of treatment for postmenopausal osteoporosis?**

Bisphosphonates.

● ● ● CONTRACEPTIVE METHODS ● ● ●

○ **What are the absolute contraindications to the use of hormonal-based contraceptive agents? Explain using the mnemonic CONTRACEPTIVE:**

Coronary disease
Obesity/hyperlipidemia type II
Neoplasm of liver
Cerebrovascular disease
Estrogen-dependent tumors
Pregnancy
Thrombophlebitis
IDDM
Vaginal bleeding undiagnosed
Enzymes of liver increasing

○ **What chemical changes may predispose patients taking oral contraceptives to weight gain?**

Increases in low-density lipoproteins, decreases in high-density lipoproteins, and sodium retention.

○ **How much is menstrual blood flow decreased by OCP use?**

On average by 60%.

○ **What are the overall risks and benefits to combined oral contraceptives?**

Risks: Increase the risk for thromboembolism, MIs, CVAs, hypertension, amenorrhea, cholelithiasis, and benign hepatic tumors.

Benefits: Regulate the menstrual cycle, decrease premenstrual symptoms, and curb the progression of endometriosis, ovarian cysts, and benign breast disease. They also decrease the risk of ovarian and endometrial cancer, decrease the incidence of ectopic pregnancy, salpingitis, and anemia. They are known to be therapeutic against rheumatoid arthritis.

○ **For women using oral contraceptives for 4 years or less, what is the reduction in the risk of ovarian cancer?**

30%. For 12 or more years of use, the risk is decreased by 80%.

○ **For women using oral contraceptives for at least 2 years, what is the reduction in the risk of endometrial cancer?**

40%. This increases to 60% for 4 or more years of use.

○ **What effect does oral contraceptive use have on the risk of developing cervical cancer?**

Oral contraceptive users as a group are at higher risk for cervical neoplasia. This increased risk may be secondary to sexual habits rather than the pill itself.

○ **What are the estrogen-mediated side effects of oral contraceptive pills?**

Headache, nausea, breast enlargement or tenderness, fluid retention, chloasma, and telangiectasia.

○ **What are progestin-/androgen-mediated side effects of oral contraceptive pills?**

Depression, fatigue, acne, oily skin, and increased appetite.

○ **What is the incidence of venous thrombosis among oral contraceptive users?**

10–20/100,000 users. Much higher incidence in smokers.

○ **How effective is breast-feeding alone in preventing pregnancy?**

98% for the first 6 months in women who have not resumed their menses.

○ **How does DepoProvera work?**

High levels of progestin suppressing FSH and LH levels and eliminating the LH surge. This inhibits ovulation.

○ **What is the effect of progestin on the uterus?**

It results in a shallow atrophic endometrium and a thick cervical mucus. These both result in decreased sperm transport.

○ **What is the delay in return to fertility after DepoProvera?**

6 months to 1 year.

○ **What is the risk of ectopic pregnancy in women with an IUD in place?**

5%. Hormone-based IUD users have a 6- to 10-fold increase in ectopic rates compared with copper IUD users.

○ **How long after exposure can emergency oral contraceptives be given?**

Up to 72 hours. It is most effective if initiated in 12 to 24 hours. Emergency contraception provides a 75% reduction in the risk of pregnancy. Patients should have a negative pregnancy test prior to treatment.

○ **What is the total dose of estrogen that should be used in __combined__ emergency oral contraceptive pills?**

200 μg of ethinyl estradiol—2 doses of 100 μg taken 12 hours apart.

○ **Besides emergency contraceptive pills, what other contraceptive method can be used to prevent pregnancy after unprotected intercourse?**

Copper IUD.

○ **How long after the removal of Norplant capsules must patients wait to become pregnant?**

Ovulation usually occurs within 3 months.

○ **How long after delivery should a postpartum tubal ligation be performed? Why?**

It is common practice to wait 8 to 12 hours postpartum before inducing anesthesia for tubal ligation. This time interval is useful to allow the patient to reach cardiovascular stability and increase the likelihood of gastric emptying.

● ● ● INFERTILITY ● ● ●

○ **What percentage of American couples are infertile?**

15% to 20% of women older than 35 years in the United States are infertile.

○ **What is the difference between primary and secondary infertility?**

Primary—no conception or history of conception. Secondary—at least one prior episode of conception (even if did not result in term pregnancy and birth).

○ **What percentage of infertility is due to the male factor?**

40%. Problems with the cervix, uterus, fallopian tubes, peritoneum, or ovulation account for the remaining 60%.

○ **What are the numbers for a normal semen analysis?**

1 mL in volume (>20,000,000 sperm) with >50% motility.

○ **How long do sperm stay in the vagina postcoitus?**

At least 72 hours; however, sperm are motile only for 6 hours. When performing a rape kit, it is important to test for acid phosphatase. This enzyme is present for 24 hours and confirms that ejaculation has occurred.

○ **What hormone is a marker of changes in basal body temperature?**

Progesterone.

○ **In the evaluation of infertility, what procedure can be both diagnostic and therapeutic?**

Hysterosalpingogram. It is typically performed between cycle days 6 and 10.

● ● ● **UNCOMPLICATED PREGNANCY** ● ● ●

○ **What percentage of pregnant women get "morning sickness"?**

50% to 70%. It generally occurs in the first trimester (up to week 14–16).

○ **How should morning sickness be treated?**

Frequent small meals, carbohydrates, IV hydration, and antiemetics as last resort.

○ **What is hyperemesis gravidarum?**

Excessive vomiting during pregnancy that results in starvation (ketonuria), dehydration, and acidosis.

○ **What is pica?**

This is a craving for eating nonfoods, such as laundry starch and clay, during pregnancy. If severe, it can result in nutritional deficiencies and anemia. It is also possible that the agent ingested may be toxic to the developing fetus.

○ **Does the presence of a thick endometrial stripe on ultrasound indicate an intrauterine pregnancy?**

The endometrium can be thickened due to the hormonal stimulation associated with either an ectopic or intrauterine pregnancy, so this is not a consistent sign of a normal pregnancy.

○ **When can an intrauterine gestational sac be identified by an abdominal ultrasound?**

In the fifth week. A fetal pole can be identified in the sixth week and an embryonic mass with cardiac motion in the seventh week.

○ **For a gestational sac to be visible on ultrasound, what must the β-hCG level be?**

At least 6500 mIU/mL for a transabdominal ultrasound, and 2000 mIU/mL for a transvaginal ultrasound.

○ **What secretes β-hCG? Why?**

Placental trophoblasts secrete β-hCG to maintain the corpus luteum, which in turn maintains the uterine lining. The corpus luteum is maintained through the sixth to eighth week of pregnancy, by which time the placenta begins to produce its own progesterone to maintain the endometrium.

○ **How soon after implantation can β-hCG be detected?**

2 to 3 days.

○ **At what rate do β-hCG levels rise?**

They double every 48 hours.

○ **At what gestational age does hCG peak?**

8 to 10 weeks.

○ **Name four physiologic actions of hCG:**

1. Maintenance of corpus luteum and continued progesterone production
2. Stimulation of fetal testicular testosterone secretion promoting male sexual differentiation
3. Stimulation of the maternal thyroid by binding to TSH receptors
4. Promotes relaxin secretion by the corpus luteum

○ **What does a progesterone level of 25 ng/mL or higher indicates about a pregnancy?**

A viable, uterine pregnancy. Serum progesterone is produced by the corpus luteum in the pregnant patient and remains constant for the first 8 to 10 weeks of pregnancy.

○ **Which routine screenings should be performed on pregnant women?**

Hepatitis B and C, syphilis, rubella, chlamydia, gonorrhea, and other STDs. Women in high-risk categories should also be screened for HIV.

○ **By which week of gestation can a mother feel fetal movement? What is the term used to describe this?**

16th to 20th week of gestation; termed "quickening."

○ **Which week of gestation can fetal heart tones be detected by Doppler?**

12th week.

○ **When can one auscultate the fetal heart?**

Ultrasound: 6 weeks

Doppler: 10 to 12 weeks

Stethoscope: 18 to 20 weeks

○ **What immunizations are contraindicated during pregnancy?**

In general, live virus vaccines are contraindicated during pregnancy. These include measles, mumps, rubella, oral polio, and varicella. On the other hand, all toxoids, immunoglobulins and killed virus vaccines are considered safe in pregnancy and should not be withheld, if indicated.

○ **What are the drug-labeling categories for use during pregnancy?**

The FDA lists five categories of labeling:

Category A: Safe for use in pregnancy.

Category B: Animal studies have demonstrated the drug's safety and human studies do not reveal any adverse fetal effects.

Category C: The drug is a known animal teratogen, but no data are available about human use; or there are no data in either humans or animals.

Category D: There is a positive evidence of human fetal toxicity, but benefits in selected situations makes use of the drug acceptable despite its risks.

Category X: The drug is a definite human and animal teratogen and should not be used in pregnancy.

○ **In general, at what time during pregnancy is the fetus most susceptible to teratogens?**

During the embryonic period, which lasts from 2 to 8 weeks postconception. This is the time of organogenesis.

○ **Name the anticoagulant safe in pregnancy:**

Heparin. Warfarin is contraindicated.

○ **What is the known effect of folic acid deficiency in pregnancy?**

Folate deficiency is associated with neural tube defects (i.e., spina bifida, anencephaly).

○ **What effect does pregnancy have on BUN and creatinine?**

Both are decreased. This is the result of increased renal blood flow and increased glomerular filtration rate.

○ **Why should pregnant women rest in the left lateral decubitus position?**

To avert supine hypotension syndrome due to compression of the IVC by the uterus.

○ **What is the normal P_{CO_2} in pregnancy?**

30 to 34 mm Hg from chronic mild hyperventilation, presumably as a result of progesterone.

○ **What is the predominant change in the lung volumes in pregnancy?**

Decrease in functional residual capacity by as much as 15% to 25%. Tidal volume increases by 40%.

○ **What WBC count is expected during pregnancy?**

WBC counts of 15,000 to 20,000 are considered normal during pregnancy.

○ **What are the normal physical changes in the cervix during pregnancy?**

Softening and cyanosis.

○ **What are the expected changes in cervical mucous and vaginal flora during pregnancy?**

Thick tenacious mucous forms a plug blocking the cervical canal. Increased cervical and vaginal secretions result in thick, white odorless discharge. The pH is between 3.5 and 6.0 resulting from increased production of lactic acid from the action of *Lactobacillus acidophilus*.

○ **What is the average weight gain in pregnancy?**

11 kg (25 lbs). Only 30% of the maternal weight gain is attributed to the placenta and fetus. Another 30% is attributed to blood, amniotic fluid, and extravascular fluid. Another 30% is attributed to maternal fat.

○ **In general terms, what is the physiology of the maternal immune system in pregnancy?**

Pregnancy represents a 50% allograft from the paternal contribution. As a result, there is a general suppression of immune function.

○ **What are the normal changes in the auscultative heart examination during pregnancy?**

Exaggerated split S1 with increased volume of both components. Systolic ejection murmurs heard at the left sternal border are present in 90% of patients, soft and transient diastolic murmurs are heard in 20%, and continuous murmurs from breast vasculature are heard in 10%. The significance of murmurs in pregnancy must be carefully evaluated and clinically correlated. Harsh systolic murmurs and all diastolic murmurs should be taken seriously and worked up before being attributed to pregnancy.

○ **Why is pregnancy termed a "hyperparathyroid state"?**

The fetomaternal unit has the primary goal of transporting calcium across the placenta (by active transport) for fetal skeletal development. This consumes most of the maternal calcium. With this increase in calcium need, parathyroid hormone levels are increased by 30% to 50% to bring calcium from the maternal bone, kidney, and intestine into the serum.

○ **A pregnant patient complains that her contact lenses are painful to wear recently. Is this normal?**

Yes. Corneal thickness increases in pregnancy and can cause discomfort when wearing lenses fitted before pregnancy.

○ **What kind of changes occur in the cardiovascular system of a pregnant patient?**

Cardiac output increases by 30% in the first trimester and then 50% by the second trimester.

Stroke volume increases 25% and hemoatocrit drops due to hemodilution.

Plasma volume increases by 50% and pulse increases 12 to 18 bpm.

Systolic and diastolic blood pressure decrease by 10 to 15 mm Hg in the second trimester, then gradually returns to prepregnant levels in the third trimester.

○ **What happens to the bladder anatomy during pregnancy?**

The bladder is displaced superiorly and anteriorly.

○ **What kind of changes occur in the gastrointestinal system of a pregnant patient?**

Gastric emptying and GI motility decrease leading to GERD and constipation. In the third trimester, GERD can also be the result of increased intraabdominal pressure. Alkaline phosphatase increases. Peritoneal signs such as rigidity and rebound are diminished or absent.

○ **Can iodinated radiodiagnostic agents be used in pregnant patients?**

No. They should be avoided because concentration in the fetal thyroid can cause permanent loss of thyroid function. Nuclear medicine scans, pulmonary angiography with pelvic shielding, and impedance plethysmography are preferred.

○ **What radiation dose increases the risk of inhibited fetal growth?**

10 rad. Typical abdominal and pelvic films deliver 100 to 350 mrad. A shielded chest X-ray should deliver under 10 mrad to the fetus. Do not withhold necessary X-rays.

○ **When does labor begin?**

Labor begins with the onset of regular, rhythmic contractions that lead to serial dilatation and effacement of the cervix. Thus, to say labor has begun, one must observe changes in the cervix. The presence of contractions alone does not qualify for the onset of labor.

○ **What are the four stages of labor and delivery?**

Stage I: Onset of labor to complete dilation of the cervix

Stage II: Cervical dilation to birth

Stage III: Birth to delivery of the placenta

Stage IV: Placenta delivery to stability of the mother (about 6 hours)

○ **How long is the average latent phase of labor?**

In a nullipara, the average is 6.4 hours; in the multipara, the average is 4.8 hours

○ **What is the rate of cervical dilation (active phase) in primiparous and multiparous women?**

The active phase begins when the uterus is regularly contracting and the cervix is 3 to 4 cm dilated. The minimal dilation is 1 cm/h for primiparous and 1.5 cm/h for multiparous women.

○ **What are the six movements of delivery?**

1. Descent
2. Flexion
3. Internal rotation
4. Extension
5. External rotation
6. Expulsion

○ **How long may a patient push once fully dilated?**

Provided that the fetal heart pattern is reassuring and maternal expulsive forces remain effective, a second stage may last up to 2 hours (average nullipara is 40 minutes, multipara 20 minutes); up to 3 hours is appropriate if the patient has regional analgesia/anesthesia. Beyond these time limits, one sees an increase in fetal acidosis and lower Apgar scores, as well as a greater risk of maternal postpartum hemorrhage and febrile morbidity.

○ **What is "effacement" of the cervix?**

Effacement refers to the foreshortening and thinning of cervix as it is drawn upwards (intra-abdominally). It is usually expressed in percentages by which cervical length has been reduced (from 0%, or uneffaced, to 100%, or fully effaced).

○ **What agents may be used to ripen the cervix?**

Both chemical and physical agents have been used. Oxytocics, prostaglandins (especially PGE2), progesterone antagonists (RU-486), and dehydroepiandrosterone are such pharmacologic agents. Laminaria and foley catheter balloons are examples of physical dilators.

○ **What other uterotonic agents are there besides oxytocin?**

Vasopressin (antidiuretic hormone), prostaglandins (PGE2 and PGF2α) and thromboxane are natural oxytocics. Ergot alkaloids (e.g., Methergine) and the synthetic prostaglandin 15-methyl-F2-α-PG are used clinically to increase uterine contractions, especially for postpartum uterine atony.

○ **Does epidural analgesia affect the course of labor?**

Studies showed that epidural analgesia does not slow the progress of labor in the first stage of labor. However, the second stage of labor appears to be prolonged for an average of 20 to 25 minutes. There is no evidence that this prolongation is harmful to the fetus.

○ **What is a "walking epidural"?**

An intrathecal opioid or epidural opioid plus an ultralow dose of local anesthetic, followed by continuous infusion of opioid and local anesthetics, for labor analgesia. These regimens cause no or minimal motor block on the lower extremities, and allow the mother to ambulate in the early first stage of labor.

○   **What complications are seen with precipitous labors?**

There is a higher incidence of fetal trauma (intracranial hemorrhage and fractured clavicle) and long-term neurologic injury. The mother is at higher risk for pelvic lacerations and postpartum hemorrhage (including, somewhat paradoxically, from uterine atony).

○   **What is the most common cause of a prolonged active phase of labor?**

Cephalopelvic disproportion caused by contraction of a narrowed midpelvis.

○   **What is the first step in the evaluation of a protraction or arrest disorder of labor?**

Assess fetopelvic size. If disproportion is suspected, augmentation should not be undertaken.

○   **At term, what percentage of fetuses are in vertex presentation?**

95%.

○   **What is the largest risk for breech presentation?**

Prematurity; 25% of fetuses are breech at 28 weeks, but most correct by term.

○   **What are the three types of breech presentation?**

Frank breech: Thighs flexed, legs extended
Complete breech: At least one leg flexed
Incomplete (footling) breech: At least one foot below the buttocks with both thighs extended

○   **What is the most common breech position?**

Frank breech.

○   **What is the modified Ritgen maneuver?**

It describes the elevation of the fetal chin achieved by placement of the delivering hand between the maternal coccyx and perineal body, while the other hand guides the crowning vertex. This technique assists in extension of the fetal head and allows the clinician to control delivery.

○   **What is the difference between high forceps, mid forceps, and low forceps deliveries?**

High forceps refers to the use of forceps when a baby is not yet in the birth canal (rarely used).
Mid forceps refers to the use of forceps when a baby is in the birth canal and within reach (used in cases of fetal distress).
Low forceps refers to the outlet and forcep is used when the baby's head is at the pelvic floor (most often used to shorten labor when the mother is tiring or to control normal labor).

○   **How can ruptured membranes be diagnosed?**

Nitrazine paper will turn blue and a ferning pattern will be seen under the microscope in the presence of amniotic fluid. Also, look for pooling of amniotic fluid in the posterior fornix.

○ **What are the degrees of perineal tears that may occur with delivery? Describe.**

First degree: Perineal skin or vaginal mucosa

Second degree: Submucosa of vagina or perineum

Third degree: Anal sphincter

Fourth degree: Rectal mucosa

○ **What are the advantages and disadvantages of a mediolateral episiotomy?**

Such an episiotomy allows for greater room without lacerating the external sphincter ani or rectum. However, these episiotomies are associated with a greater blood loss and postpartum pain, greater likelihood for suboptimal healing, and subsequent dyspareunia.

○ **What are the advantages and disadvantages of a midline (median) episiotomy?**

These are easier to repair, associated with a lower blood loss, usually heal better (less postpartum discomfort and better cosmetic result), and less subsequent dyspareunia.

The principal disadvantage to such an episiotomy, compared to a mediolateral one, is the greater propensity to extend into the external anal sphincter or rectum resulting in possible rectal dysfunction or rectal prolapse in the future.

○ **How can fetal lung maturity be assessed?**

The L/S ratio; if the ratio of lecithin to sphingomyelin is more than 2:1, then the fetal lungs are mature.

○ **What are the benefits of antepartum corticosteroids in premature babies?**

Increased lung compliance, increased surfactant production, less respiratory distress syndrome, less intraventricular hemorrhage, less necrotizing enterocolitis, and less neonatal mortality.

○ **What is the normal fetal heart rate?**

120 to 160 bpm. If bradycardia is detected, position the mother on her left side and administer oxygen and an IV fluid bolus.

○ **Are accelerations normal?**

Yes and no. Rapid heart rate can indicate fetal distress; 2 accelerations every 20 minutes are normal. An acceleration must be at least 15 bpm above baseline and last at least 15 seconds.

○ **What causes variable decelerations?**

Transient umbilical cord compression. These often change with maternal position.

○   **A baby is born with a pink body, blue extremities, and a heart rate of 60. The neonate is mildly irritable (grimaces) and has weak respirations and no muscle tone. What is this patient's Apgar?**

$1 + 1 + 1 + 1 + 0 = 4$

Apgar points	0	1	2
Color	Blue	Extremities blue	All pink
Heart rate	Ø	<100	>100
Irritability	Ø	Mild grimace	Strongly irritable
Respiratory effort	None	Weak	Cry
Muscle tone	Flaccid	Weak	Strong

● ● ● **COMPLICATED PREGNANCY** ● ● ●

○   **What percentage of pregnancies are ectopic?**

1.5%. Ectopic pregnancies are the leading cause of death in the first trimester.

○   **What is the risk of a repeat ectopic pregnancy?**

10% to 15%.

○   **What are the risk factors for ectopic pregnancy? Explain using the mnemonic ECTOPIC:**

Endometriosis
Congenital anomaly of tubes
Tubal surgery
Old abdominal scar
PID
In vitro fertilization
Contraceptive pills

○   **When and how does an ectopic pregnancy most commonly present?**

6 to 8 weeks into the pregnancy. Patients usually present with amenorrhea and sharp, generally unilateral abdominal or pelvic pain.

○   **In an ectopic pregnancy, is an adnexal mass a common finding?**

No. An adnexal mass is actually found in less than 50% of cases. Abdominal pain is the most frequent symptom. Amenorrhea is the second most common symptom.

○   **What is the most common site of implantation in an ectopic pregnancy?**

The ampulla of the fallopian tube (95%). Less common sites are abdomen, uterine cornua, cervix, and ovary.

○ **How do hCG levels differ in women with ectopic pregnancies versus intrauterine pregnancy?**

In 85% of women with ectopic pregnancy, the hCG level is lower than expected.

○ **Which is the <u>most common</u> sign of an ectopic pregnancy by transvaginal ultrasound: adnexal mass or absence of an intrauterine pregnancy?**

The absence of an intrauterine pregnancy at an hCG level >2000 mIU/mL is highly predictive of an ectopic pregnancy. An adnexal mass or gestational sac in the adnexal is less reliable finding and is not always seen in early ectopic pregnancies. Follow-up ultrasound is always recommended in high-risk patients to ensure intrauterine pregnancy.

○ **Who is eligible for methotrexate treatment of an ectopic pregnancy?**

Patients who are hemodynamically stable with unruptured gestations <4 cm in diameter by ultrasound.

○ **What is the mode of action of methotrexate?**

Methotrexate is a folic acid antagonist.

○ **What criteria are used for assuring the success of methotrexate?**

With a single-dose therapy, the hCG levels should fall by 15% between days 4 and 7 after therapy and continue to fall weekly until undetectable.

○ **What are the indications for laparotomy for the treatment of ectopic pregnancy?**

Common indications for laparotomy include an unstable patient, large hemoperitoneum, cornual pregnancy, and lack of appropriate surgical tools for laparoscopy. A large ectopic (>6 cm) and fetal heart tones in the adnexa may also be considered as indications for laparotomy.

○ **A patient who is 3 months pregnant presents to your office with pelvic pain. On examination, a retroverted and retroflexed uterus is found. What is the diagnosis?**

Incarceration of the uterus. Patients typically complain of rectal and pelvic pressure. Urinary retention may be found. The knee–chest position or rectal pressure may correct the problem.

○ **What are the differences between spontaneous, threatened, incomplete, complete, and missed abortions?**

Spontaneous abortion is the loss of the fetus before the 20th week of gestation.

Threatened abortion is uterine cramping or bleeding in the first 20 weeks of gestation without the passage of products of conception or cervical dilatation.

Incomplete abortions are partial abortions in which part of the products of conception are aborted and part remain within the uterus. The cervix is dilated on examination, and dilation and curettage is necessary to remove the remainder of tissue.

Complete abortion is when all the products of conception have been passed, the cervix is closed, and the uterus is firm and nontender.

Missed abortion is defined as no uterine growth, no cervical dilation, no passage of fetal tissue, and minimal cramping or bleeding. Diagnosis is made by the absence of fetal heart tones and an empty sac on ultrasound.

○   **What percentage of pregnancies result in spontaneous abortions? What is the number one cause of natural abortions?**

15% to 20%. Genetic defects (50%), usually the result of an abnormal number of chromosomes.

○   **Name three independent risk factors for spontaneous abortion:**

Increasing parity, maternal age, and paternal age.

○   **What is the effect of smoking and drinking on the abortion rate?**

Women who smoke more than 14 cigarettes daily have a 1.7 times greater chance of a spontaneous abortion. Those who drink alcohol at least 2 days a week have a twofold greater risk for spontaneous abortion.

○   **How do spontaneous abortions most commonly present?**

Abdominal pain followed by vaginal bleeding typically before 8 to 9 weeks of gestation.

○   **What is the chance of spontaneous abortion once fetal cardiac activity is established at eight weeks of gestation?**

3% to 5%.

○   **In what percentage of patients will spontaneous labor occur within 3 weeks of fetal death?**

80%. It may be helpful to induce labor with vaginal suppositories due to the psychological effects of carrying a dead baby.

○   **At what gestational age is suction or vacuum curettage used to terminate the pregnancy?**

7 to 13 weeks of gestation.

○   **What is the most common cause of postabortal pain, bleeding, and low-grade fever?**

Retained gestational tissue or clot.

○   **What is the most likely diagnosis in a patient whose uterus is larger than expected from the history of gestation, has vaginal bleeding, and passes grape-like tissue from the vagina?**

Hydatidiform mole.

○   **How does age influence the incidence of hydatidiform moles?**

Compared to women aged 25 to 29 years, women older than 50 years have a 300- to 400-fold increase in risk and women younger than 15 years have a 6-fold increase. Similarly, increased paternal age (above 45 years of age) also confers an increased risk of a complete molar pregnancy, although the increase is much lower and adjusted for maternal age.

○   **How is human chorionic gonadotropin (hCG) useful in the evaluation of gestational trophoblastic disease?**

Both molar pregnancies and gestational choriocarcinomas produce BhCG due to their trophoblastic origin. The tumor marker correlates well with the volume of disease and can be followed as a marker during therapy.

○ **With what endocrine abnormalities are moles and other gestational trophoblastic neoplasms associated?**

Hyperthyroidism.

○ **Describe the characteristics of gestational choriocarcinoma:**

Gestational choriocarcinomas contain both cytotrophoblast and syncytiotrophoblast elements. They are considered invasive molar pregnancies. Invasive moles are pathologically similar to complete hydatidiform moles but invade beyond the normal placentation site into the myometrium. Penetration into the venous system can result in venous metastases to the lower genital tract and lungs.

○ **Why is induction of labor with oxytocin or prostaglandins not recommended for the evacuation of molar pregnancies?**

Uterine contractions against an undilated cervix theoretically carries an increased risk for the dissemination of trophoblast throughout the systemic circulation.

○ **What is the most common presentation of twins?**

Vertex–vertex. If the first twin is vertex and the second breach, it is still possible to attempt a vaginal delivery because the extra space afforded after the birth of the first baby allows room to manipulate the position of the second.

○ **What is the average gestational age at delivery for twins, triplets, and quadruplets?**

Twins: 36–37 weeks

Triplets: 33–34 weeks

Quadruplets: 30–31 weeks

3 or more fetuses reduced to twins: 35–36 weeks

○ **What are the risk factors for elevated maternal serum α-fetoprotein? Explain using the mnemonic MSAFP (elevated MSAFP):**

Multiple gestations

Spina bifida (NTDs)

Abdominal wall defects (Omphalocele, gastroschisis)

Fetal death

Placental anomalies

○ **What conditions are suggested by an elevated maternal serum α-fetoprotein?**

Neural tube defects (an encephalopathy), ventral abdominal wall defects, fetal demise, multiple fetuses. A low α-fetoprotein is indicative of Down syndrome.

○ **What are the baseline congenital anomaly risks in the general population?**

Regardless of family history or teratogenic exposure, the background risk for major congenital anomalies is 3% to 5%. These include abnormalities that, if uncorrected, affect the health of the individual. Some examples are pyloric stenosis, cleft lip and palate, and neural tube defects.

The background rate for minor congenital anomalies is 7% to 10%. These include strabismus, polydactyly, misshapen ears, etc. If uncorrected, they do not significantly affect the health of the individual.

○   **Why is the Rh status of a pregnant patient important?**

If the mother is Rh negative and the fetus is Rh positive, there is a risk of developing Rh isoimmunization and fetal anemia, hydrops, and/or fetal loss.

○   **Which type of blood test is used to determine if a patient needs RhoGAM therapy?**

A Kleihauer-Betke checks for fetomaternal bleeding.

○   **When should RhoGAM (anti-Rh immunoglobulin) be used?**

Within 3 days of the birth of an Rh+ child (if the mother is Rh−). It should also be used in the event of any mixing of fetal and maternal blood (e.g., trauma). RhoGAM is safe because it does not pass the placenta barrier.

The standard dose of RhoGAM is 300 mg.

○   **Should Rh-negative women with ectopic pregnancies be given RhoGAM?**

The administration of mini-RhoGAM (50 μg) is recommended with any failed pregnancy up to 12 weeks (with full dose RhoGAM after 12 weeks).

○   **A young patient has a threatened abortion in the first trimester. Laboratory studies reveal she is Rh negative and her husband is Rh positive. What is the recommended management of this patient?**

The patient will need 50 μg of Rh immunoglobulin (RhoGAM) IM. After the first trimester, the dose is increased to 300 μg IM.

○   **What are some common causes of polyhydramnios?**

Maternal causes include diabetes, Rh incompatibility, and other hematological diseases. Fetal causes are anencephaly, duodenal atresia, tracheoesophageal fistula, and pulmonary disorders.

○   **What is the most common medical complication of pregnancy?**

Urinary tract infections.

○   **What is the treatment for gestational diabetes?**

Diet, insulin, and exercise. Do not give patients oral hypoglycemics because these cross the blood–brain barrier.

○   **What level of serum glucose in a patient with gestational diabetes warrants hospital admission?**

Persistent hyperglycemia (>200 mg).

○   **When should you be most concerned about a pregnant patient with underlying heart disease?**

During weeks 18 to 24, when the female body experiences a maximal increase in cardiac output (40%).

○   **What are some of the common misconceptions about the management of asthma during pregnancy?**

Dyspnea is common in pregnancy with or without underlying asthma. Medications should be used sparingly. Uncontrolled asthma causes more fetal harm than medications.

○ **What are the factors during pregnancy that increase the risk of aspiration of stomach contents?**

Increased intragastric pressure from the gravid uterus, progesterone-induced relaxation of the lower esophageal sphincter, delayed gastric emptying in labor, and depressed mental status from analgesia.

○ **Is appendicitis more common during pregnancy?**

No (approximately 1 out of 850). However, the outcome is worse. Prompt diagnosis is important because the incidence of perforation increases from 10% in the first trimester to 40% in the third.

○ **During which trimester of pregnancy is acute appendicitis most common?**

The second trimester.

○ **How is the appendix typically displaced during pregnancy?**

Superiorly and laterally. Diagnosis of appendicitis in pregnant patients may be further complicated by the fact that a normal pregnancy can itself cause an increased WBC. In a pregnant patient, pyuria with no bacteria suggests appendicitis. Pregnant patients may lack GI distress, peritoneal signs on examination, and fever may be absent or low grade.

○ **What viral or protozoal infections require extensive work-up during pregnancy? Define ToRCH:**

Toxoplasma gondii
Rubella
Cytomegalovirus
Herpes genitalis

○ **What foods put a pregnant woman at risk for mercury poisoning?**

The only real human exposure to organic mercury is through consumption of fish, primarily from predatory fish such as shark, swordfish, pike, and bass.

○ **What is the recommended fish consumption for pregnant women to avoid mercury poisoning?**

Fish consumption by pregnant women should be limited to 350 g per week. Fetuses are more susceptible to toxic effects of mercury than their maternal hosts. Large exposures to methyl mercury have resulted in infants with microcephaly, mental retardation, cerebral palsy, and blindness.

○ **Why is ephedrine usually the first choice to treat maternal hypotension?**

Ephedrine does not produce significant uterine vascular constriction, and therefore, it does not result in decreased uterine blood flow.

○ **What causes dependent and nondependent edema in pregnant women?**

Compression of veins by the growing uterus causes dependent edema, whereas hypoalbuminemia can cause nondependent edema.

○ **Define pregnancy-induced hypertension:**

An increase in the systolic pressure > 30 mm Hg or an increase in diastolic pressure > 15 mm Hg over baseline, measured on two separate occasions at least 6 hours apart.

○ **What are the pharmacotherapeutic options for the treatment of hypertension of pregnancy?**

Methyldopa, labetalol, hydralazine, and clonidine. Antihypertensive treatment is indicated if the systolic BP is >170 mm Hg or the diastolic is >110 mm Hg. Although many choices to treat earlier. Other options not used as frequently include nifedipine, atenolol, prazosin, and minoxidil.

○ **What are the nonpharmacotherapeutic options for the treatment of hypertension of pregnancy?**

Sodium restriction to 2 to 3 g/d; abstaining from alcohol and tobacco; weight reduction; moderate activity as tolerated but rigorous activity should be limited; more frequent prenatal visits and ultrasound surveillance is recommended to monitor for signs of fetal anomalies/stress or preeclampsia.

○ **Define preeclampsia:**

Hypertension (a systolic pressure > 160 mm Hg or a diastolic pressure > 110 mm Hg) after 20 weeks of estimated gestational age with generalized edema or proteinuria of 5 g or more in a 24-hour period.

○ **Who is more likely to have preeclampsia: primiparous or multiparous women?**

Primiparous. Other risk factors include pregnancies associated with a large placenta, patients with a history of HTN, renal disease, family history of preeclampsia, older women, women with multiple gestations, and women with prior vascular disease.

○ **Which two drugs are used to treat eclampsia?**

Magnesium sulfate, 4 to 6 g bolus IV followed by a 2 g/h infusion, and hydralazine, 10 to 20 mg IV. Labetalol may also be used.

○ **Should blood pressure be lowered acutely in a preeclampsia patient?**

No. Dangerous hypertension (>170/110) should be gradually lowered with hydralazine, 10 mg IV followed by a drip.

○ **How should hydralazine be dosed for a preeclamptic patient?**

Hydralazine should be given in 5 mg boluses every 20 minutes until adequate BP control (90/110 diastolic) is achieved or a total of 20 mg is reached.

○ **What is the major cause of death in women with eclampsia?**

Intracranial hemorrhage.

○ **What are the warning signs of impending seizure in a patient with preeclampsia?**

Headache, visual disturbances, hyperreflexia, and abdominal pain.

○ **What is the treatment for eclampsia?**

Delivery!!! Until you are able to deliver you can use magnesium sulfate, valium, and hydralazine. Phenytoin or diazepam can be used for seizures resistant to magnesium therapy.

○ **How long should treatment continue after delivery for a woman with <u>preeclampsia</u>?**

24 hours. The cure for preeclampsia is delivery. Antihypertensives and antiseizure medication (IV magnesium sulfate) should be continued until there is no longer a risk to the mother.

○ **If a patient had an eclamptic seizure prior to delivery, can they have additional after delivery?**

Yes. Up to 10 days postpartum.

○ **At what point does magnesium become toxic?**

Respiratory arrest occurs at levels >12 mEq/L. Loss of reflexes occurs at levels >8 mEq/L and can therefore be used as a guide for treatment.

○ **What is the antidote for magnesium toxicity?**

Calcium gluconate (1 g IV push); magnesium should be stopped if the DTRs disappear.

○ **What does HELLP stand for?**

Hemolysis
Elevated
Liver enzymes
Low **P**latelet levels

The HELLP syndrome is a very severe form of preeclampsia. Signs and symptoms include RUQ pain/tenderness, nausea, vomiting, edema, jaundice, GI bleeding, and hematuria in addition to the symptoms of preeclampsia.

○ **What is the difference between placenta previa and abruptio placenta?**

Placenta previa is the implantation of the placenta in the lower uterine segment thus covering the cervical os. Presentation is <u>painless</u> vaginal bleeding with a soft nontender uterus.

Abruptio placenta is the premature separation of the placenta from the uterine wall. Abruptio placenta causes <u>painful</u> uterine bleeding.

Both are complications of third trimester pregnancies.

○ **A patient presents in her third trimester complaining of vaginal bleeding but no pain or contractions. How should you diagnose this patient?**

With a transabdominal ultrasound. Since 95% of placenta previas can be diagnosed this way, a vaginal examination should be avoided until placenta previa has been ruled out via ultrasound. Abruptio placentae is generally accompanied by pain, shock, or an expanding uterus. It is not easily diagnosed on ultrasound.

○ **What are the risk factors for placenta previa?**

Previous cesarean section, previous placenta previa, multiparity, multiple induced abortions, maternal age over 40 years, and multiple gestations.

○ **What are the risk factors for placental abruption?**

Smoking, trauma, cocaine, hypertension, alcohol, PROM, trauma, previous abruptio placentae, and retroplacental fibroids.

○ **What are the presenting signs and symptoms of abruptio placentae?**

Placental separation before delivery is associated with vaginal bleeding (78%) and abdominal pain (66%) as well as with tetanic uterine contractions, uterine irritability, and possibly fetal death.

○ **What physical examination findings may be discovered in abruptio placenta?**

Rapidly increasing fundal height secondary to bleeding into the uterus or a higher than expected fundal height.

○ **What are the etiologies for uterine rupture (both gynecologic and obstetric)?**

Oxytocin stimulation, cephalopelvic disproportion, grand multiparity, abdominal trauma, prior hysterotomy, previous cesarean section, myotomy, curettage, or manual removal of the placenta.

○ **What is the number one risk factor for uterine rupture?**

Previous cesarean section.

○ **What are the common signs of uterine rupture?**

Fetal distress, unrelenting pain, hypotension, tachycardia, and vaginal bleeding. Fetal distress is usually the first sign of uterine rupture.

○ **What two findings on physical examination are indicative of uterine rupture?**

Loss of uterine contour and palpable fetal part.

○ **Why is the incidence of thromboembolism increased in pregnancy?**

Venous stasis from the uterine pressure on the inferior vena cava, increase in clotting factors, increased fibrinogen, and decreased fibrinolysis.

○ **What are some of the risk factors for thromboembolism in pregnancy?**

C-section, multiparity, bed rest, obesity, increased maternal age, and surgical procedures.

○ **What are the predisposing factors for amniotic fluid embolism?**

Older maternal age, multiparity, C-section, amniotomy, and insertion of intrauterine fetal monitoring devices.

○ **How does amniotic fluid enter maternal circulation?**

Through uterine tears or injury or through endocervical veins.

○ **What are the major consequences of amniotic fluid embolism?**

Cardiorespiratory collapse and DIC. Treatment is supportive.

○ **What is the mortality rate in amniotic fluid embolism?**

About 80%.

○ **How does cocaine adversely affect pregnancy?**

Cocaine is especially toxic during pregnancy. The most common complication caused by cocaine during pregnancy is abruptio placentae, which may result in fetal death. In addition, brain anomalies, intestinal atresia, and limb reduction defects have been described. Investigators have also reported increases in congenital heart defects in exposed infants. Cocaine may cause these effects by vasoconstrictions and subsequent infarction.

○ **Does methadone have the same adverse affect as cocaine in pregnancy?**

Not even close. In fact, one study compared cocaine-abusing women to women being treated with methadone and found a much higher complication rate in the cocaine-abuse group. Methadone is not thought to be a teratogen.

○ **What is neonatal abstinence syndrome, and what agents cause it?**

It is caused by maternal heroin addiction or maternal methadone treatment during pregnancy. It results from neonatal withdrawal and consists of tremulousness, hyperreflexia, high pitch cry, sneezing, sleepiness, tachypnea, yawning, sweating, fever, and seizures. The onset of symptoms is at birth.

○ **What are the signs and symptoms of fetal alcohol syndrome?**

Infants suffer from intrauterine growth restriction, mental retardation, and develop a characteristic facies, which consists of short palpebral fissures, a flat midface, a thin upper lip, and hypoplastic philtrum. Alcohol abuse is the most common preventable cause of mental retardation during pregnancy.

○ **At what time during gestation is the fetus most susceptible to alcohol toxicity?**

Probably in the second and third trimesters. In a study of 60 women, those who were heavy drinkers but stopped after the first trimester had children with normal mentation and behavioral patterns.

○ **What are the major adverse effects of smoking during pregnancy?**

Smoking causes intrauterine growth restriction and increases the incidence of preterm delivery in a dose-dependent manner. The incidence of placenta previa, abruptio placentae, and spontaneous abortion also appears to be increased in smokers.

○ **What are the indications for cardiotocographic monitoring in a pregnant trauma patient?**

All women past 20 weeks gestation with indirect or direct abdominal trauma require 4 hours of monitoring. Loss of beat-to-beat variability, uterine contractions, or fetal bradycardia or tachycardia demands immediate obstetrical consultation.

○ **When monitoring a pregnant trauma victim, whose vital signs are the most sensitive, those of the mother or those of the fetus?**

The fetal heart rate is more sensitive to inadequate resuscitation. Remember that the mother may lose 10% to 20% of her blood volume without a change in vital signs, whereas the baby's heart rate may increase or decrease above 160 or below 120, indicating significant fetal distress. The most common pitfall is failure to adequately resuscitate the mother.

○ **What are maternal risk factors for shoulder dystocia?**

Diabetes, maternal obesity, postterm babies, and mothers with excessive weight gain.

Intrapartum risk factors include a prolonged second stage of labor, oxytocin use (augmentation or induction), and midforceps deliveries.

○ **What is the best known fetal risk factor for shoulder dystocia?**

Fetal weight. The risk is approximately 0.2% if the fetus weighs 2500 to 3000 g but rises to about 10% if the baby weighs 4000 to 5000 g and up to 20% if the baby weighs more than 4500 g. In diabetic patient's these latter weight-associated risks are approximately doubled.

○ **What is the difference between a classic C-section and a newer C-section?**

A classic C-section is a vertical incision in the uterus. This type of C-section predisposes women to future uterine rupture. Hence, subsequent deliveries should be made via C-section as well.

The newer C-sections are low transverse incisions; they have a much lower rate of uterine rupture with subsequent deliveries.

○ **What percentage of women can have vaginal births after low transverse incision C-sections (aka VBAC)?**

75%. Vaginal birth is contraindicated after a <u>classic</u> C-section.

○ **What is the average blood loss for vaginal delivery and for cesarean section?**

400 to 600 mL for vaginal delivery and 800 to 1000 mL for cesarean section.

○ **Why is a rapid cesarean delivery an important part of maternal resuscitation?**

Removing the fetus relieves aortocaval compression. With uterine contraction after delivery, some blood may enter the circulation and may help increase venous return. Cardiac output produced by chest compression may be more adequate without the fetus.

○ **What happens if some placenta or fetal membranes are left inside the uterus?**

Retained tissue or products of conception may lead to postpartum hemorrhage. It also increases the risk of postpartum endometritis.

● ● ● **POSTPARTUM** ● ● ●

○ **What is the puerperium?**

The puerperium refers to the time just after birth and lasts about 6 weeks. It is the time it takes the uterus to return to its nonpregnant state.

○ **What are the causes of immediate postpartum hemorrhage?**

Uterine atony, followed by vaginal/cervical lacerations, and retained placenta or placental fragments.

○ **What is the most common cause of postpartum hemorrhage?**

Uterine atony.

○ **What factors predispose one to uterine atony?**

Fetal macrosomia, polyhydramnios, abnormal labor progress, amnionitis, oxytocin stimulation, and multiple gestations.

○   **What is routinely done to decrease the risk of postpartum hemorrhage?**

Uterine massage and oxytocin. Lacerations are sutured. In severe cases, where bleeding cannot be stopped, the hypogastric vessels are ligated or a hysterectomy is performed.

○   **What is lochia?**

Lochia refers to the uterine discharge that follows delivery. It consists of necrotic decidua, blood, inflammatory cells, and bacteria. This discharge lasts about 5 weeks.

○   **A patient presents 3 days postpartum with a fever, malaise, and lower abdominal pain. On examination, a foul lochia and tender boggy uterus are present. What is the most likely diagnosis?**

Endometritis. This typically occurs 1 to 3 days postpartum. It is felt that the mechanism of infection is from ascending cervicovaginal flora.

○   **Is endometritis more common after vaginal delivery or C-section?**

The rate of endometritis is 5 to 10 times greater after C-section.

○   **What is the treatment for endometritis?**

Admission and IV broad-spectrum antibiotics.

○   **Why is the risk of a thromboembolic event increased in the postpartum time?**

While immediate platelet count changes are variable, platelet counts reach a peak at 2 weeks postpartum. Fibrinogen levels remain elevated for at least 1 week as do factors VII, VIII, IX, and X. In addition, there is greater vessel trauma and less mobility.

○   **What postpartum immunizations are part of standard care?**

Rubella and rubeola immunization vaccinations should be administered to all susceptible postpartum women. In theory, diphtheria and tetanus toxoid boosters may also be administered if indicated. The non-isoimmunized Rh-negative patient should also receive anti-D immune globulin if her child is Rh positive.

○   **How common are "postpartum" blues?**

50% to 70% of mothers will have postpartum blues.

○   **How common is postpartum depression?**

Only 4% to 10% of postpartum mothers will have true postpartum depression.

○   **When does ovulation resume postpartum?**

In nonlactating women, ovulation may occur as early as 27 days postpartum. The average is 10 weeks. In women exclusively breast-feeding, ovulation may be delayed for the duration of active breast-feeding, although the mean is 6 months.

○   **When may coitus resume following delivery?**

Most physicians instruct their patients to abstain from coitus for 6 weeks. From a physiologic standpoint, once uterine involution and perineal healing are complete, coitus may resume.

○   **What is Sheehan syndrome?**

Anterior pituitary necrosis following postpartum hemorrhage and hypotension. It results in amenorrhea, decreased breast size, and decreased pubic hair.

● ● ● REFERENCES ● ● ●

Beckmann C, Ling F, Smith R, Barzansky B, Herbert W, Laube D. *Obstetrics and Gynecology.* 5th ed. Philadelphia, PA: Lippincott, Williams & Wilkins; 2007.

Bickley L. *Bates' Guide to Physical Examination and History Taking.* 9th ed. Philadelphia, PA: Lippincott, Williams & Wilkins; 2007.

Decherney A, Nathan L, Goodwin TM, Laufer N. *Current Diagnosis and Treatment Obstetrics & Gynecoogy.* 10th ed. Lange Series. New York, NY: McGraw-Hill; 2007.

DeGowin R, LeBlond R, Brown D. *DeGowin's Diagnostic Evaluation. The Complete Guide to Assessment, Examination, and Differential Diagnosis.* 8th ed. New York, NY: McGraw-Hill; 2004.

Lemcke D, Pattison J, Marshall L, Cowley D. *Current Care of Women Diagnosis & Treatment.* Lange Series. New York, NY: McGraw-Hill; 2004.

Saslow D, et al. American Cancer Society Guidelines for Breast Screening with MRI as an Adjunct to Mammography. *CA Cancer J Clin.* 2007;57:75–89. http://caonline.amcancersoc.org/cgi/content/full/57/2/75#T1.

Gilbert D, Sande M, Moellering R Jr, Eliopoulous G. *The Sanford Guide to Antimicrobial Therapy.* 38th ed. Antimicrobial Therapy, Inc., Sperryville, VA; 2008.

Smith R, Saslow D, et al. American Cancer Society Guidelines for Breast Cancer Screening: Update 2003. *CA Cancer J Clin.* 2003;53:141.

Centers for Disease Control. Cervical Cancer Screening Guidelines, Table 1. http://www.cdc.gov/std/hpv/ScreeningTables.pdf. Accessed June 2009.

UpToDate (online 17.1). www.uptodateonline.com. Accessed May 2009, June 2009.

CHAPTER 9

Musculoskeletal

John Oliphant, MHP, MSEd, RPAC, ATC

● ● ● GENERAL ORTHOPEDIC CONCEPTS ● ● ●

○ **By definition, a <u>sprain</u> involves injury to what types of connective tissue?**

Those tissues that give support to joints: ligaments and joint capsules.

○ **How are sprains classified?**

First degree: Minor stretching or partial tear of ligaments/capsule without instability when the joint is stressed

Second degree: Significant stretching and partial tear of ligaments/capsule allowing for partial opening of the joint when stressed

Third degree: Complete tear of ligaments/capsule with complete opening of joint when stressed

○ **By definition, a <u>strain</u> involves injury to what two types of connective tissue?**

Muscle or tendon.

○ **What is a valgus deformity? Varus deformity?**

- Valgus deformity is the angulation of an extremity at a joint with the more distal part angled away from the midline.
- Varus deformity is the angulation of an extremity at a joint with the more distal part angled toward the midline.

○ **Are dislocations and sprains more common in children or adults?**

Dislocations and ligamentous injuries are uncommon in prepubertal children as the ligaments and joints are quite strong as compared to the adjoining growth plates. Excessive force applied to a child's joint is more likely to cause a fracture through the growth plate than a dislocation or sprain.

○ **Which type of Salter-Harris fracture has the worst prognosis?**

Type V (compression injury of the epiphyseal plate). **(See Figure 9-1.)**

○ **Which type of Salter-Harris fracture is most common?**

Type II (a triangular fracture involving the metaphysis and an epiphyseal separation). **(See Figure 9-1.)**

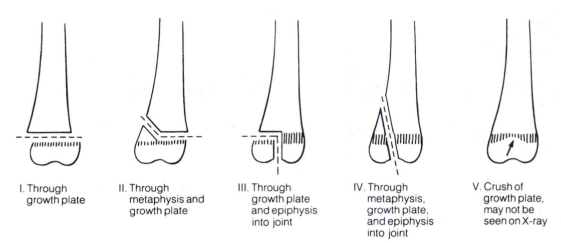

I. Through growth plate

II. Through metaphysis and growth plate

III. Through growth plate and epiphysis into joint

IV. Through metaphysis, growth plate, and epiphysis into joint

V. Crush of growth plate, may not be seen on X-ray

Figure 9-1 (Reproduced, with permission, from Stone CK, Humphries RL. *Current Diagnosis & Treatment Emergency Medicine.* 6th ed. New York, NY: McGraw-Hill; 2008, Fig. 26-2.)

○ **What is a stress fracture?**

A stress or fatigue fracture is caused by small, repetitive forces that usually involve the metatarsal shafts, the distal tibia, and the femoral neck (though many other bones may be affected). These fractures may not be seen on initial radiographs.

○ **After a fracture, what are the three stages of healing?**

1. Inflammatory
2. Reparative
3. Remodeling

○ **The end of the reparative phase is usually marked by clinical union of the fracture. How is clinical union defined?**

- The fractured bones do not shift on clinical examination
- The fracture site is nontender
- The patient can use the limb without significant pain

○ **A pneumatic tourniquet can be inflated on an extremity to a level higher than a patient's systolic blood pressure for how long without damaging underlying vessels or neurons?**

2 hours.

○ **What basic disorder contributes to the pathophysiology of compartment syndrome?**

Increased pressure within closed tissue spaces compromising blood flow to muscle and nerve tissue. There are three prerequisites to the development of compartment syndrome:

1. Limiting space
2. Increased tissue pressure
3. Decreased tissue perfusion

○   **What are the two basic mechanisms for elevated compartment pressure?**

1. External compression—by circumferential casts, dressings, burn eschar, or pneumatic pressure garments

2. Volume increase within the compartment—hemorrhage into the compartment, IV infiltration, or edema secondary to injury or due to postischemic swelling

○   **What intracompartmental pressure level raises concern?**

Normal pressure is less than 10 mm Hg. It is generally agreed that pressure greater than 30 mm Hg mandates emergency fasciotomy. The treatment for compartment pressures between 20 and 30 mm Hg is controversial and may require surgical consultation, especially if the patient is unreliable, i.e., with an altered level of consciousness.

○   **How do you clinically differentiate between acute compartment syndrome, neurapraxia, and arterial occlusion?**

- The patient will have normal pulses in neuropraxia
- Decreased pulses in compartment syndrome (though this is a very rare and insensitive finding)
- No pulses in arterial occlusion
- Stretching the muscles will cause great pain in compartment syndrome but not in neuropraxia

○   **What fracture is most commonly associated with compartment syndrome?**

The tibia, which often results in anterior compartment syndrome.

○   **What are the early signs and symptoms of compartment syndrome?**

- Tenderness and pain out of proportion to the injury
- Pain with active and passive motion
- Hypesthesia and paresthesia

○   **What are the six Ps of compartment syndrome?**

Pain

Pallor

Pulselessness

Paresthesia

Pressure

Paralysis

○   **What four Cs determine muscle viability?**

Color

Consistency

Contraction

Circulation

○   **What are the late signs and symptoms of compartment syndrome?**

- Tense, indurated, and erythematous compartment
- Slow capillary refill
- Pallor and pulselessness

○ **What conditions are in the differential diagnosis of a limp or gait abnormality in a child?**

- Legg-Calvé-Perthes disease (avascular necrosis of the femoral head)
- Osgood-Schlatter disease
- Avulsion of the tibial tubercle
- Infection
- Toxic transient tenosynovitis
- Patellofemoral subluxation

- Chondromalacia patella
- Slipped capital femoral epiphysis
- Septic arthritis
- Metatarsal fracture
- Proximal stress fracture
- Toddler fracture (spiral tibia fracture)

• • • DISORDERS OF THE SHOULDER AND UPPER ARM • • •

○ **What are the four muscles of the rotator cuff?**

1. Supraspinatus
2. Infraspinatus
3. Teres minor
4. Subscapularis

○ **Which bone is most often fractured at birth?**

The clavicle.

○ **What is the most common type of shoulder dislocation?**

Anterior dislocation.

○ **A patient cannot actively abduct her shoulder due to pain and weakness. What injury does this suggest?**

A rotator cuff tear.

○ **What is the most common joint dislocation?**

Anterior shoulder dislocations account for half of all joint dislocations.

○ **What nerve is usually injured in glenohumeral dislocation?**

Axillary nerve.

○ **What is the most reliable method of diagnosing a posterior shoulder dislocation?**

Performing a physical examination and ordering a scapular Y-view X-ray. A posterior dislocation of the shoulder is often missed with a standard radiographic shoulder series.

○ **In a humeral shaft fracture, what nerve is most commonly injured?**

The radial nerve.

○ **A patient presents with a complaint of pain at the site of the deltoid insertion with radiation into the back of the arm (C5 distribution). On examination, there is increased pain with active abduction from 70° to 120°. X-rays reveal calcification at the tendinous insertion of the greater tuberosity. What is the likely diagnosis?**

Supraspinatus tendonitis.

○ **What is the most common tendon affected in calcified tendonitis?**

The supraspinatus.

○ **What humerus position puts the shoulder in greatest risk of dislocating anteriorly?**

Abduction and external rotation.

○ **Shoulder separations happen at what joint?**

The acromioclavicular joint.

○ **Shoulder dislocations happen at what joint?**

The glenohumeral joint.

○ **What is the best way to position a patient's arm to palpate the subacromial bursa?**

With the humerus held in passive extension.

○ **What muscle forms the anterior wall of the axilla?**

The pectoralis major.

○ **What muscle forms the posterior wall of the axilla?**

The latissimus dorsi.

○ **What muscle is most frequently absent (either totally or partially) due to a congenital anomaly?**

The pectoralis major.

○ **What portion of the bicep is most commonly torn from its bony attachment?**

The long head of the biceps.

○ **Winging of the scapula indicates a weakness of what muscle?**

The serratus anterior muscle.

○ **A positive drop arm test is suggestive of what condition?**

A tear in the rotator cuff (especially the supraspinatus muscle).

○ **What is the likely diagnosis in a patient with significantly restricted range of motion at the shoulder joint 4 weeks after a painful shoulder injury?**

Adhesive capsulitis (frozen shoulder).

○ **What other injuries may occur with an anterior dislocation of the shoulder?**

- Axillary nerve injury
- Axillary artery injury (geriatric patients)
- Compression fracture of the humeral head (Hillsack deformity)
- Rotator cuff tear
- Fractures of the anterior glenoid lip
- Fractures of the greater tuberosity of the humerus

○   **What type of shoulder dislocation is pictured in the radiograph Figure 9-2?**

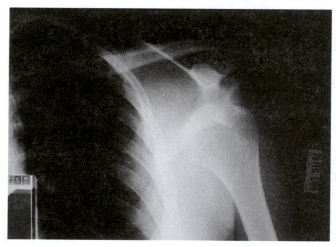

Figure 9-2   (Photo contributed by Kevin J. Knoop, MD MS, reproduced with permission from Knoop KJ, Stack LB, Storrow AB. *Atlas of Emergency Medicine.* 3rd ed. New York, NY: McGraw-Hill; 2010, Fig. 11.5)

This shows an anterior shoulder dislocation. Note the humeral head is anterior and inferior to the glenoid fossa

● ● ● DISORDERS OF THE ELBOW AND FOREARM ● ● ●

○   **What is "nursemaid elbow"?**

A subluxation of the radial head. During forceful retraction, fibers of the annular ligament that encircle the radial neck become trapped between the radial head and the capitellum. On presentation, children hold their arm in slight flexion and pronation.

○   **A patient has a fracture of the proximal third of the ulna. What additional injury should be ruled out?**

A dislocation of the radial head. An anterior dislocation is most common. A proximal ulna fracture with a radial head dislocation is often called a Monteggia fracture.

○   **What is the significance of the fat pad sign seen on a lateral radiograph of the elbow following an injury?**

This indicates the presence of an effusion or hemarthrosis of the elbow joint, suggestive of an occult fracture of the radial head, supracondylar fracture of the humerus, or proximal ulnar fracture.

○   **What is the order of appearance of the ossification centers in the elbow? At what approximate age do they appear?**

Remember the acronym **CRITOE**:

- **C**apitellum (3–5 months)
- **R**adial head (4–5 years)
- **I**nternal (medial) epicondyle (5–7 years)
- **T**rochlea (8–9 years)
- **O**lecranon (9–10 years)
- **E**xternal (lateral) epicondyle (11–12 years)

○ **What is the most common site of bursitis?**

The olecranon bursa of the elbow.

○ **What is the usual mechanism of injury in a supracondylar distal humeral fracture?**

A fall on an outstretched arm.

○ **What artery is commonly injured with a supracondylar distal humeral fracture?**

Brachial artery.

○ **What nerve is commonly injured with a supracondylar fracture?**

The median nerve.

○ **Why is a displaced supracondylar fracture of the distal humerus in a child considered an emergency?**

Because of the high potential for neurovascular compromise, which may lead to ischemic injury or nerve palsy.

○ **What nerve injury is associated with a medial epicondyle fracture?**

Ulnar nerve.

○ **What is the most commonly missed fracture in the elbow region?**

A radial head fracture. Like a scaphoid (navicular) fracture in the wrist, radiographic signs of a radial head fracture may not show up for days after the injury. A positive fat pad sign may be the only finding suggestive of this injury.

○ **Which epicondyle is involved in tennis elbow?**

The lateral epicondyle.

○ **Which epicondyle is involved in golfer elbow?**

The medial epicondyle.

○ **Does damage to the olecranon bursa tend to produce diffuse or localized swelling?**

Localized as shown in Figure 9-3.

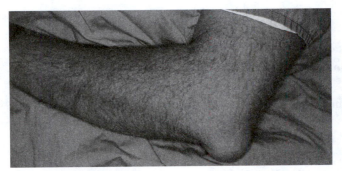

Figure 9-3 (Photo contributed by Selim Suner, MD MS, reproduced with permission from Knoop KJ, Stack LB, Storrow AB. *Atlas of Emergency Medicine*. 3rd ed. New York, NY: McGraw-Hill; 2010, Fig. 12.17.)

○ **Which bone articulates with the humerus in the olecranon fossa?**

The ulna.

○ **What are the three bony articulations of the elbow?**

1. The humeroulnar joint
2. The humeroradial joint
3. The radioulnar joint

○ **Where can the ulnar nerve be best palpated at the elbow joint?**

In the sulcus between the medial epicondyle and the olecranon fossa.

○ **What are the primary muscles that produce active elbow flexion?**

The brachialis and biceps muscles.

○ **What are the primary muscles that produce active elbow extension?**

The triceps muscles.

○ **Besides flexion and extension, what other motions happen at the elbow joint?**

Supination and pronation.

○ **What motor neurons are being evaluated with biceps, brachioradialis, and triceps reflex testing?**

• Biceps reflex—C5
• Brachioradialis reflex—C6
• Triceps reflex—C7

• • • DISORDERS OF THE WRIST AND HAND • • •

○ **What tendons are involved in de Quervain tenosynovitis?**

The abductor pollicis longus and the extensor pollicis longus and brevis tendons.

○ **What is Finkelstein test?**

A test used to determine whether a patient has de Quervain tenosynovitis. If pain is elicited when the patient grasps his thumb with the fingers of the same hand and deviates his wrist in the ulnar direction, then the test is positive.

○ **What is the most common type of peripheral nerve compression?**

Carpal tunnel syndrome, which involves compression of the median nerve at the wrist. This syndrome is more often diagnosed in female patients than in male patients. Clinically, the patient will have pain and weakness, which worsen at night. Splinting the wrist in a neutral position or corticosteroid injections may provide relief. If conservative measures do not work, surgical decompression can be performed.

○ **Which fingers are potentially affected by carpal tunnel syndrome?**

The first, second, third, and the radial side of the fourth finger.

○   **Describe Tinel and Phalen tests:**

Both test for carpal tunnel syndrome:

Tinel test: Tapping the volar aspect of the wrist over the median nerve with the hand hyperextended produces pain and/or paresthesias in the distribution of the median nerve

Phalen test: Full flexion at the wrist for 1 minute leads to paresthesia along distribution of median nerve

○   **What injury is often referred to as gamekeeper thumb?**

Instability of the ulnar collateral ligament of the MCP joint of the thumb. This may be due to chronic valgus stresses on the joint or more commonly an acute injury (such as a fall during skiing) that results in a sudden valgus stress. Often, an acute injury of the ulnar collateral ligament of the thumb is referred to as "skier thumb."

○   **What is a felon and how is it treated?**

A felon is a subcutaneous infection in the pulp space of the fingertip, usually due to *Staphylococcus aureus*. Treat by incising the pulp space.

○   **What is the most commonly fractured carpal bone?**

The scaphoid bone (navicular).

○   **How is a scaphoid (navicular) fracture diagnosed?**

The initial radiograph frequently appears to be normal. If the patient has tenderness in the anatomical snuff box or pain with axial loading of the thumb, a scaphoid (navicular) fracture should be presumed and the hand splinted. A follow-up radiograph 10 to 14 days after the injury may then reveal the fracture.

○   **What is the most feared complication of a scaphoid (navicular) fracture?**

Avascular necrosis. The more proximal the fracture, the more commonly avascular necrosis occurs.

○   **What is Kienbock disease?**

Avascular necrosis of the lunate with collapse of the lunate secondary to fracture. As with a scaphoid (navicular) fracture, initial wrist X-rays may not demonstrate the fracture. Therefore, tenderness over the lunate warrants immobilization.

○   **What is a boutonnière deformity and how does the injured finger appear?**

It is a rupture of the extensor apparatus of the PIP joint of a finger. The injured finger appears flexed at the PIP joint and extended at the DIP joint.

○   **How is a boutonnière deformity initially treated?**

By splinting the PIP joint in full extension.

○   **Describe Dupuytren contracture:**

A nodular thickening and contraction of the palmar fascia.

○   **Describe Galeazzi fracture/dislocation:**

Displaced fracture of the distal radius with a dislocation of the distal ulna or a fracture of the distal ulnar physis.

○   **What are Kanavel four cardinal signs of infectious digital flexor tenosynovitis?**

1. Tenderness along the tendon sheath
2. Finger held in flexion
3. Pain on passive extension of the finger
4. Finger swelling

○   **What fracture has likely occurred to the individual in Figure 9-4?**

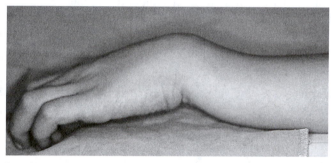

Figure 9-4 (Photo contributed by Cathleen M. Vossler, MD, reproduced with permission from Knoop KJ, Stack LB, Storrow AB. *Atlas of Emergency Medicine.* 3rd ed. New York, NY: McGraw-Hill; 2010, Fig. 11.19.)

A Colles fracture, which is a complete fracture of the distal radius in which the fragment is displaced dorsally as shown in the radiograph in Figure 9-5.

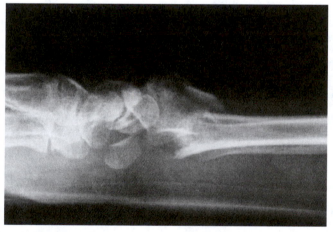

Figure 9-5 (Reproduced, with permission, from Brunicardi FC, Andersen DK, et al. *Schwartz's Priniciples of Surgery.* 8th ed. New York, NY: McGraw-Hill; 2007, Fig. 13.12.)

○   **Active adduction of the thumb tests which nerve?**

Ulnar nerve.

○   **What is the best X-ray view for diagnosing lunate and perilunate dislocations?**

Lateral X-ray views of the wrist.

○ **A patient presents with an injury to his second (index) finger after forced flexion. He reports an inability to actively extend the tip of his finger (but he can extend it passively) (see Figure 9-6). What is the likely injury?**

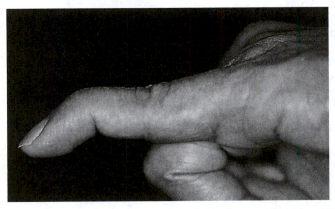

Figure 9-6 (Reproduced, with permission, from Knoop KJ, Stack LB, Storrow AB. *Atlas of Emergency Medicine.* 3rd ed. New York, NY: McGraw-Hill; 2010, Fig. 11.51.)

Mallet finger, which is a result of either a rupture of the distal extensor tendon or an avulsion fraction of the tendon insertion on the distal phalanx with a dorsal plate avulsion.

○ **What nerve provides sensations to both the dorsum and volar aspects of the hand?**

Ulnar. Radial is primarily dorsum, and median is primarily volar.

○ **A patient presents with a small, soft bump on the dorsum of her wrist. The mass has a jelly-like consistency and is not significantly point tender. What is the likely diagnosis?**

A ganglion cyst.

○ **In the wrist, what bone is dislocated most often?**

Lunate. It is also the second most commonly fractured bone in the wrist.

○ **How is a perilunate dislocation diagnosed?**

By AP and lateral X-rays. The lunate remains in alignment with the radial fossa, while the other carpal bones appear displaced.

○ **On an X-ray of the hand, the AP view shows a triangular shaped lunate. Diagnosis?**

Lunate dislocation. Lateral films will reveal what resembles a cup spilling water.

○ **A patient presents with a snapping sensation in the wrist and a click. The X-ray of the patient's hand reveals a 3 mm space between the scaphoid and the lunate. What is your diagnosis?**

Scaphoid dislocation.

○ **In a boxer fracture, how much angulation of the fifth metacarpal neck is acceptable?**

Less than 40°.

○ **What ligament in the hand is commonly injured in a fall while skiing?**

Thumb MCP joint ulnar collateral ligament rupture (gamekeeper thumb).

○ **Why is it important to get radiographic studies after an acute dislocation?**

To rule out other injuries including ligament avulsion, articular fracture, or other signs that might indicate the presence of gross joint instability.

○ **Atrophy of the thenar eminence of the palm may indicate entrapment of what nerve?**

The median nerve.

○ **Atrophy of the hypothenar eminence of the palm may indicate entrapment of what nerve?**

The ulnar nerve.

○ **The median nerve passes through the carpal tunnel at the wrist. Where does the ulnar nerve pass through at the wrist?**

The tunnel of Guyon.

○ **What other important structure passes through the tunnel of Guyon?**

The ulnar artery.

○ **What do you call an infection that occurs on the posterior distal aspect of a finger, may wrap around the border of the finger nail, and often starts with a hangnail?**

A paronychia.

○ **How should one treat a paronychia that has formed an abscess?**

Incision and drainage of the abscess. Antibiotics may be used as well if an associated cellulitis has developed or in the rare situation where systemic signs and symptoms are present.

○ **Do most median nerve injuries occur as a result of acute macrotrauma or chronic microtrauma?**

Most median nerve injuries are a result of repetitive movements over time producing chronic micro trauma.

● ● ● DISORDERS OF THE BACK/SPINE ● ● ●

○ **What is the leading cause of disability for patients younger than 45 years?**

Chronic lower back pain. Most patients with lower back pain do not need surgery and will recover from their injury within 6 weeks.

○ **What must be checked in a patient with Down syndrome before medical clearance can be given for participation in sports?**

Atlantoaxial instability must be ruled out by means of cervical radiographs and possibly CT scans with the head in various positions; 10% to 20% of children with Down syndrome have unstable atlantoaxial joints.

○ **What vertebrae most commonly sustains a thoracolumbar wedge fracture in the elderly?**

L1.

○ **A patient in a motor vehicle accident sustains a hyperextension injury to the neck. Plain films reveal a C2 bilateral facet fracture through the pedicles. What is the common name for this type of fracture?**

A hangman fracture.

○ **Injury to what cervical area results in Horner syndrome (ptosis, miosis, and anhidrosis)?**

Disruption of the cervical sympathetic chain at C7 through T2.

○ **What spinal level corresponds to the dermatomal innervation of the perianal region? The nipple line? The index finger? The knee? The lateral foot?**

- Perianal region: S2-S4
- Nipple line: T4
- Index finger: C6
- Knee: L4
- Lateral foot: S1

○ **A patient has difficulty squatting and standing due to weakness. What is the most likely spinal pathology?**

L4 root compression with involvement of quadriceps muscles.

○ **What is the most common site of lumbar disk herniations?**

Most clinically important lumbar disk herniations are at the L4-L5 or L5-S1 intervertebral levels. Evaluate these patients by checking for weakness of ankle and great toe dorsiflexors (L5). Also check pinprick sensation over the medial aspect of the foot (L5) and the lateral portion of the feet (S1).

○ **What is the eponym for a C1 burst fracture from vertical compression?**

Jefferson fracture.

○ **Where is the most common site of cervical disk herniation?**

Cervical disk herniations are most common at C6-C7, but also may occur at C5-C6 and other levels.

○ **Define spondylolysis:**

A defect in the pars interarticularis.

○ **Define spondylolisthesis:**

The forward movement of one vertebral body on the vertebra below. Spondylolysis can lead to spondylolisthesis as seen in the Figure 9-7.

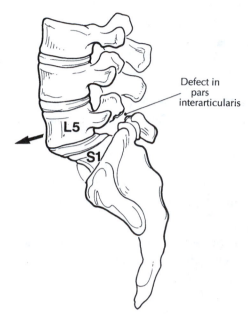

Defect in
pars
interarticularis

Figure 9-7 (Reproduced, with permission, from Chen MYM, Pope TL Jr, Ott DL. *Basic Radiology.* New York, NY: McGraw-Hill; 2004, Fig. 13.12.)

○ **A patient presents with back pain and complaints of incontinence. On examination, loss of anal reflex and decreased sphincter tone is noted. What is your diagnosis?**

Cauda equina syndrome. The most consistent finding is urinary retention. On physical examination, you should expect saddle anesthesia (numbness over the posterior superior thighs as well as numbness of the buttocks and perineum).

○ **A patient has an avulsion fracture of the spinous process of C7 with a history of a hyperflexion mechanism. What is the diagnosis?**

Clay shoveler fracture—a fracture involving the spinous process of C6, C7, or T1. The mechanism is usually flexion or a direct blow.

○ **A patient suffers a bilateral interfacetal dislocation as a result of excessive flexion. What is your concern?**

Ligament disruption has occurred causing the C-spine to be unstable.

○ **Stable or unstable: clay shoveler fracture?**

Stable.

○ **Stable or unstable: fracture of the posterior arch of C1?**

Stable.

○ **While providing medical coverage at a soccer game, a player goes down complaining of neck pain after a hard collision with another player and the ground. She does not lose consciousness, has full sensation and motor function in her extremities, but has significant point tenderness directly over her cervical vertebrae. How should you remove this player from the field?**

Apply a stiff extrication collar, strap her to a backboard, and transport her to the hospital via ambulance for imaging studies. She may have a nondisplaced cervical fracture that could shift causing spinal cord damage if she is allowed to move freely.

○ **From what spinal nerve roots does the brachial plexus originate?**

C5 through T1.

○ **Someone with a C5 disk herniation causing right-sided nerve root impingement will likely have pain in what part of his/her body besides the neck?**

The right shoulder.

○ **At what level does spinal stenosis most commonly occur?**

L3-4 and L4-5 interspaces.

○ **In patients with significant lumbar spinal stenosis, does walking lead to worsening or improving leg pain?**

Worsening.

○ **In what gender does scoliosis most commonly occur?**

Females.

○ **In males, when is kyphosis most common?**

During adolescences.

○ **In women, when is kyphosis most common?**

After menopause when osteoporosis and vertebral body fractures may lead to kyphosis.

○ **The C7 neurologic area is responsible for sensation in what part of the body?**

The third finger.

○ **Of cervical, thoracic, and lumbar intervertebral disks, which has the lowest rate of herniation?**

Thoracic.

○ **Fifty percent of cervical rotation takes place between what two cervical vertebrae?**

C1 (atlas) and C2 (the axis). The remaining 50% is split up fairly evenly among the remaining five cervical vertebrae.

○ **The 12th ribs articulate with what vertebrae?**

The 12th thoracic vertebrae. Generally, the 12 sets of ribs articulate posteriorly with the thoracic vertebrae assigned the same number (i.e., 1st ribs articulate with T1, 2nd ribs with T2, etc.).

○ **What condition must be ruled out in a middle-aged man with profound limitation in spinal mobility?**

Ankylosing spondylitis.

● ● ● DISORDERS OF THE HIP AND PELVIS ● ● ●

○ **Describe the leg position of a patient with a femoral neck fracture:**

Shortened, abducted, and slightly externally rotated.

○ **Describe the leg position of a patient with an anterior hip dislocation:**

Mildly flexed, abducted, and externally rotated.

○ **Describe the leg position of a patient with a posterior hip dislocation:**

Shortened, adducted, flexed, and internally rotated.

○ **What mechanism of injury typically leads to posterior hip dislocations and what are some common complications?**

The mechanism of injury is force applied to a flexed knee directed posteriorly. This dislocation is associated with sciatic nerve injury and avascular necrosis of the femoral head.

○ **Describe the leg position of a patient with an intertrochanteric hip fracture:**

Shortened, externally rotated, and abducted.

○ **Describe a typical patient with a slipped capital femoral epiphysis:**

An obese boy, 10 to 16 years old, with groin or knee discomfort increasing with activity. He may also have a limp. The slip can occur bilaterally and best observed on a lateral view of the hip.

○ **What is the Young classification system for pelvic fractures?**

The Young system divides pelvic fractures into four categories depending on the type and direction of force:

1. Lateral compression (LC)

2. Anterior–posterior compression (APC)

3. Vertical sheer (VS)

4. Combination mechanical mixed (CM)

○ **Describe a lateral compression pelvic fracture (LC):**

This fracture is usually caused by a motor vehicle collision in which the car and patient are broadsided. The lateral force from the collision causes a sacral fracture, iliac wing fracture, or a sacroiliac ligamentous injury and a transverse fracture of the pubic rami. There is no ligamentous injury at the pubic symphysis.

○ **Describe an anterior–posterior compression pelvic fracture (APC):**

APCs are usually caused by a head-on motor vehicle collision. They always include a disruption of the pubis symphysis and usually involve a disruption (of different degrees) of the sacroiliac joint.

○ **Describe a vertical sheer pelvic fracture (VS):**

VSs are usually caused by a fall. They involve an injury of the sacroiliac ligaments and either a disruption of the pubis symphysis or vertical fractures through the pubic rami. The iliac wing is vertically displaced.

○ **What life-threatening injury is associated with pelvic fractures?**

Severe hemorrhage, usually retroperitoneal. Up to 6 L of blood can be accommodated in this space.

○ **What pelvic fracture is most likely to involve severe hemorrhage?**

Vertical sheer fractures.

○ **Which pelvic fracture is most likely to involve bladder rupture?**

Lateral compression fractures.

○ **Which pelvic fracture is most likely to involve urethral injury?**

Anterior–posterior compression fracture.

○ **Which fracture is associated with avascular necrosis of the femoral head?**

Femoral neck fractures.

○ **Describe the common features of a slipped femoral capital epiphysis:**

The injury usually occurs in adolescence. The condition typically presents with anterior proximal thigh pain and a painful limp. Frequently, hip motion is limited, particularly internal rotation. Evaluation is aided by AP and frog-leg lateral radiographs of both hips.

○ **Which type of hip dislocation is most common: anterior, posterior, lateral, or medial?**

Posterior hip dislocations are the most common, accounting for approximately 90% of all hip dislocations.

○ **A fracture of the acetabulum may be associated with damage to what nerve?**

The sciatic nerve.

○ **Describe the signs and symptoms of pressure on the first sacral root (S1):**

Symptoms of S1 injury include pain radiating to the midgluteal region, posterior thigh, posterior calf, and down to the heel and sole of the foot. Sensory signs are localized to the lateral toes. S1 root compression typically involves the plantar flexor muscles of the foot and toes. The ankle reflex is decreased or absent.

○ **What is the most commonly missed hip fracture?**

Femoral neck fracture.

○ **What is the most common site of aseptic necrosis?**

The hip.

○ **What must be done to effectively palpate the coccyx and sacrococcygeal joint?**

A rectal examination.

○ **What test can be done on newborn infants to check for a congenitally dislocating hip?**

Ortolani click test. The child is positioned on his/her back and the hips are flexed, abducted, and externally rotated. The involved hip is unable to be abducted as far as the uninvolved side and there is a palpable click when the hip is reduced.

○ **What is the primary hip flexor muscle?**

The iliopsoas muscle.

○ **What is the primary hip extensor muscle?**

The gluteus maximus muscle.

○ **What is the primary hip abductor muscle?**

The gluteus medius muscle.

○ **What is the primary hip adductor muscle?**

The adductor longus muscle.

○ **Point tenderness and a boggy feeling over the greater trochanter may be indicative of what?**

Trochanteric bursitis.

○ **What are the superior and inferior attachments of the inguinal ligament?**

The superior attachment is at the anterior, superior iliac spines and the inferior attachment is at the pubic tubercles.

○ **What nerve lies midway between the ischial tuberosities and greater trochanters and can best be palpated with the hip in a flexed position?**

The sciatic nerve.

○ **How are the femoral nerve, artery, and vein positioned in relationship to each other?**

Moving from lateral to medial just inferior to the inguinal ligament, first comes the nerve, then the artery, and the most medial structure of the three is the vein.

● ● ● DISORDERS OF THE KNEE AND LOWER LEG ● ● ●

○ **What long bone is most commonly fractured?**

The tibia.

○ **A 43-year-old female runner complains that she has diffuse, aching <u>anterior</u> knee pain that is worsened when she walks up or down stairs or when she squats down. There has been no acute trauma, but she has been increasing her running mileage. No effusion is present. What is the probable diagnosis?**

Patellofemoral pain syndrome.

○ **What is the most significant complication of a proximal tibial metaphyseal fracture?**

Arterial involvement, especially when there is a valgus deformity.

○ **Why "tap" a knee with an acute hemarthrosis?**

Tapping the knee relieves pressure and pain for the patient and will allow you to ascertain whether fat globules are present, indicating a fracture.

○ **What are the four compartments of the leg?**

1. Anterior
2. Lateral
3. Deep posterior
4. Superficial posterior

○ **What is the most common site of compartment syndrome?**

The anterior compartment of the leg.

○ **What are the most common lower extremity fractures in children?**

Tibial and fibular shaft fractures, usually secondary to twist forces.

○ **What radiograph would one order for a suspected patellar fracture in a child?**

Standard radiographs including patellar or "sunrise views," plus radiographs of the uninvolved knee for comparison.

○ **What are the differences between an avulsion fracture of the tibial tubercle and Osgood-Schlatter disease (which also involves the tibial tubercle)?**

- Avulsion fractures present with an <u>acute</u> inability to walk. A lateral view of the knee is most diagnostic. Treatment is often surgical.
- Osgood-Schlatter disease is an overuse injury, which gradually develops in growing children. It is exacerbated by running, jumping, and kneeling activities. Treatment involves ice, padding, stretching, NSAIDS, rest, and occasionally immobilization.

○ **True/False: Osgood-Schlatter disease often requires surgical intervention:**

False. It is usually a self-limiting condition with symptoms resolving by early adulthood. An enlarged, but painless tibial tuberosity often persists.

○ **What is a toddler fracture?**

A spiral fracture of the tibia without fibular involvement. This type of fracture in toddlers is a common cause of limping or refusal to walk.

○   **With a complete rupture of the medial collateral ligament, what would be felt by the examiner during a valgus stress of the knee?**

Excessive laxity with no firm endpoint.

○   **A female basketball player plants her foot to make a quick change of direction while running down the court. She feels a popping sensation and falls to the ground in pain. Later that day she has a large effusion. Which knee ligament did she likely tear?**

Anterior cruciate ligament.

○   **Which test is more sensitive when used to determine an anterior cruciate ligament tear in the knee: the anterior drawer test or the Lachman test?**

The Lachman test is more sensitive because the stabilizing effect of the hamstrings is eliminated. While the knee is held at 20° flexion and the distal femur is stabilized, the lower leg is pulled forward. Significant anterior laxity compared to the other knee is evidence of an anterior cruciate ligament tear.

○   **What lower extremity joint is most commonly affected with pseudogout?**

The knee. The causative agent is calcium pyrophosphate crystals.

○   **What nerve may be injured in a distal femoral fracture?**

Peroneal nerve.

○   **Which is more common, a medial or a lateral tibial plateau fracture?**

The lateral tibial plateau is most commonly fractured. If AP and lateral films are negative and you are suspicious of a tibial plateau fracture, follow-up with oblique views.

○   **What nerve may be injured with a knee dislocation?**

The peroneal nerve.

○   **Does a torn meniscus or torn cruciate ligament produce a more dramatic appearing knee effusion?**

A torn cruciate ligament due to its greater vascular supply.

○   **Are the anterior and posterior cruciate ligaments named based on the location of their attachments to the femur or tibia?**

The tibia.

○   **Is the lateral or medial meniscus injured more frequently and why?**

The medial meniscus is injured far more frequently due to its more firm fixation to the tibia and joint capsule as well as its attachment to the medial collateral ligament. Because the lateral meniscus is smaller, attached more loosely to the tibia, and not attached to the lateral collateral ligament, it has more ease of movement and is less prone to injury.

○   **A patient presents with a large area of swelling localized to the front of the knee, between the patella and the skin after a fall directly on her patella. The likely diagnosis is what?**

Prepatellar bursitis.

○ **Do patellar dislocations usually result in the patella going medially or laterally from its normal position?**

Laterally.

○ **Do patellar dislocations occur more commonly in males or females?**

Females.

○ **What four muscles make up the quadriceps?**

1. Vastus lateralis
2. Vastus intermedius
3. Vastus medialis
4. Rectus femoris

○ **What three muscles make up the hamstrings?**

1. Semimembranosus
2. Semitendinosus
3. Biceps femoris

○ **What condition is often a result of avascular necrosis of a segment of subchondral bone, typically involving the lateral surface of the medial femoral condyle?**

Osteochondritis dissecans. This condition may also give rise to loose bodies within the joint.

● ● ● DISORDERS OF THE ANKLE AND FOOT ● ● ●

○ **What is the most common type of ankle injury?**

Sprains account for the majority of all ankle injuries. Of these, most involve the lateral complex. The anterior talofibular ligament is the most commonly injured of the lateral ankle ligaments.

○ **Where are the most common sites of <u>stress</u> fractures in the foot?**

Second and third metatarsals.

○ **A 21-year-old female patient complains of pain and a clicking sound located at the posterior lateral malleolus. A fullness beneath the lateral malleolus is found. What is the probable diagnosis?**

Peroneal tendon subluxation with associated tenosynovitis.

○ **What is the most helpful physical examination test for determining if an anterior talofibular ligament injury has occurred?**

An anterior drawer test will reveal pain and/or laxity if an anterior talofibular ligament injury has occurred.

○ **What are the signs and symptoms for compartment syndrome involving the anterior compartment of the leg?**

Pain on active and passive dorsiflexion and plantar flexion of the foot, and hypesthesia/paresthesia of the first web space of the foot.

○ **What metatarsal fracture is often associated with a disrupted tarsal–metatarsal joint?**

Fracture of the base of the second metatarsal. Treatment may require open reduction and internal fixation.

○ **What fracture is frequently missed when a patient complains of an ankle injury?**

Fracture at the base of the fifth metatarsal, caused by plantar flexion and inversion. Radiographs of the ankle may not include the fifth metatarsal.

○ **Achilles tendon ruptures occur most commonly in what gender and age group?**

Middle-aged men. It occurs most commonly on the left side.

○ **A stress fracture of the second or third metatarsal is suspected but not detected on initial X-rays. How many days after the initial examination should a second X-ray be ordered?**

14 to 21 days.

○ **What tarsal bone is most commonly fractured?**

The calcaneus (60%).

○ **What is the most common injury mechanism that results in a calcaneus fracture?**

A fall from a significant height.

○ **What guidelines are often used to determine if a patient who has suffered an ankle injury needs X-rays?**

The Ottawa ankle rules.

○ **What is the tarsal–metatarsal joint also called?**

Lisfranc joint.

○ **The second metatarsal is the locking mechanism for the midpart of the foot. A fracture at the base of the second metatarsal should raise suspicion of what?**

A disrupted joint. Treatment may require open reduction and internal fixation (ORIF).

○ **What is a Jones fracture?**

An avulsion fracture at the base of the fifth metatarsal, usually secondary to plantar flexion and inversion. Also called a ballet fracture, it is the most common metatarsal fracture.

○ **The mortise view of the ankle is important in the diagnosis of:**

Medial (deltoid) ligament disruption of the ankle.

○ **What potential complication is of concern in distal tibial (medial malleolus) fractures that are treated without surgery?**

Nonunion at the fracture site.

○ **What is the most common presentation of a Charcot joint?**

A swollen ankle and a "bag of bones" appearance on X-ray.

○ **What is the most common cause of a Charcot joint?**

Diabetic peripheral neuropathy.

○ **What nerve is located in the tarsal tunnel?**

The tibial nerve.

○ **What ligament is commonly injured after an inversion ankle sprain?**

The anterior talofibular ligament.

○ **What joint is most commonly affected with gout?**

The great toe MCP joint.

○ **Describe the signs and symptoms of tarsal tunnel syndrome:**

Insidious onset of paresthesia as well as burning pain and numbness on the plantar surface of the foot. Pain radiates superiorly along the medial side of the calf. Rest decreases pain.

○ **The strong ligaments on the medial side of the ankle are collectively known by what name?**

The deltoid ligament.

○ **What ankle motion can lead to injury to the deltoid ligaments?**

Excessive eversion.

○ **Extreme pain on the undersurface of the foot from the calcaneus anteriorly that is often worse with the first few steps of the day or after a prolonged period of standing is likely due to what condition?**

Plantar fasciitis.

○ **What are the characteristics of a Morton foot?**

The second toe is longer than the first, which can lead to an increased risk of overuse injuries.

○ **What group of muscles on the lateral part of the lower leg must be strong to prevent excessive ankle inversion?**

The peroneal muscles.

○ **What are the characteristics of a cavus foot (pes cavus)?**

A high medial longitudinal arch, limited tarsal mobility, poor shock absorption qualities, excessive callus build up on the ball, and/or heel area caused by increased stresses in these areas.

○ **What two plantar flexing muscles attach into the Achilles tendon?**

The gastrocnemius and soleus muscles.

○ **What is the common name for a laterally deviated first toe or hallucis valgus?**

Bunion.

○   **What are the characteristics of a pes planus foot?**

Flat foot, lowered medial longitudinal arch, often associated with excessive foot pronation.

○   **What type of serious ankle injury is seen in the radiograph in Figure 9-8?**

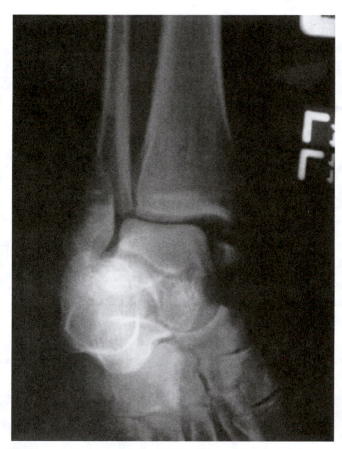

Figure 9-8 (Reproduced, with permission, from Brunicardi FC, Andersen DK, et al. *Schwartz's Principles of Surgery.* 8th ed. New York, NY: McGraw-Hill; 2007, Fig. 42-49.)

A bimalleolar ankle fracture involving the distal tibia and fibula.

● ● ● INFECTIOUS DISEASE ● ● ●

○   **Where is the most common site of infectious arthritis in adults?**

The knee (although it can occur in other joints such as the hip, ankle, and wrist).

○   **What is the most common bacteria implicated in infectious arthritis in adults?**

Staphylococcus aureus.

○   **Where is the most common site of osteomyelitis of the vertebral column?**

The lumbar spine.

○ **What are the different types of osteomyelitis?**
  - Acute hematogenous osteomyelitis
  - *Salmonella* osteomyelitis
  - Chronic hematogenous osteomyelitis
  - Exogenous osteomyelitis

○ **What bacterial organism is most commonly the cause of osteomyelitis?**

Staphylococcus aureus.

○ **What is the most common mechanism that infectious organisms use to reach the bone leading to osteomyelitis?**

By hematogenous spread.

○ **What other mechanisms of pathogen transmission can result in osteomyelitis?**
  - Spread of organisms from contiguous soft tissue infection
  - Direct inoculation of the pathogen into the bone from trauma or surgery

○ **What is the best way to determine the organism(s) that may be causing osteomyelitis?**

Bone biopsy of the suspected infection site with sample sent for culture and sensitivity.

○ **What are the most common findings of osteomyelitis on X-ray?**

Periosteal elevation and demineralization.

○ **Where does acute hematogenous osteomyelitis most commonly affect children?**

The long bones.

○ **Where does acute hematogenous osteomyelitis most commonly affect adults?**

The vertebrae.

○ **What must be done if the patient with osteomyelitis does not respond to antibiotic therapy?**

A surgical decompression of the infected area.

○ **What patients are at risk for developing *Salmonella* osteomyelitis?**

Patients with sickle cell anemia.

● ● ● **NEOPLASTIC DISEASE** ● ● ●

○ **What five primary carcinomas most commonly metastasize to the bone?**
  1. Prostate
  2. Breast
  3. Lung
  4. Kidney
  5. Thyroid

○ **What part of the body is most commonly the site of metastatic tumors?**

The spine.

○ **In what age group are cancerous bone lesions generally metastatic and not primary tumors?**

In patients older than 60 years, most bone lesions are metastatic.

○ **What is more common: benign or malignant tumors of the bone and soft tissue?**

Benign tumors are more common.

○ **What are lipomas?**

Benign, soft, freely movable, nontender masses in the soft tissue.

○ **What are chondrosarcomas?**

Malignant tumors of the cartilage.

○ **What are osteosarcomas?**

Malignant tumors of the bone.

○ **With what is nocturnal bone pain often associated?**

Malignancy, but some benign bone lesions can produce nocturnal pain as well.

○ **What part of the skeletal system is affected by Ewing sarcoma, multiple myeloma, and lymphoma of the bone?**

The marrow elements.

○ **What is osteoid osteoma?**

A fairly common benign bone tumor that often occurs in the proximal femur and can present as hip pain that is often worse at night and responds well to NSAIDS.

○ **What population is most likely to develop osteoid osteoma?**

Teenagers.

○ **What has likely occurred if a patient has had dull achy pain for some time associated with a malignant bony lesion and then suddenly has intense pain at the same location after some moderate stress on that bone?**

The patient may have experienced a pathologic fracture.

○ **What is the most common malignant bony lesion of the foot and where is it usually found?**

Ewing sarcoma is the most common malignant bony lesion of the foot, often affecting the tarsal bones or the diaphysis of the metatarsals when it occurs. Despite this, Ewing sarcoma is seen much more frequently in the proximal femur, tibia, fibula, humerus, and pelvis than it is in the foot.

○ **What is the best way to confirm the diagnosis when a suspicious bony lesion is seen in an imaging study (X-ray, CT, MRI, bone scan, etc.)?**

A bone biopsy must be done (often as an open procedure).

○ **What is the most common primary malignant bone tumor that proliferates through the bone marrow and often results in extensive skeletal destruction, osteopenia, and pathologic fractures?**

Multiple myeloma.

● ● ● OSTEOARTHRITIS ● ● ●

○ **Which is more common osteoarthritis or rheumatoid arthritis?**

Osteoarthritis is the most common type of arthritis.

○ **What structure is progressively damaged and eroded over time leading to osteoarthritis?**

Articular cartilage.

○ **Which joints of the hands are most commonly affected by osteoarthritis?**

The distal interphalangeal (DIP) joints of the fingers are most commonly affected by osteoarthritis.

○ **What are the bony prominences (caused by osteophytes) at the DIP joints in patients with osteoarthritis called?**

Heberden nodes.

○ **What are some of the common risk factors for developing osteoarthritis?**
- Advancing age
- Obesity
- Repetitive micro joint trauma
- Acute major joint trauma

○ **What are the most common symptoms and signs of osteoarthritis?**
- Joint stiffness
- Joint pain
- Joint deformity

○ **What effect on function can osteophytes have in advanced osteoarthritis?**

The osteophytes can cause a physical obstruction resulting in significantly decreased range of motion in the affected joints.

○ **Does osteoarthritis typically produce a mild or major joint effusion?**

The effusions that occur with osteoarthritis are typically mild.

○ **What findings would commonly be seen on the weightbearing X-rays of a patient with severe osteoarthritis of the knees?**

- Decreased joint space between the femur and tibia (may be bone-on-bone), especially in the medial compartment
- Osteophytes or spurs at the joint margins
- Sclerosis of the bone

○ **What lifestyle changes can help patients with osteoarthritis decrease their symptoms and slow the progression of the condition?**

- Weight loss if the patient is overweight so as to decrease the stress on the joints
- Avoidance of activities that place heavy impact, torsion, or other stresses on the joints
- Gentle exercise that encourages motion of the joints (gentle yoga, water exercises, exercise bikes, etc.)
- Shock absorbing footwear or shoe inserts to minimize the stress transferred to the weight-bearing joints

○ **What types of medication may provide some relief for patients suffering with osteoarthritis?**

- Acetaminophen
- Salicylates
- NSAIDS
- Topical analgesic liquids, creams, balms, and patches
- Glucosamine and chondroitin*
- Intra-articular corticosteroid injections
- Intra-articular hyaluronan injections (for knee joints)

○ **What surgical treatment options exist for those with severe joint pain and dysfunction that have failed conservative management of their osteoarthritis?**

- Joint replacement surgery (arthroplasty) can provide significant pain reduction and increased function for many patients. There have been especially good outcomes for those undergoing arthroplasty of the hips, knees, and shoulders.
- Joint fusion surgery (arthrodesis) may be a good option to reduce joint pain in some patients, especially those suffering from severe ankle or wrist osteoarthritis. Joint motion will be lost.

● ● ● OSTEOPOROSIS ● ● ●

○ **What leads to increased fracture rates among those with osteoporosis?**

Decreased bone volume. The bone that remains is generally normal.

○ **How many general types of osteoporosis are there?**

There are two types. Type 1 occurs only in postmenopausal women due to loss of estrogen levels while type 2 can occur in either gender and is associated with advancing age.

○ **What bones are most commonly fractured in patients with type 1 osteoporosis?**

The vertebrae and distal radius.

○ **What type of bone is primarily affected by type 1 osteoporosis?**

Trabecular bone.

*At the time of publication of this book, these substances were still being investigated in several studies to determine true efficacy.

○ **What bones are most commonly fractured in patients with type 2 osteoporosis?**

The hip and pelvis.

○ **What type of bone is affected by type 2 osteoporosis?**

Both trabecular and cortical bone.

○ **What test is generally used to diagnose osteoporosis?**

A DEXA scan (dual energy X-ray absorptiometry).

○ **What percentage of bone loss must occur before decreased bone density is visible with traditional X-rays?**

More than 30%.

○ **What nutritional supplements when combined with resistance exercises and a physically active lifestyle might help prevent the development of osteoporosis?**

Calcium and vitamin D.

○ **What class of medication is commonly used to treat patients with confirmed osteoporosis?**

Bisphosphonates.

○ **When patients have decreased bone mineral density, but not decreased enough to be diagnosed with osteoporosis, what other condition might they be diagnosed with?**

Osteopenia.

● ● ● RHEUMATOLOGIC CONDITIONS ● ● ●

○ **Describe the classic bony changes that occur in the hands of someone suffering from rheumatoid arthritis:**

Ulnar deviation and subluxation at the MCP joints.

○ **Describe the classic bony changes that occur in the feet of someone suffering from rheumatoid arthritis:**

Claw toes and hallux valgus.

○ **Describe the systemic manifestations that can occur with rheumatoid arthritis:**

- Vasculitis
- Pericarditis
- Pulmonary disease

○ **Besides a positive rheumatoid factor, what other laboratory values are commonly seen in patients with rheumatoid arthritis?**

- Elevated erythrocyte sedimentation rate (ESR)
- Elevated C-reactive protein (CRP)

○   **Needle-shaped crystals found within the synovial fluid of a painful joint are associated with what condition?**

Gout.

○   **What is the chemical composition of the crystals found in the joint of a patient suffering from gout?**

Uric acid.

○   **What is the treatment for acute gout?**

Indomethacin or other NSAIDs. For those intolerant of NSAIDS, colchicines is effective as well, but many patients experience nausea, vomiting, and/or diarrhea.

○   **What medications have been most commonly used to prevent future gout attacks by decreasing uric acid levels?**

Probenecid and allopurinol.

○   **What joint is most commonly the site of an initial gout attack?**

The first metatarsal phalangeal joint.

○   **Examination using polarized microscopy of synovial fluid aspirated from a painful, swollen joint showing positively birefringent rhomboid-shaped crystals is associated with what condition?**

Pseudogout.

○   **What is the chemical composition of the crystals found in the joint of someone suffering from pseudogout?**

Calcium pyrophosphate dihydrate.

○   **What joints are most commonly affected by pseudogout?**
- Knee
- Wrist
- Elbow

○   **What is the recommended treatment for pseudogout that is affecting one or two joints?**

Joint aspiration followed by intra-articular glucocorticoid injection. Adjuvant treatment with NSAIDS or colchicine may also be used.

○   **What autoimmune disorder commonly affects women of childbearing age, may affect multiple organs, and commonly presents with a facial rash, photosensitivity, arthralgias, and antinuclear antibodies?**

Systemic lupus erythematous (SLE).

○   **The joints of what body parts are most effected by SLE?**

Hands, wrists, and knees.

○ **What is Felty syndrome?**

Rheumatoid arthritis with splenomegaly and neutropenia. It is a late complication of rheumatoid arthritis.

○ **If a patient presents with multiple joint arthralgias as well as excessive dryness of the mouth and eyes, what condition must be ruled out?**

Sjögren syndrome.

○ **A middle-aged female patient presents with swelling, stiffness, and pain in her fingers, wrists, and knee joints as well as taut, shiny skin. What is her likely diagnosis?**

Scleroderma.

○ **A 65-year-old female patient presents to an urgent care center with complaints of fatigue, fever, a 10 lb weight loss, as well as pain and stiffness in her neck, shoulders, and pelvic area. What condition do you suspect?**

Polymyalgia rheumatica.

○ **What condition is characterized by inflammation of striated muscles in the proximal limbs, neck, and pharynx and elevated enzymes including CPK, AST, ALT, and LDH?**

Polymyositis.

○ **What condition is far more common in women and is characterized by diffuse muscle tenderness, heightened sensitivity to touch in many different areas of the body, fatigue, and often depression?**

Fibromyalgia.

○ **Describe the three general subcategories of juvenile rheumatoid arthritis (JRA):**

1. Pauciarticular-onset JRA is diagnosed in those patients with involvement of less than five joints after 6 months of illness. This is the most common type of JRA and actually has several subgroups.

2. Polyarticular-onset JRA is diagnosed in patients with involvement of more than four joints after 6 months of illness. This is the second most common type of JRA and also has several subgroups.

3. Systemic-onset JRA (formerly called Still disease) is associated with arthritis in any number of joints, rash, and intermittent fever. This is the least common form of JRA.

○ **What condition is characterized by inflammation of the medium- (and sometimes small) sized arteries, occurs most commonly in middle-aged men, presents with fever, fatigue, weakness, weight loss, abdominal pain, arthralgias, arthritis, skin lesions, renal insufficiency, hypertension, edema, and oliguria?**

Polyarteritis nodosa (PAN).

○ **What condition is a seronegative arthritis that is often seen in combination with urethritis and conjunctivitis? This condition is often precipitated by a sexually transmitted disease (often linked to *Chlamydia trachomatis*) or gastroenteritis and may present with lesions in multiple locations (mouth, penis, extremities), swollen toes, and heel pain.**

Reactive arthritis (formerly known as Reiter syndrome).

● ● ● **REFERENCES** ● ● ●

Becker MA. Prevention of recurrent gout. In: Basow D, ed. UpToDate. Waltham, MA: UpToDate; 2009.

Becker MA. Treatment of acute gout. In: Basow D, ed. UpToDate. Waltham, MA: UpToDate; 2009.

Becker MA. Treatment of calcium pyrophosphate crystal deposition disease. In: Basow D, ed. UpToDate. Waltham, MA: UpToDate; 2009.

Beutler A, Stephens MB. General principles of fracture management: bone healing and fracture management. In: Basow D, ed. UpToDate. Waltham, MA: UpToDate; 2009.

Bloom J, Burroughs KE. Metacarpal neck fractures. In: Basow D, ed. UpToDate. Waltham, MA: UpToDate; 2009.

Booher JM, Thibodeau GA. *Athletic Injury Assessment*. 3rd ed. St. Louis, MO: Mosby; 1994.

Chorley J. Elbow injuries in the young athlete. In: Basow D, ed. UpToDate. Waltham, MA: UpToDate; 2009.

DeLaney TF, et al. Clinical presentation, staging, and prognosis of the Ewing's sarcoma family of tumors. In: Basow D, ed. UpToDate. Waltham, MA: UpToDate; 2009.

Goldenberg DL. Clinical manifestations and diagnosis of fibromyalgia in adults. In: Basow D, ed. UpToDate. Waltham, MA: UpToDate; 2009.

Griffen L. *Essentials of Musculoskeletal Care*. 3rd ed. Rosemont, IL: American Academy of Orthopaedic Surgeons; 2005.

Hoppenfeld S. *Physical Examination of the Spine and Extremities*. East Norwalk, CT: Appleton-Century-Croft/Prentice-Hall; 1976.

Hunder GG, Stone JH. Clinical manifestations of and diagnosis of polyarteritis nodosa. In: Basow D, ed. UpToDate. Waltham, MA: UpToDate; 2009.

Lehman TJ. Classification of juvenile rheumatoid arthritis. In: Basow D, ed. UpToDate. Waltham, MA: UpToDate; 2009.

Nigrovic PA. Overview of hip pain in childhood. In: Basow D, ed. UpToDate. Waltham, MA: UpToDate; 2009.

O'Connell CB, Zarbock SF. *A Comprehensive Review for the Certification and Recertification Examinations for Physician Assistants*. Baltimore, MD: Lippincott William & Wilkins; 2004.

Sexton DJ. Overview of osteomyelitis. In: Basow D, ed. UpToDate. Waltham, MA: UpToDate; 2009.

Thomas CL. (Editor). *Taber's Cyclopedic Medical Dictionary*. Philadelphia, PA: F.A. Davis; 1993.

Yu DT. Reactive arthritis (formerly Reiter syndrome). In: Basow D, ed. UpToDate. Waltham, MA: UpToDate; 2009.

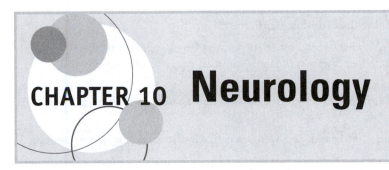

Michel Statler, MLA, PA-C

○ **What are the reversible causes of dementia?**

While normal pressure hydrocephalus, brain tumors, hypothyroidism, and vitamin B12 deficiency are reversible causes of dementia, they are less commonly seen. Nevertheless, diagnostic studies should be used to rule them in or out as the underlying cause of dementia since early diagnosis will help to stop or even reverse any cognitive impairment.

○ **What is the most common cause of dementia in Western countries?**

Alzheimer disease is the most common cause of dementia, followed by vascular dementia and dementia associated with Parkinson disease.

○ **What are the risk factors for Alzheimer disease?**

Increasing age, Down syndrome (Trisomy 21), and family history. Familial Alzheimer disease is associated with an autosomal dominant inheritance with mutations in the gene for amyloid precursor proteins on chromosome 21.

○ **What are the characteristic pathologic features associated with Alzheimer disease?**

Alzheimer disease is characterized by abnormal metabolism and deposition of β-amyloid proteins resulting in the formation of neuritic or senile plaques and neurofibrillary tangles.

○ **What is often the first sign of Alzheimer disease?**

Family members often note impairment in recent memory when patients become disoriented to time and then to place.

○ **What are the manifestations of the late stages of Alzheimer disease?**

As the disease progresses, patients develop psychiatric symptoms, such as delusions, hallucinations, and paranoia. Patients may also develop seizures.

○ **What are the clinical features common to subcortical dementia?**

Subcortical dementias are characterized by movement disorders in conjunction with memory loss and apathy. Language and visuospatial functions are preserved.

○ **What are the causes of subcortical dementia?**

Parkinson disease, hypothyroidism, normal pressure hydrocephalus, multiple sclerosis, and vascular dementia.

○ **What type of neurologic deficits are found with cortical dementias?**

Cortical dementias are associated with loss of higher cortical functions, such as language. Patients have varying degrees of aphasia, agnosia, and apraxia. Alzheimer disease is the most common type of cortical dementia.

○ **Which medications are recommended to improve the cognitive dysfunction associated with Alzheimer disease?**

Acetylcholinesterase inhibitors, such as donepezil (Aricept) or rivastigmine (Exelon), address the deficits associated with degeneration of cholinergic neurons.

○ **Which medications are indicated for the management of the behavioral disturbances seen in association with Alzheimer disease?**

Antipsychotic medications, such as haloperidol (Haldol) or risperidone (Risperdal), can be used to address hallucinations, delusions, or aggression. Antidepressants and anxiolytics can also be used to address symptoms of depression and anxiety, respectively.

○ **What is the underlying pathophysiology of normal-pressure hydrocephalus?**

Normal-pressure hydrocephalus is called a communicating or nonobstructive form of hydrocephalus since the flow or cerebrospinal fluid (CSF) is not obstructed. Hydrocephalus develops due to impaired absorption of CSF by the arachnoid granulations along the superior sagittal sinus in the subarachnoid space.

○ **A 62-year-old man presented with the progressive gait difficulty. The patient reports unsteadiness with standing and trouble initiating walking even though he denies any muscle weakness. His wife notes that his thinking is "slower" and he is becoming more forgetful. A non-contrast CT scan of the head (see Figure 10-1) was obtained during the diagnostic evaluation. What is the most likely diagnosis?**

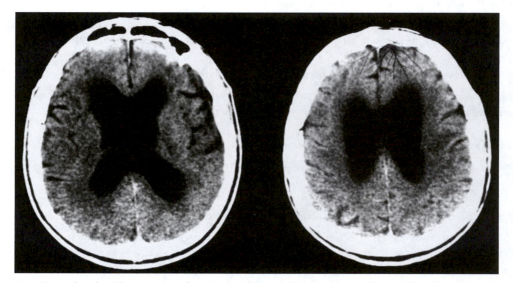

Figure 10-1 (Reproduced, with permission, from Simon RP, Greenberg DA, Aminoff MJ. *Clinical Neurology.* 6th ed. New York, NY: McGraw-Hill; 2009, Fig. 1-16.)

Normal-pressure hydrocephalus (NPH). Gait difficulties are often the initial presentation of NPH. Patients describe feeling as if they are glued to the floor; once they are able to start moving, their gait is slow and shuffling. Early symptoms of NPH also include mental slowness, memory impairments, and apathy; aphasia and agnosia are uncommon.

○ **What is the characteristic triad of normal-pressure hydrocephalus?**

Dementia, incontinence, and gait ataxia (often described as a "magnetic" gait).

○ **What are the common symptoms associated with dementia with Lewy bodies?**

Dementia with Lewy bodies is characterized by fluctuating cognitive impairment, visual hallucinations, and signs of parkinsonism (i.e., bradykinesia, tremor, and rigidity). Lewy bodies are intraneuronal cytoplasmic inclusions that contain similar proteins that are found in Alzheimer disease and Parkinson disease.

○ **What class of medications should be avoided in patients with Lewy body dementia?**

Antipsychotic medications should be avoided since they will exacerbate the extrapyramidal symptoms.

○ **What are the risk factors associated with vascular (or multi-infarct) dementia?**

Risk factors for multi-infarct dementia include a history of hypertension, diabetes, atrial fibrillation, peripheral vascular disease, or other evidence of advanced atherosclerotic disease.

○ **What is an important historical distinction between vascular dementia and Alzheimer disease?**

The onset of symptoms can be helpful to distinguish between the two disorders. Alzheimer disease has a slowly progressive loss of cognitive function, whereas patients with multi-infarct dementia have acute episodes of neurologic deterioration that progress in an irregular stepwise manner with each ischemic insult.

○ **What is an associated symptom with dementia secondary to Huntington disease?**

Huntington disease is an autosomal dominant inherited condition characterized by a movement disorder (choreiform movements) in addition to progressive memory loss.

○ **What is the most common neurologic complication associated with AIDS?**

AIDS dementia is more common in patients who are severely immunocompromised; however, it can also be a presenting symptom.

○ **What are the associated physical examination findings with AIDS dementia?**

Behavioral changes (social withdrawal) and motor symptoms can be seen. Ataxia, increased muscle tone, and hyperreflexia can all be seen during the early stage of the disease; however, the motor symptoms become much more pronounced as the disease progresses to later stages.

○ **What are the typical findings on cerebrospinal fluid analysis for a patient with AIDS dementia?**

Mild to moderate elevations in protein levels (≤ 200 mg/dL), modest mononuclear pleocytosis (≤ 50 cells/μL), and the presence of oligoclonal IgG bands.

○ **What are the common, underlying characteristics associated with cerebral palsy?**

Cerebral palsy refers to a chronic condition characterized by impaired muscle tone, strength, and coordination of movements. It is associated with a cerebral injury that can occur either before birth, during birth, or in the perinatal period.

○ **What are the most common causes of cerebral palsy?**

Intrauterine hypoxia, intrauterine bleeding, infections, toxins, congenital malformations, neonatal infections, neonatal hypoglycemia, and kernicterus; the underlying etiology is never identified in about 25% of cases.

○ **What is the most common clinical manifestation seen in cerebral palsy?**

The most common manifestation of cerebral palsy is spasticity of the limbs, which can involve one or more limbs. Spasticity can present as a monoplegia, hemiplegia, paraplegia, or quadriplegia.

○ **What associated movement disorder can be seen in patients with cerebral palsy?**

Choreoathetosis, or twisting and jerking involuntary movements, can be seen in a small percentage of patients.

○ **What type of neurologic deficits can be associated with cerebral palsy?**

Associated neurologic deficits can include seizures, which can be seen in about 50% of patients; varying levels of mental retardation can also be seen, ranging from mild to severe. Patients can have various language, speech, hearing, and vision problems in isolation or in combination with other deficits.

○ **What physical examination findings can be seen with cerebral palsy?**

Spasticity, hyperreflexia, choreoathetosis, and ataxia.

○ **In addition to findings consistent with cerebral palsy, which additional physical examination findings are associated with a congenital infection with cytomegalovirus (CMV) or rubella?**

The presence of congenital cataracts, retinopathy, and congenital heart defects suggest an infection with CMV or rubella.

○ **What is the cause of Bell palsy?**

Bell palsy is an idiopathic lower motor neuron type of facial weakness.

○ **What are the signs and symptoms commonly associated with Bell palsy?**

Additional signs and symptoms include impaired taste, lacrimation, or hyperacusis; the clinical presentation varies depending on the location of the lesion. For example, a lesion distal to the sternomastoid foramen will produce purely a motor deficit, whereas a lesion in the petrous temporal bone will produce an ipsilateral facial weakness with impaired taste, lacrimation, and hyperacusis.

○ **What is Ramsay Hunt syndrome?**

Ramsay Hunt syndrome is a facial nerve palsy associated with a herpes zoster infection of the geniculate ganglion. Patients have an eruption of an erythematous vesicular rash involving the ear, palate, pharynx, and neck.

○ **What is synkinesia?**

Synkinesia is a complication associated with Bell palsy in which there are abnormal facial movements attributed to problems with regeneration of the nerve. Active movement of one part of the face is associated with involuntary movement of another part of the face. For example, the patient's eye might close when he smiles.

○ **How can you tell the difference between a central facial palsy and a peripheral facial palsy?**

A peripheral facial palsy is a lower motor neuron lesion affecting the entire side of the face ipsilateral to the lesion. A central facial palsy is an upper motor neuron lesion affecting the lower part of the face contralateral to the lesion. Central facial palsies are often associated with motor weakness of the upper extremity on the same side as the facial palsy.

○ **What are the predisposing factors associated with Guillain-Barré syndrome?**

Minor illnesses, gastrointestinal infections with *Campylobacter jejuni*, recent immunizations, and surgical procedures.

○ **What are the signs and symptoms associated with Guillain-Barré syndrome?**

Guillain-Barré syndrome is characterized by an ascending symmetrical lower extremity weakness. Bulbar muscles can also be involved, resulting in facial weakness and dysphagia. If the diaphragm is involved, patients will present with respiratory insufficiency. Deep tendon reflexes will be depressed or absent. Patients may also complain of sensory loss, which is in a "glove-and-stocking" distribution. Sensory losses are generally less severe than muscle weakness.

○ **What clinical findings would help to rule out Guillain-Barré syndrome as a diagnosis for a patient with the new onset of weakness?**

Pertinent negatives would include a markedly asymmetrical pattern of weakness, bowel or bladder incontinence at the onset of symptoms, a well-defined sensory level, and/or a CSF white blood cell count >50.

○ **What is a characteristic finding on cerebrospinal fluid (CSF) analysis for patients with Guillain-Barré syndrome?**

The CSF will show an elevation in protein levels without an elevation in the white cell count.

○ **Does early treatment with intravenous immunoglobulin (IVIG) or plasmapheresis accelerate the recovery for patients diagnosed with Guillain-Barré syndrome?**

Yes, IVIG or plasmapheresis will shorten the recovery time as well as decrease the likelihood of long-term neurologic disability.

○ **What is the prognosis for patients with Guillain-Barré syndrome?**

Approximately 70% to 75% of patients have a full recovery; 25% of patients have mild, residual neurologic deficits, and 5% of patients will die. Advanced age, respiratory insufficiency requiring ventilator support, and rapid progression of symptoms are all associated with a poorer prognosis.

○ **What are the clinical features of chronic inflammatory demyelinating polyneuropathy?**

The clinical presentation is the same as Guillain-Barré syndrome; however, the course is progressive and characterized by relapses. Predominant features include muscle weakness affecting the upper and lower extremities, distal greater than proximal, decreased or absent deep tendon reflexes, and distal sensory deficits (glove-and-stocking distribution).

○ **What role do corticosteroids have in the treatment of Guillain-Barré syndrome?**

Corticosteroids are associated with adverse outcomes and may actually delay recovery and are therefore contraindicated in the treatment of Guillain-Barré syndrome (an acute inflammatory polyneuropathy); chronic inflammatory demyelinating polyneuropathy, however, is responsive to corticosteroids. Accordingly, treatment with prednisone for 2 to 4 weeks, followed by a tapered dosage is indicated.

○ **What medical conditions can be associated with myasthenia gravis?**

Thyrotoxicosis, disseminated lupus erythematous, tumors of thymus, and rheumatoid arthritis.

○ **What is the hallmark of myasthenia gravis?**

Fluctuating weakness and fatigability of voluntary muscle activity, with involvement of ocular, bulbar, limb, or respiratory muscles. Bulbar involvement presents as dysarthria and dysphagia.

○ **What is the underlying pathophysiology of myasthenia gravis?**

Myasthenia is characterized by auto-antibodies to acetylcholine at neuromuscular junction. Accordingly, there is a block in neuromuscular transmission as well as a decrease in the number of functioning receptors, which account for the fatigable weakness.

○ **What are the two subtypes of myasthenia gravis?**

Ocular and generalized. The ocular type is characterized by diplopia and ptosis, which are two of the most common presenting symptoms of myasthenia. Patients with ocular symptoms often progress to the generalized subtype. Generalized myasthenia presents with weakness of the upper and/or lower extremities and overall fatigability.

○ **What type of conditions or medications are associated with exacerbations of myasthenia gravis?**

Minor infections, pre-menses, pregnancy, stress, and hot weather can all lead to an exacerbation; medications that are associated with exacerbations include quinine, quinidine, procainamide, propranolol, phenytoin, lithium, tetracycline, and aminoglycoside antibiotics.

○ **A 32-year-old female patient presents with diplopia and ptosis, which are both worse by the end of the day. She also notes dysarthria if she has been talking a lot. What diagnostic test is indicated for the evaluation of this patient?**

The most commonly used test is the edrophonium or Tensilon test. Up to 10 mg can be given as an intravenous dose to look for improvement in muscle strength. The effects of the Tensilon test are transient.

○ **What additional diagnostic studies can be used for a patient with suspected myasthenia gravis?**

Acetylcholine receptor antibodies are elevated in up to 90% of patients; repetitive nerve stimulation will show a decrement in response amplitude. A single fiber EMG, which is a specialized EMG that analyzes individual muscle fiber's firing pattern, is the most sensitive test.

○ **What is the treatment of choice for myasthenia gravis?**

The treatment of choice is pyridostigmine (Mestinon).

○ **What are additional treatment options for the management of myasthenia gravis?**

Thymectomy will provide symptomatic relief or remission. Corticosteroids for patients who are nonresponders to anticholinesterase medications. For patients with progressive disease who do not respond to thymectomy, anticholinesterases, corticosteroids and azathioprine can be used.

○ **What is myasthenic crisis?**

Patients in myasthenic crisis have significant impairment in respiratory function, requiring intubation and ventilator support. Plasmapheresis is also indicated.

○ **What underlying conditions are associated with Lambert-Eaton syndrome?**

Lambert-Eaton is associated with malignancies, especially oat cell carcinoma. It can also be associated with pernicious anemia.

○ **How does the clinical presentation of Lambert-Eaton syndrome differ from that of myasthenia gravis?**

Although both conditions are associated with muscle weakness, extraocular muscle function is preserved in Lambert-Eaton syndrome.

○ **What are the different types of diabetic neuropathy?**

Mixed (sensory, motor, and autonomic) in 70%; primary sensory in 30%.

○ **What is the classic presentation of a diabetic sensory neuropathy?**

The classic presentation is a symmetric stocking-glove sensory loss distribution. The lower extremities are generally affected first, followed by the upper extremities. Patients complain of numbness, tingling, and other paresthesias. Patterns of loss can be assessed with monofilament testing.

○ **What is the clinical presentation of mononeuropathy simplex and multiplex?**

Mononeuritis simplex involves a superficial nerve, whereas mononeuritis multiplex presents with asymmetric involvement of multiple superficial nerves. The lower extremities are more commonly affected; acute onset of pain associated with cramping. Pain is typically worse at night.

○ **What symptoms are associated with autonomic dysfunction secondary to diabetes mellitus?**

Postural hypotension, impaired temperature regulation, gastroparesis, alternating diarrhea and constipation, urinary hesitancy, overflow incontinence, and impotency.

○ **What is the treatment for diabetic polyneuropathy?**

Maintaining optimal glucose control is key; painful paresthesias can be treated with gabapentin, carbamazepine, clomipramine, or topical capsaicin ointment.

○ **What complications are associated with a diabetic sensory polyneuropathy?**

Complications include foot ulcerations; due to sensory neuropathy patients are unaware of minor traumas to the feet which can progress to ulcerations.

○ **What complication of diabetes is characterized by degenerative changes in the tarsal and tarsometatarsal joints of the foots?**

Charcot joint, a neuropathic joint disease.

○ **What are the common causes of acute or new onset headaches?**

Headaches associated with an acute onset include subarachnoid hemorrhage, meningitis, or encephalitis, and ophthalmologic conditions such as acute-angle closure glaucoma or acute iritis.

○ **What are the common causes of subacute headaches that generally develop over weeks to months?**

Causes of headache associated with a subacute onset include temporal (or giant cell) arteritis, intracranial mass lesions (primary or metastatic tumors, abscesses), and neuralgia (trigeminal neuralgia (or tic douloureux)), glossopharyngeal neuralgia, or postherpetic neuralgia.

○ **What are the common causes of chronic headaches that can occur intermittently over years?**

Migraines, cluster headaches, and tension headaches. Chronic headaches can also be associated with degenerative disease in the cervical spine.

○ **What are the pain-sensitive structures associated with headache?**

Intracranial pain-sensitive structures are arteries, venous sinuses, meninges, and cranial nerves. Extracranially, the periosteum of the skull, skin and subcutaneous tissues, muscles, eyes, ears, paranasal sinuses, and oropharynx are all pain-sensitive structures.

○ **What are the common precipitating factors for migraine headaches?**

Common precipitating factors include meats with nitrite preservatives (i.e., hot dogs or bacon), tyramine-containing cheeses, chocolate, monosodium glutamate, fasting, menses, medications (oral contraceptives), and bright lights.

○ **A 64-year-old female patient presents with a bilateral headache associated with scalp tenderness and stiffness in her jaw with eating. What is the most likely diagnosis?**

Giant cell (temporal) arteritis. Other associated symptoms include malaise, myalgias, arthralgias, and fever; symptoms are consistent with polymyalgia rheumatica.

○ **What diagnostic studies are used in the evaluation of temporal arteritis?**

The erythrocyte sedimentation rate (ESR) will be elevated, often as high as 100 mm/h. A temporal artery biopsy will be diagnostic for the presence of giant cells.

○ **What is the treatment of giant cell arteritis?**

Prednisone, 40 to 60 mg/day for 102 months, and then the dose can be tapered gradually over 1 to 2 years.

○ **What complication is associated with temporal arteritis?**

Blindness can develop in half of the patients with temporal arteritis if left untreated.

○ **A 56-year-old man presents with a mild to moderate dull headache (HA) that has steadily progressed over the past month. The HA is worse when he gets up in the morning or with coughing and sneezing. He also notes the recent onset of nausea and vomiting. What is the most likely diagnosis?**

An intracranial tumor. Patients with brain tumors do not always have a headache as an initial symptom. However, when patients do develop HA, the pain is dull and aggravated by position changes or coughing and sneezing, which increase intracranial pressure. Any patient presenting with a HA associated with a focal neurologic deficit (i.e., weakness, visual field deficit) needs to undergo a neuroimaging study.

○ **A 67-year-old woman complains of intermittent episodes of pain in her cheek and jaw that feel like a "lightning bolt hit her face." The pain is triggered by eating or touching her face. Her physical examination is unremarkable. What is the most likely diagnosis?**

Trigeminal neuralgia, or tic douloureux, is associated with severe facial pain in the distribution of the trigeminal nerve; most commonly affecting V2 or V3. Episodes of pain may be triggered by any sort of sensory stimulus to the face, i.e., touching, chewing, talking, shaving, cold weather, or wind.

○ **What is the first-line treatment for the patient described in the previous question?**

First-line treatment would be carbamazepine with dosing between 400 and 1200 mg/day.

○   **A 26-year-old woman complains of a dull, throbbing right-sided headache (HA) that lasts for hours but is relieved by sleep. The HA is associated with nausea, vomiting, and a sensitivity to light and sound. She gets similar HA at least once a month and says that prior to the HA, there are "holes in her vision" along with "zigzag lines." What is the most likely diagnosis?**

Classic migraine headache. While classic migraine HA are less common, they are associated with an aura that is usually a visual disturbance (i.e., scintillating scotomata).

○   **What is the clinical presentation of a common migraine headache?**

Common migraines, now referred to as migraine without aura, occur more frequently than classic migraines. About 70% of all migraine-type headaches are common migraines or migraine without aura. Common migraines are associated with unilateral pulsatile pain with nausea, vomiting, phonophobia, and photophobia. There is usually a strong family history of migraine headaches.

○   **What is the abortive treatment for migraine headaches?**

Mild analgesics, such as nonsteroidal anti-inflammatory medications or acetaminophen, are effective in relieving headache pain. Other first-line options are the 5-HT agonists or triptans, i.e., sumatriptan. For analgesics and triptans to be effective, they must be administered at the onset of the headache. Antiemetics are helpful as well.

○   **What are the contraindications for the use of 5-HT agonists or triptans?**

Poorly controlled hypertension, coronary artery, or peripheral vascular disease.

○   **What are the indications for the use of prophylactic medications in the management of migraine headaches?**

Frequent headaches (more than one per week), headaches that are difficult to control, or for patients who cannot tolerate triptans or ergot alkaloids.

○   **What classes of medications are effective for prophylactic management of migraines?**

Beta-blockers, tricyclic antidepressants, anticonvulsants, calcium channel blockers, and ergot alkaloids.

○   **What is the recommended treatment for migraines during pregnancy?**

Migraines during pregnancy should be treated with opiates, i.e., meperidine. All other migraine treatments have risks of teratogenicity or complications with the pregnancy.

○   **What signs and symptoms are seen in conjunction with a basilar migraine?**

Basilar migraines are associated with visual disturbances (scintillating scotomata, visual acuity loss, and visual field deficits), nausea/vomiting, impaired consciousness (syncope, confusion, stupor, coma), bilateral paresthesias, vertigo, dysarthria, and ataxia.

○   **A 39-year-old man presents with intermittent episodes of severe headaches around the left eye and temple. The headaches awaken him nightly for several days in a row then he is headache-free for a couple of months before another "round" begins. What is the most likely diagnosis?**

Cluster headaches present with severe nonthrobbing headaches that typically occur at the same location and the same time each day. Headaches generally last for a few minutes up to a couple of hours. The headaches occur daily for weeks to months before they spontaneously resolve; patients may be pain-free for months to years.

○ **What are the associated signs and symptoms seen with cluster headaches?**

Conjunctival injection, lacrimation, and nasal congestion on the same side as the headache; Horner syndrome (anhidrosis, miosis, and ptosis) can also be seen on the affected side.

○ **What are the abortive therapy options to treat cluster headaches?**

100% oxygen, sumatriptan, or dihydroergotamine.

○ **What is the role of corticosteroids in the treatment of cluster headaches?**

Prednisone can be initiated at the beginning of a cluster cycle to effectively eliminate the patient's symptoms; most patients will be pain-free within 2 days.

○ **What are the presenting signs and symptoms associated with tension headaches?**

Patients describe a nonthrobbing, bilateral headache ("tight band") without the associated visual disturbances, nausea, and vomiting seen in conjunction with migraine headaches.

○ **What types of medications are effective in the treatment of tension headaches?**

Acetaminophen, nonsteroidal anti-inflammatory drugs, and ergotamine can be helpful for acute headaches; tricyclic antidepressants and beta-blockers can be used for prophylaxis.

○ **What is the differential diagnosis for fever, headache, and nuchal rigidity?**

Bacterial meningitis, aseptic meningitis, encephalitis, and brain abscess.

○ **What are the most common pathogens associated with bacterial meningitis in a neonate?**

Group B *Streptococcus, E. coli, Listeria.*

○ **What are the most common pathogens associated with bacterial meningitis in adults 20 to 50 years of age?**

Streptococcus pneumoniae, Neisseria meningitidis, and *Hemophilus influenzae.*

○ **What are the most common bacterial pathogens for adults who are older than 50 years of age or immunocompromised?**

S. pneumoniae, Listeria, and gram-negative bacilli.

○ **What risk factors are associated with bacterial meningitis?**

Exposure during delivery (*E. coli,* group B *Streptococcus*); colonization from respiratory tract, sinusitis, otitis (*S. pneumoniae*); crowded conditions (military, college (*N. meningitidis*)); head trauma (*Staphylococcus*), and neurosurgical procedures (*Staphylococcus,* gram-negative organisms).

○ **What are the presenting signs and symptoms associated with bacterial meningitis?**

Fever, nuchal rigidity, headache, altered mental status, photophobia, nausea, and vomiting; cranial nerve palsies and seizures can be seen in 40% of patients.

○ **Which pathogen associated with bacterial meningitis presents with a petechial and purpuric rash?**

N. meningitidis.

○ **What are the signs of meningeal irritation?**

Kernig and Brudzinski signs are used to assess for meningeal irritation. Kernig is performed by having the patient supine with the hip and knee flexed; pain and resistance to extension of the knee is considered a positive sign. Brudzinski is performed with the patient supine; flexion of the hips and knees with forward flexion of the neck is considered a positive sign. These signs may not be present in very young or very old patients or in patients who have severe impairment in consciousness.

○ **What is the key to establishing the diagnosis of bacterial meningitis?**

Cerebrospinal fluid analysis is the key; gram stain will identify the organism in 60% to 90%. Perform LP with CSF analysis first unless contraindicated.

○ **What are the contraindications to performing a lumbar puncture for a patient with suspect bacterial meningitis?**

Papilledema, focal deficits, or altered mental status are consistent with elevations in intracranial pressure. Obtain blood cultures, then begin empiric antibiotic therapy depending upon the patient's age and the most likely organisms before the CT scan.

○ **What are the cerebrospinal fluid (CSF) findings in bacterial meningitis?**

Elevated WBC (>1000 cells/mm^3), decreased CSF glucose (<45 mg/dL), and elevated CSF protein levels (>500 mg/dL). Serum glucose levels should be checked at the time of lumbar puncture to correlate the CSF and serum glucose levels. The CSF-to-blood glucose ratio is normally 0.6; in bacterial meningitis, this ratio is less than 0.4.

○ **What is the recommended antibiotic treatment for a newborn (<1 month old) with bacterial meningitis?**

Ampicillin and cefotaxime.

○ **What is the recommended antibiotic treatment for an 18-year-old patient with bacterial meningitis?**

Cefotaxime (or ceftriaxone) and vancomycin.

○ **What is the recommended antibiotic treatment for a 60-year-old adult with bacterial meningitis?**

Ampicillin, cefotaxime (or ceftriaxone), and vancomycin

○ **What role do corticosteroids play in bacterial meningitis?**

Dexamethasone has been shown to decrease the morbidity and mortality, in particular sensorineural hearing loss.

○ **What complications are associated with bacterial meningitis?**

Impaired mental status/cognition, cerebral edema, seizures, focal neurologic deficits, sensorineural hearing loss, and brain abscess.

○ **What type of prophylaxis is indicated for meningitis secondary to *N. meningitides* or *H. influenzae*?**

Prophylaxis with rifampin (600 mg BID × 2 days) is indicated for any close contacts of patients with meningococcal meningitis or meningitis due to *H. influenzae*.

○ **What type of vaccination is required for the prevention of bacterial meningitis?**

Meningococcal vaccination is indicated for the military personnel and travelers to endemic areas (i.e., the "meningitis belt" in Africa); it is not routinely given in the United States.

○ **What is the most common cause of aseptic meningitis?**

The most common of aseptic meningitis are enteroviruses (90%); herpes simplex virus (HSV), varicella zoster virus (VZV), mumps, HIV, EBV, and West Nile virus can also cause aseptic meningitis.

○ **What are the uncommon causes of aseptic meningitis?**

Uncommon causes include malignancy due to direct invasion of the meninges from leukemia, lymphomas, and breast, pulmonary, or gastrointestinal malignancies. Medication reactions are another uncommon cause; may be associated with NSAIDs, antibiotics, or IVIG. Considered a diagnosis of exclusion once other causes are ruled out; symptoms will resolve with discontinuation of medication.

○ **What is the current gold standard in the diagnosis of aseptic meningitis?**

Viral cultures are the current gold standard; however, they can take from 4 to 8 weeks to obtain results. Reverse transcriptase polymerase chain reaction assays (RT-PCR) are a more sensitive and specific test. The turnaround time for results is approximately 34 hours, but RT-PCRs are not routinely available at present, but they have the potential to become new gold standard.

○ **What are the cerebrospinal fluid (CSF) findings in aseptic meningitis?**

The WBC is modestly elevated with a predominance of lymphocytes (100–1000 cells/mm^3); CSF protein is usually normal but can be slightly elevated (less than 80–100 mg/dL); CSF glucose to blood glucose ratio is normal.

○ **What is the most common cause of encephalitis?**

Herpes simplex virus type 1 is the most common; arboviruses (West Nile Virus. St. Louis, eastern equine, western equine) can also cause this; uncommon causes include varicella zoster virus, Epstein-Barr virus, and HIV.

○ **What are the presenting signs and symptoms consistent with encephalitis?**

Headache, progressive alterations in mental status, and focal neurological deficits (cranial nerve palsies, hemiparesis); seizures are common.

○ **What will CSF studies show in patients with encephalitis?**

CSF findings will be similar to findings seen with aseptic meningitis. There will be increased WBC (less than 250/mm^3) of predominantly lymphocytes; CSF glucose will be normal.

○ **What is the recommended treatment for encephalitis?**

Acyclovir 10 mg/kg q8h IV × 14 days along with seizure prophylaxis.

○ **What is the prognosis for patients diagnosed with encephalitis?**

14% mortality at 1 year; HSV encephalitis can be fatal if untreated; poor neurologic recovery associated with diffuse cerebral edema or intractable seizures at time of presentation.

○ **What is the most common cause of meningitis in patients with AIDS?**

Cryptococcus neoformans.

○ **What is the most common involuntary movement disorder?**

Essential tremor.

○ **What is the etiology of essential tremor?**

The underlying etiology is unknown; about 50% of patients have a positive family history that is consistent with an autosomal dominant pattern of inheritance.

○ **What factors can cause an exacerbation of a physiologic postural tremor?**

Anxiety, sleep deprivation, alcohol withdrawal, drug intoxication (i.e., bronchodilators, tricyclic antidepressants), carbon monoxide poisoning, and thyrotoxicosis.

○ **What are the clinical features of essential tremor?**

Bilateral involvement of the upper extremities with sparing of the legs; tremor is usually symmetric although one side can be affected more than the other; can also see voice tremors and head tremors (yes–yes or no–no).

○ **What are the recommended treatments for essential tremor?**

Propranolol and primidone.

○ **How can essential tremor be differentiated from Parkinson disease?**

Resting tremor, bradykinesia, rigidity, and micrographia are all absent.

○ **What type of hyperkinetic movement disorder is characterized by rapid, nonpatterned, dancelike movements?**

Chorea.

○ **What is the most common cause of Parkinson disease?**

Idiopathic degeneration of dopamine-producing neurons in the substantia nigra.

○ **What is the peak age of onset of Parkinson disease?**

The peak is in the early 60s; onset ranges from 35 to 85 years of age.

○ **What are the risk factors for Parkinson disease?**

Male gender, history of prior head injury, exposure to pesticides, and positive family history.

○ **What factors are associated with a decreased incidence of Parkinson disease?**

Smoking, coffee consumption, use of NSAIDs, and estrogen replacement in women who are postmenopausal.

○ **What medications are associated with parkinsonism symptoms?**

Conventional antipsychotics; haloperidol and perphenazine have the highest risk.

○ **What signs and symptoms are associated with Parkinson disease?**

Rigidity, bradykinesia, shuffling gait, and resting tremor.

○ **What is cogwheel rigidity?**

Brief interruptions in muscle resistance during assessment of passive movement.

○ **What is a festinating gait?**

The patient appears to accelerate in an attempt to catch up with the center of gravity due to flexed posture and loss of postural reflexes; classic sign of parkinsonism.

○ **What type of nonmotor symptoms are seen in association with Parkinson disease?**

Depression, sleep disturbances, cognitive impairments, and autonomic dysfunction.

○ **What are the signs of autonomic dysfunction in Parkinson disease?**

Orthostatic hypotension, urinary urgency, constipation, and excessive sweating.

○ **What is the first-line treatment of Parkinson disease?**

Levodopa-carbidopa or a dopamine agonist.

○ **What complications are associated with levodopa-carbidopa treatment?**

Motor fluctuations ("on–off" phenomena) and dyskinesias.

○ **Which class of drugs is indicated in the management of a patient with Parkinson disease who has a debilitating tremor as the predominant symptom?**

Anticholinergics.

○ **What are the indications for the surgical treatment of Parkinson disease?**

Intractable tremor and drug-induced motor fluctuations or dyskinesias.

○ **What is the preferred surgical procedure for Parkinson disease?**

Deep brain stimulation.

○ **What is the pattern of inheritance for Huntington disease?**

Autosomal dominant; due to a mutation on chromosome 4p.

○ **What is inheritance with anticipation?**

The trend for earlier age of diagnosis for subsequent generations; most pronounced if disease inherited from the father.

○ **What is the usual age of onset for Huntington disease?**

Fourth or fifth decade of life.

○ **What is the average lifespan for a patient with Huntington disease once there is the onset of symptoms?**

15 years.

○ **What are the primary symptoms associated with Huntington disease?**

Chorea, dementia, dysarthria, and gait disturbances.

○ **How do clinical features change as Huntington disease progresses to an advanced stage?**

Choreiform movements become less prominent; dystonia, rigidity, spasticity, bradykinesia, and myoclonus may begin.

○ **What type of behavioral issues are common with Huntington disease?**

Depression, suicidal ideations, aggressiveness, psychosis, and dementia.

○ **What is the treatment for the choreiform movements associated with Huntington disease?**

Dopamine-blocking agents, such as haloperidol or chlorpromazine, can be used to treat chorea. However, they are not routinely used because they may actually aggravate motor symptoms.

○ **What is the age of onset for multiple sclerosis?**

Usually between 20 and 40 years of age.

○ **What are the diagnostic criteria for multiple sclerosis?**

At least two or more documented episodes of neurologic symptoms and examination findings affecting distinct areas of the central nervous system; symptoms must last at least 24 hours and the interval between episodes needs to be separated by at least 1 month.

○ **What is the underlying etiology for multiple sclerosis?**

The cause is unknown; however, several viral autoimmune and genetic factors have been implicated.

○ **What is the most common clinical type of multiple sclerosis?**

Relapsing remitting.

○ **What are the common presenting symptoms associated with multiple sclerosis?**

Paresthesias, gait disorders (unsteadiness, disequilibrium), lower extremity weakness, and incoordination.

○ **What common physical examination findings are seen with multiple sclerosis?**

Spasticity, hyperreflexia, ataxia, extensor response (positive Babinski), impaired rapid alternating movements, impaired vibration, and proprioception.

○ **What is dysdiadochokinesia?**

The inability to perform rapid alternating movements.

○   **What is internuclear ophthalmoplegia?**

Impairment of adduction with eye movements; bilateral involvement is a pathognomic sign of multiple sclerosis.

○   **A 28-year-old female patient presents with a 1-week history of diplopia and vertigo. Three months earlier, she had an episode of blurred vision that resolved spontaneously after 2 days. Physical examination was remarkable for nystagmus and bilateral horizontal gaze palsy on adduction. The remainder of her neurologic examination was normal. An MRI was obtained (see Figure 10-2). What is the most likely diagnosis?**

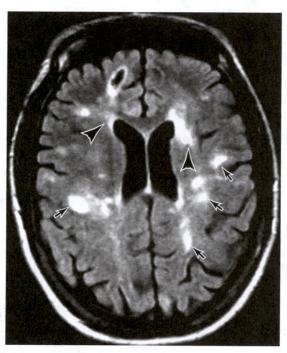

Figure 10-2   (Reproduced, with permission, from Simon RP, Greenberg DA, Aminoff MJ. *Clinical Neurology*. 6th ed. New York, NY: McGraw-Hill; 2009, Fig. 5-2B.)

Multiple sclerosis; the initial presentation was consistent with optic neuritis. Note the signal abnormalities in the white matter, which are consistent with multiple sclerosis.

○   **A patient with multiple sclerosis describes an electric shocklike sensation that runs down her back to her legs when she flexes her neck forward. What is this phenomenon called?**

Lhermitte sign.

○   **What are the findings on examination of the cerebrospinal fluid for a patient with multiple sclerosis?**

Mild pleocytosis and the presence of oligoclonal bands.

○   **What neurophysiologic tests are indicated in the evaluation of a patient with suspected multiple sclerosis?**

Evoked potentials will show slowed conduction due to demyelination. Visual evoked potentials will evaluate the integrity of the optic nerve, brainstem evoked responses (BAERs) evaluate the integrity of the auditory nerve, and somatosensory evoked potentials (SSEPs) evaluate the integrity of peripheral sensory pathways.

○ **A 34-year-old woman develops blurred vision associated with unilateral retro-orbital pain that is worse with eye movement. On physical examination, her visual acuity is decreased but extraocular eye movements are intact. Funduscopic examination reveals mild papillitis but no exudates or hemorrhages. What is the most likely diagnosis?**

Optic neuritis.

○ **What is the treatment of choice for an acute exacerbation of multiple sclerosis?**

Corticosteroids; intravenous methylprednisone, followed by a prednisone taper.

○ **Which pharmacologic intervention is used as a disease-modifying agent in the treatment of multiple sclerosis?**

Interferon has been shown to decrease the number of lesions seen on MRI as well as the number of exacerbations experienced by the patient.

○ **What is the treatment for the spasticity associated with multiple sclerosis?**

Lioresal (Baclofen).

○ **What is the most common cause of seizures in infants and children?**

Febrile seizures are most common between the ages of 3 months and 5 years of age.

○ **What is the most common cause of seizures in adolescents and adults?**

Head trauma.

○ **What is the most common cause of seizures in adults older than 65 years?**

Cerebrovascular disease (ischemic strokes more than hemorrhagic strokes).

○ **What is the most common epilepsy syndrome associated with complex partial seizures?**

Mesial temporal lobe epilepsy syndrome (MTLE), which is characterized by sclerosis of the hippocampus. MTLE is usually refractory to anticonvulsants but responds well to surgical resection.

○ **Which epilepsy syndrome, seen in children, is characterized by cognitive impairments and multiple seizure types?**

Lennox-Gastaut syndrome.

○ **What type of seizure disorder is characterized by a sudden loss of postural muscle tone?**

Atonic seizures; may present with a sudden head drop or complete collapse associated with falling.

○ **What type of symptoms can be seen with simple partial seizures?**

Motor, sensory, autonomic, or psychic.

○ **A patient initially experiences clonic movements of the hand, which then spread to involve the forearm and upper arm. What is this phenomenon called?**

Jacksonian march; reflective of seizure involvement spreading to neighboring areas of the motor cortex.

○ **What is Todd paralysis?**

Following a motor seizure of an extremity, there is a paresis of the muscles that were involved in the seizure that can last from several minutes up to several hours.

○ **What happens to the level of consciousness during a simple partial seizure?**

Consciousness is preserved.

○ **What type of autonomic symptoms can be seen with a simple partial seizure?**

Pupillary dilation, pallor, flushing, sweating, vomiting, and urinary incontinence.

○ **What type of psychic symptoms can be seen in association with a simple partial seizure?**

Memory distortions (i.e., déjà vu), fear, detachment, depersonalization, illusions (objects may appear to grow larger or smaller).

○ **Which type of seizure disorder is characterized by focal seizure activity accompanied by impaired consciousness?**

Complex partial seizures.

○ **What are automatisms?**

Automatisms are involuntary muscle activity seen in association with complex partial seizures; typical automatisms include lip smacking and chewing and picking or fumbling with clothing.

○ **A 6-year-old child is brought to your office by her mother. The mother states that for the past 6 months she and the girl's teacher have frequently noticed the child staring into space. Each episode lasted about 15 seconds and was associated with eye blinking. What is the most likely diagnosis?**

Absence seizures.

○ **What is the recommended first-line treatment for the patient described in the previous question?**

Ethosuximide or valproic acid are recommended as first-line medications for absence seizures.

○ **A 22-year-old female patient presents with recurrent episodes of altered consciousness during which time she would smack her lips and fumble with her clothing, according to witnesses. She was not responsive during these episodes and afterwards she would remain confused for up to an hour. What is the most likely diagnosis?**

Complex partial seizure.

○ **What medications can be used as first-line treatment for the patient described in the previous question?**

Carbamazepine, phenytoin, lamotrigine, and valproic acid are all first-line treatment options for complex partial seizures.

○ **A 25-year-old male patient is brought to the emergency department by his brother. They were watching a football game when he suddenly lost consciousness and fell to the floor. He was initially rigid before beginning to "shaking all over" for about a minute or two. He was sleepy and disoriented afterwards. What is the most likely diagnosis?**

Generalized tonic–clonic seizure.

○ **What is the recommended first-line treatment for the patient described in the previous question?**

Valproic acid, lamotrigine, and topiramate.

○ **What percentage of epilepsy patients are refractory to treatment with anticonvulsants?**

Approximately 20% to 30%; these patients should be referred to neurosurgery for consideration of a possible surgical resection.

○ **What type of seizure disorder is characterized by 30 minutes of continuous seizures or frequent seizures that occur without full restoration of consciousness?**

Status epilepticus.

○ **In addition to the "ABCs," what pharmacologic intervention is recommended for the first-line treatment of status epilepticus?**

Lorazepam.

○ **What is the definition of a transient ischemic attack?**

TIAs have been redefined as the acute onset of a neurologic deficit that resolves within an hour without a residual deficit.

○ **A patient presents with the loss of vision in the left eye, which he describes as "someone pulling a shade down over his eye." The episode resolved spontaneously within 30 minutes. What is this neurologic symptom called?**

Amaurosis fugax.

○ **Amaurosis fugax is consistent with pathology involving which blood vessel?**

Ipsilateral carotid artery; debris from an atherosclerotic plaque in the internal carotid can embolize to the central retinal artery.

○ **What is the risk of stroke following a transient ischemic attack?**

10% to 15% during the first 3 months; however, most strokes occur within the first 2 days following a TIA.

○ **What are the types of stroke?**

Ischemic (more common) and hemorrhagic.

○ **What is the most common cause of ischemic stroke?**

Atherosclerosis.

○   **What is the most important risk factor for stroke secondary to atherosclerosis?**

Hypertension, systolic or diastolic; increased blood pressure can triple the risk of stroke.

○   **What cardiac conditions are associated with increased stroke risk?**

Mural thrombus postinfarction, atrial fibrillation, endocarditis, and paradoxical emboli via a patent foramen ovale.

○   **What hematologic conditions are associated with increased risk for stroke?**

Thrombocytosis, polycythemia, and sickle cell disease; hypercoagulopathy is also associated, but it is uncommon.

○   **What is a lacunar infarct?**

Lacunar infarcts are strokes that are secondary to small vessel disease.

○   **What are common locations for lacunar infarcts?**

Basal ganglia, thalamus, and pons.

○   **What are the signs of an anterior cerebral artery stroke?**

Contralateral sensorimotor deficit affecting the leg and urinary incontinence.

○   **What are the signs of a middle cerebral artery stroke?**

Contralateral sensorimotor deficit affecting the arm, central VII palsy, visual field deficit, and language disturbances.

○   **What type of language deficit is seen with a middle cerebral artery stroke affecting Broca area in the dominant hemisphere?**

Expressive (nonfluent) aphasia; presentation may vary from word-finding difficulty to total mutism.

○   **What type of language deficit is seen with a middle cerebral artery stroke affecting Wernicke area in the dominant hemisphere?**

Receptive aphasia. Patients will not be able to follow commands since their ability to understand language will be lost; speech will be fluent but nonsensical.

○   **What type of visual field deficit is seen with a middle cerebral stroke?**

Contralateral homonymous hemianopsia.

○   **What are the signs of a posterior cerebral artery stroke?**

Contralateral visual field deficit (homonymous hemianopsia with or without macular sparing), and visual agnosia; cortical blindness can be seen with bilateral involvement.

○   **What is prosopagnosia?**

The inability to recognize familiar faces; it is seen with a posterior cerebral artery stroke.

○   **What are the signs of vertebrobasilar insufficiency?**

Cranial nerve palsies (diplopia, dysarthria), hemiplegia or quadriplegia, and altered mental status.

○ **A patient presents with the acute onset of quadriplegia. He is able to communicate only by blinking or moving his eyes up and down. What is the most likely diagnosis?**

Locked-in syndrome; consistent with a pontine stroke.

○ **What is the key diagnostic study in the evaluation of an acute stroke?**

Noncontrast CT scan of the head to distinguish an ischemic from hemorrhagic stroke.

○ **A 59-year-old male patient with a history of diabetes and chronic atrial fibrillation presented with the acute onset of a left hemiparesis involving the upper arm. There is a right-sided facial nerve palsy involving the lower face. A noncontrast CT scan of the head was obtained (see Figure 10-3). What is the most likely diagnosis?**

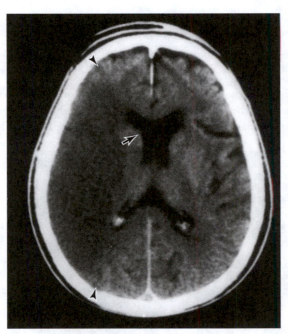

Figure 10-3 (Reproduced, with permission, from Simon RP, Greenberg DA, Aminoff MJ. *Clinical Neurology.* 6th ed. New York, NY: McGraw-Hill, 2009; Fig. 9-14A.)

Acute ischemic stroke.

○ **What vascular territory is involved in the patient described in the previous question?**

Middle cerebral artery (MCA). The wedge-shaped density changes on CT are consistent with the vascular territory for the middle cerebral artery; symptoms are also consistent with a MCA stroke.

○ **What is the recommended treatment of an asymptomatic carotid bruit?**

Aspirin.

○ **What is the recommended long-term treatment for transient ischemic attacks secondary to cardiac emboli?**

Warfarin.

○ **What is the time window to administer recombinant t-PA to treat an acute stroke if contraindications have been ruled out?**

3 hours from the onset of symptoms.

○ **What are contraindications for the use of thrombolytics in the management of an acute stroke?**

Poorly controlled hypertension (systolic BP > 185 mm Hg; diastolic BP > 110 mm Hg); major surgery within past 2 weeks; prior intracranial hemorrhage; other intracranial disease (history of trauma); history of bleeding from either the gastrointestinal or genitourinary tracts within past 3 weeks; abnormal coagulation profile.

○ **What is the most common cause of intracerebral hemorrhage?**

Hypertension.

○ **What are the most common locations for intracerebral hemorrhages?**

Basal ganglia (most common), thalamus, pons, and cerebellum.

○ **A 62-year-old, hypertensive man presented with the acute onset of a severe headache associated with nausea and vomiting. By the time he arrived in the emergency department, he was lethargic and not able to follow commands. A noncontrast CT scan of the head was done (see Figure 10-4). What is the most likely diagnosis?**

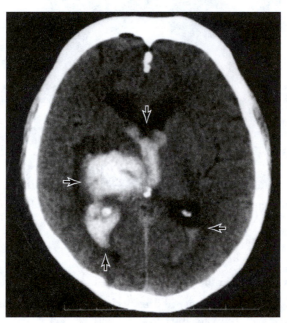

Figure 10-4 (Reproduced, with permission, from Simon RP, Greenberg DA, Aminoff MJ. *Clinical Neurology*. 6th ed. New York, NY: McGraw-Hill; 2009, Fig. 9-18.)

Intracerebral hemorrhage in the area of the thalamus with extension into the ventricles. (Primary extension into right lateral and third ventricle; although there is some extension into the occipital horn of the left lateral ventricle.)

○ **When is surgical decompression indicated in the management of an intracerebral hemorrhage?**

Cerebellar hemorrhages require decompression so as to avoid brainstem compression; surgery is not indicated for bleeds in the basal ganglia, thalamus, or pons.

○ **In addition to hypertension, what are other causes for intracerebral hemorrhages?**

Trauma, arteriovenous malformations, amyloid angiopathy, recreational drug use (amphetamines or cocaine), anticoagulation therapy, and coagulopathies.

○ **What is the most common cause of a nontraumatic subarachnoid hemorrhage?**

Congenital berry aneurysms.

○ **What additional congenital abnormalities may be seen with berry aneurysms?**

Polycystic kidney disease and coarctation of the aorta.

○ **What are the most frequent locations for intracranial aneurysms?**

Middle cerebral artery (29%), internal carotid artery (16%), anterior communicating artery (15%), basilar artery (14%), and anterior cerebral artery (9%).

○ **A 44-year-old patient presented with the "worst headache of her life." The headache came on suddenly and was associated with neck stiffness and vomiting. There was nuchal rigidity on examination, but no focal motor or sensory deficits. What is the most likely diagnosis?**

Subarachnoid hemorrhage.

○ **What is the first-line diagnostic study indicated in the evaluation of a possible subarachnoid hemorrhage?**

Noncontrast CT scan of the head; will be diagnostic in at least 90% of patients.

○ **For patients who have a suspected subarachnoid hemorrhage but a nondiagnostic CT scan, which diagnostic study is indicated?**

Lumbar puncture with cerebrospinal fluid analysis.

○ **What are the typical findings on analysis of cerebrospinal fluid (CSF) for a patient with a subarachnoid hemorrhage?**

Grossly bloody CSF and an elevated opening pressure; xanthochromia will be seen with centrifuged CSF.

○ **What is the definitive diagnostic study used in the evaluation of a subarachnoid hemorrhage?**

Four-vessel angiography.

○ **What is the recommended treatment of an intracranial aneurysm?**

Surgical clipping or endovascular placement of a coil into the aneurysm.

○ **What complications are associated with a subarachnoid hemorrhage?**

Vasospasm, hydrocephalus, recurrent hemorrhage, and seizures.

○ **What pharmacologic intervention is recommended to minimize the effects of vasospasm?**

Nimodipine, a calcium channel blocker, can help to minimize the ischemic effects associated with vasospasm.

○ **A 36-year-old patient presents with altered mental status following the acute onset of a severe headache. What is the diagnosis after viewing the CT in Figure 10-5A?**

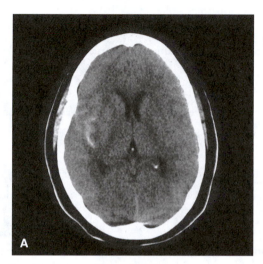

Figure 10-5A

Acute right-sided subarachnoid hemorrhage confined mostly to the sylvian fissure. The differential diagnosis is between trauma and ruptured intracerebral aneurysm. In this patient, a large right middle cerebral artery trifurcation aneurysm is confirmed by contrast angiography. (Figure 10-5B).

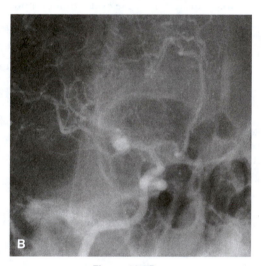

Figure 10-5B

○ **This is a 68 year old patient with new onset right homonomous hemianopsia. Based on the images shown in Figure 10-6A, what is the diagnosis?**

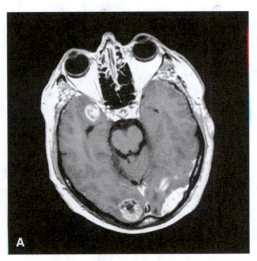

Figure 10-6A

Multiple enhancing lesions are present throughout the brain, several of which are shown here. The left occipital lesion would explain the patient's visual symptoms. The chest X-ray demonstrates a large mass in the right hilum (Fig. 10-6B), which was consistent with lung carcinoma and multiple brain metastases.

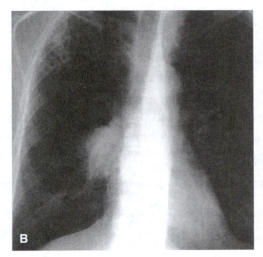

Figure 10-6B

○ **A 59-year-old man presents with a history of worsening confusion and the new onset of seizures. An MRI with gadolinium was obtained with the following results (see Figure 10-7). What is the most likely diagnosis?**

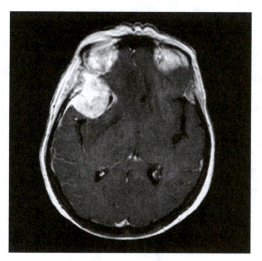

Figure 10-9

A large dural-based enhancing mass with a dural tail arises near the greater wing of the sphenoid at the junction of the right frontal and temporal lobes. The mass has characteristics of an extra-axial lesion and is consistent with a meningioma. Note that the finding of a small dural tail of enhancement along the edge of the mass is quite characteristic of meningioma along with its broad-based dural attachment.

• • • REFERENCES • • •

Aminoff MJ, Greenberg DA, Simon RP. *Clinical Neurology.* 6th ed. New York, NY: McGraw-Hill; 2005.

Fauci AS, Kasper DL, Longo DL, et al. *Harrison's Principles of Internal Medicine.* 17th ed. New York, NY: McGraw-Hill; 2008.

Fiebach NH, Kern DE, Thomas PA, Ziegelstein RC. *Barker's, Burton, and Zieve's Principles of Ambulatory Medicine.* 7th ed. Philadelphia, PA: Lippincott Williams & Wilkins; 2007.

Hay WW, Levin MJ, Sondheimer JM, Deterding RR. *Current Diagnosis and Treatment in Pediatrics.* 18th ed. New York, NY: McGraw-Hill; 2007.

Mumenthaler M, Mattle H, Taub E. *Fundamentals of Neurology: An Illustrated Guide.* New York, NY: Thieme; 2006.

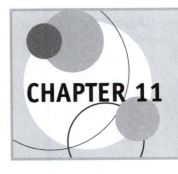

Daniel Thibodeau, MHP, PA-C

• • • ANXIETY DISORDERS • • •

○ **What are the two most common behavior problems seen by general practitioners?**

Anxiety and depression.

○ **What are the eight common <u>medical</u> causes of anxiety or anxiety attacks?**

1. Alcohol withdrawal

2. Thyrotoxicosis

3. Caffeine

4. Stroke

5. Cardiopulmonary emergencies

6. Hypoglycemia

7. Psychosensory/psychomotor epilepsy

8. Pheochromocytoma

○ **What age is the average onset of separation anxiety?**

Age 9. Children with separation anxiety fear leaving home, going to sleep, being alone, going to school, and losing their parents; 75% develop somatic complaints in order to avoid attending school.

○ **Do patients with mild anxiety attacks require medication?**

In general, no. Patients who experience greater frequency of events and/or impairment normal function may require medication. Tricyclic antidepressants are a first-line treatment but are reserved due to their side effects.

○ **A 24-year-old man presents complaining of pleuritic pain, palpitations, dyspnea, dizziness, and tingling in his arms, legs, and lips. What is the potential diagnosis?**

Hyperventilation syndrome. This is frequently associated with anxiety. Decreased carbonate levels in the blood cause the tingling. This should always be a diagnosis of exclusion.

○ **A 20-year-old woman complains of sudden episodes of palpitations, diaphoresis, lightheadedness, a fear of losing control, a sense of being choked, tremors, and paresthesias. What is the diagnosis?**

Panic disorder. Panic disorders need not be linked to any events, although they are commonly associated with agoraphobia, social phobia, mitral prolapse, and late nonmelancholic depression.

○ **Which gender is more likely to suffer from panic attacks?**

Women are twice as more likely than men. Median onset is in the mid-twenties.

○ **What percentage of patients with panic disorder also suffer from major depression?**

50%. Patients who suffer from panic attacks generally have a low self-esteem as well.

○ **Describe a patient with generalized anxiety disorder:**

Patients afflicted with this disorder appear apprehensive, restless, irritable, and are easily distracted. Patients can also experience muscle tension and fatigue, as well as various autonomic symptoms, such as palpitations, shortness of breath, chest tightness, nausea, or diffuse weakness and numbness.

○ **Name a few substances that might mimic generalized anxiety when ingested:**

Nicotine, caffeine, amphetamines, cocaine, and anticholinergics. Alcohol and sedative withdrawal can also mimic this disorder.

○ **What are some risk factors for PTSD?**

Women (twice compared to men), prior history of trauma, and a family history of anxiety disorder.

○ **What is the most common symptom of a patient with PTSD?**

Reexperiencing the traumatic event by either flashback, nightmares, or intrusive memories. Other symptoms can be avoidance and hyperarousal. Insomnia is also a major problem.

○ **John has just come back from the war in Iraq and has been diagnosed with PTSD. What would be the first-line medication for John?**

Selective serotonin reuptake inhibitors (SSRIs), particularly sertraline and paroxetine.

○ **Can a person acquire posttraumatic stress disorder (PTSD) if he/she did not actually witness a disturbing event?**

Yes. According to the DSM-IV, one can experience PTSD if an event, such as a violent personal assault, a serious accident, or the serious injury of a close friend or family member, is learned of indirectly. PTSD can also occur after a person hears of a life-threatening disease affecting a friend or family member.

○ **A 28-year-old woman who was raped 6 months ago has been psychologically sound thus far. She now suddenly develops recurrent flashbacks of the rape, nightmares, intense fear, avoidance of all men, a diminished memory of the rape, and an exaggerated startle response. Is this woman experiencing PTSD?**

Yes. This is delayed onset PTSD. The onset of symptoms occurs at least 6 months after the provoking event.

○ **What is the most common phobia in men?**

Social phobia.

○ **What is social phobia?**

It is a marked and persistent fear of one or more social or performance situations in which the person is exposed to unfamiliar people or possible scrutiny by others.

○ **What is the most common specific phobia in children?**

Animal phobia.

○ **What is the most common nonpharmacologic treatment for most phobias?**

Behavioral or cognitive-behavioral psychotherapy.

• • • ATTENTION-DEFICIT DISORDERS • • •

○ **What is the most common behavioral, emotional, and cognitive disorder in the youth population?**

Attention-deficit/hyperactivity disorder (ADHD).

○ **What are some of the signs and symptoms of ADHD?**

Inattentiveness, distractibility, impulsivity, and hyperactivity that is out of the reasonable boundaries for patients within their developmental stage.

○ **What comorbid diseases could you also find in a patient with ADHD?**

Oppositional defiant disorder, conduct disorder (greater severity), mood disorders, and childhood anxiety are some of the more common diseases.

○ **The sibling to a female patient with ADHD is at a higher risk for what other disorders?**

Conduct, mood, anxiety, and antisocial disorders, substance abuse, and, of course, ADHD. Relatives of women with ADHD are at a higher risk for these disorders compared to relatives of men.

○ **What class of drugs is commonly prescribed for the treatment of ADHD?**

Stimulants, specifically methylphenidate. **ADHD** (causes or associations) (Mnemonic: DEFICIT):

Diet (malnutrition)

Exposed to toxin (lead poisoning)

Fetal alcohol syndrome

Iron deficiency

Congenital (genetics or metabolic)

Infection (brain or ears)

Traumatic brain injuries

○ **What accounts for the most referrals to child psychiatrists?**

Attention-deficit/hyperactivity disorder (ADHD). ADHD accounts for 30% to 50% of child psychiatric outpatient cases.

• • • AUTISTIC DISORDERS • • •

○ **Which gender has a greater prevalence of autism?**

Men are three to four times more likely.

○ **What are some early signs of autism?**

In early stages of childhood, the children are often mute (50%). In later stages, the child has social deficits and difficulty with social interaction, eye contact, and defective imitation.

○ **What percentage of autistic children will be able to function independently?**

20%.

○ **What is this percentage in adults?**

Only 1% to 2%.

○ **What chromosomal abnormality do autistic patients commonly have?**

A fragile X syndrome (8%).

• • • EATING DISORDERS • • •

○ **What are the two types of anorexia nervosa?**

1. Restriction
2. Binge/purging

○ **What percentage of patients with anorexia are women?**

90%.

○ **Besides vomiting (purging), what are the other methods for weight loss that patient's with anorexia use?**

Use of laxatives and diuretics.

○ **What are some signs on examination that may be present in anorexia?**

Emaciated appearance, hypotension (orthostatic sometimes), bradycardia, lanugo, salivary gland hypertrophy, peripheral edema, and dental enamel erosion.

○ **What are some commonly seen laboratory abnormalities in anorexia?**

- Hematology—Leukopenia
- Chemistry
  - Elevated—liver functions, HCO_3, carotene, and cholesterol
  - Lower—chloride, potassium, zinc, estrogen, T_3, and T_4

○ **What is the most common psychiatric comorbidity in anorexia?**

Anxiety disorders.

○ **What are the two types of bulimia?**

1. Purging type
2. Non-purging—associated with fasting and/or excessive exercising; without the use of laxatives or diuretics

○ **What is the most common age of onset for bulimia?**

18 to 20 years; 98% to 100% are women.

○ **What is the only medication that is approved for the treatment of bulimia nervosa?**

Fluoxetine 60 mg daily.

○ **What are some of the more common physical examination and laboratory abnormalities associated with bulimia?**

Physical examination—dehydration appearance, dental erosion, oropharyngeal irritation, gastrointestinal bleeding

Laboratory—electrolyte abnormalities, metabolic alkalosis, decreased serum chloride and potassium; metabolic acidosis in patients taking laxatives

○ **What findings in a female patient who presents with parotid gland swelling and eroding tooth enamel might you expect?**

Bulimia, which is associated with elevated serum amylase and hypokalemia. The enlarged parotid is referred to as the "chipmunk appearance."

● ● ● **MOOD DISORDERS** ● ● ●

○ **What is an adjustment disorder?**

It is the development of emotional or behavioral symptoms in response to stressors, which occur within 3 months of the onset of stressors.

○ **What are some risk factors for individuals with adjustment disorder?**

Prior stress, childhood experience that was stressful and mood or eating disorders. Any family unity disruption (divorce, death [especially the father], living with in-laws) and prior exposure to war without PTSD.

○   **What is the behavioral and pharmacologic therapy for a patient with an adjustment disorder?**

Psychodynamic psychotherapy and antidepressants (SSRIs).

○   **What are the two required symptoms for the diagnosis of depression?**

Depressed mood and loss of interest or pleasure for at least a 2-week period of time.

○   **What are some risk factors for depression?**

A family history of depression, or alcoholism, a recent negative life experience, personality disorder, early childhood trauma, and postpartum depressive states.

○   **What are some signs and symptoms of a major depressive event?**

Depressed mood, anhedonia, change in appetite and sleep, change in energy, body activity, feelings of worthlessness, decreased concentration, and suicidal ideation.

○   **A patient is being evaluated for depression. Would there be any reason to evaluate the patient's thyroid?**

Yes. Up to 40% of patients with depression will have lower T_4 levels on initial evaluation. Most of these patients benefit with thyroid supplementation.

○   **Is there a correlation with the number of depressive episodes and prediction for future episodes?**

Yes. The more major depressive episodes a patient has, the more likely they are to have more. In an average lifetime, most patients will suffer about five major depressive events.

○   **Which class of drugs is commonly used as a first-line treatment for depression?**

Selective serotonin reuptake inhibitors (SSRIs).

○   **What are some second-line treatment options for depression?**

Monoamine oxidase inhibitors (MAO) and TCAs. Be careful as these medications have several side effects.

○   **When would electroconvulsive therapy (ECT) be considered for treatment of depression?**

During an urgent need, when the risk of ECT outweighs pharmacological therapy, when ECT has been beneficial in the past, and strong patient preference.

○   **What are the eight common medical causes of depression?**

1. Stroke
2. Viral syndromes
3. Corticosteroids
4. Cushing disease
5. Antihypertensive medication
6. SLE
7. Multiple sclerosis
8. Subcortical dementias, such as Huntington and Parkinson diseases, and HIV encephalopathy

○ **Major depression and bipolar affective disorders account for what percentage of suicides?**

50%. Another 25% are due to substance abuse and another 10% are attributed to schizophrenia.

○ **Name some symptoms of major depression:**

IN SAD CAGES:

Interest
Sleep
Appetite
Depressed mood
Concentration
Activity
Guilt
Energy
Suicide

○ **What is dysthymia?**

Dysthymia is a chronic disorder that lasts for more than 2 years. The severe symptoms of depression, such as delusions and hallucinations, are absent. Patients with dysthymia have some good days; they react to their environment and they have no vegetative signs; 10% of patients with dysthymia develop major depression.

○ **Who is at a greater risk for mood disorders, men or women?**

Women (7:3).

○ **What are some risk factors for dysthymia?**

More common in first-degree relatives or in those with history of major depression; age of onset before 45 years.

○ **What are some of the symptoms of dysthymia?**

Low self-esteem, low self-confidence, social withdrawal, loss of pleasure or interest, chronic fatigue or tiredness, feelings of guilt, difficulty thinking, and decreased activity.

○ **What is the common class of drugs that are given for dysthymia?**

SSRIs.

○ **What percentage of patients with dysthymia recovers after 2 years?**

40%.

○ **Which has an earlier onset, bipolar disorder or unipolar disorder?**

Bipolar. Onset of bipolar disorder is usually in the patient's twenties or thirties; onset of unipolar disorder is usually between ages 35 to 50 years.

○   **Differentiate between bipolar I, bipolar II, and hypomania:**

Bipolar I: Mania and major depression

Bipolar II: Hypomania and major depression

Cyclothymic: Hypomania and mania without severe impairment or psychotic features

○   **Are the majority of affective disorder patients bipolar or unipolar?**

Unipolar (80%).

○   **Which is most commonly the first episode of bipolar disease, mania or depression?**

Mania. Depression is rarely the first symptom. In fact, only 5% to 10% of patients who develop depression first go on to have manic episodes.

○   **First-degree relatives of bipolar patients have a greater risk for which mental illnesses?**

Unipolar disorders and alcoholism.

○   **Are bipolar patients at risk for suicide?**

Yes. In fact, they are two to three times more likely to commit suicide compared to general population.

○   **Other than classic mania, what can lithium be used to treat?**

Bulimia, anorexia nervosa, alcoholism in patients with mood disorders, leucocytosis in patients on antineoplastic medication, cluster headaches, and migraine headaches.

○   **Postural tremor is a major side effect of lithium. How is this side effect controlled?**

Minimize the dose during the workday and give small doses of β-blockers.

○   **Should people who are physically active have their lithium dosage increased or decreased?**

Increased. Lithium, a salt, is excreted more than sodium in sweat.

○   **True/False: A patient starting lithium will be expected to gain weight:**

True. All psychotropic medications cause weight gain, hence, lithium's usefulness in combating anorexia nervosa.

○   **What is the potential complication associated with treating manic depression and congestive heart failure simultaneously?**

Lithium toxicity. A low-salt diet and/or sodium-losing diuretics can cause lithium retention and toxicity.

○   **Lithium toxicity begins at what level?**

14 mg/L. Above this level, nausea, diarrhea, vomiting, rigidity, tremor, ataxia, seizures, delirium, coma, and death can occur.

○   **Name some vegetative symptoms:**

Loss of appetite, lack of concentration, chronic fatigue, agitation, restlessness, inability to sleep, and weight loss.

● ● ● PERSONALITY DISORDERS ● ● ●

○ **Is there a genetic link to patients with antisocial personality disorder?**

Yes. Patients who have a father with an antisocial disorder or alcoholism are more likely to have it even if the father wasn't around to raise the child.

○ **True/False: patients with antisocial personality disorders have a higher rate of substance abuse:**

True.

○ **A 24-year-old man who has a history of antisocial personality disorder along with a substance abuse history. Provided he stops his addiction, what can you tell the patient about his long-term prognosis?**

Most patients will have some improvement and 30% to 40% will significantly improve their symptoms as they reach the mid-thirties and forties age.

○ **A 30-year-old patient that you are seeing in your clinic. She has expressed that she does not interact in social situations because of a fear of not being liked. In addition, she is obsessed with thoughts of wondering if people like her. This causes the patient to feel socially inept and inferior. What is her diagnosis?**

Avoidant personality disorder.

○ **Which gender is more likely to have avoidant personality disorder?**

Women.

○ **Are patients with avoidant personality disorders able to function in a normal environment?**

It depends. Some patients are able to survive if they are able to control the conditions in which they exist. Others who are not able to keep control of these external factors will have more problems and this will directly impact their ability to function normally.

○ **Which personality disorder accounts for up to 30% of all personality disorders?**

Borderline personality disorder.

○ **What is the most common clinical symptom of a patient with a borderline personality disorder?**

Chronic boredom. Other symptoms include severe mood swings, volatile relationships, continuous and uncontrollable anger, and impulsiveness.

○ **What is a commonly reported historical fact that most patients with borderline personality disorder admit to in their childhood?**

Sexual, physical, and/or emotional abuse.

○ **Are suicidal gestures common in borderline personality patients?**

Yes. In fact, the more that they occur, the more serious they become with 10% of these cases becoming successful.

○ **A 27-year-old woman who is a controlling individual. She will ask friends to do things that she herself thinks are unpleasant, and tries to draw attention toward herself with superficial sexuality–type behaviors. When rejected, she will display disappointment to the point of throwing a childish temper tantrum. What is the patient's diagnosis?**

Histrionic personality disorder.

○ **True/False: Histrionic patients are often introverts:**

False. They are quite extroverted and at times neurotic.

○ **What are some other psychiatric disorders that accompany patients with histrionic personalities?**

Depression and anxiety can be common diagnoses.

○ **What is a narcissistic personality disorder?**

It is a pattern of behavior that exhibits grandiosity, a feeling of being greater than what is reality, requires excessive admiration, and is critical of others who challenge the patient. There is also a lack of empathy toward others.

○ **Which gender is more common in a narcissistic personality?**

Men.

○ **Which diagnoses can be confused with narcissistic personality disorder?**

Hypomania can often mimic this as well as antisocial personality.

○ **Is psychopharmacologic therapy beneficial in a narcissistic personality?**

No.

○ **What is the prognosis for a narcissistic patient?**

Many of the patients will actually worsen as they get older, typically in their forties. Depression is also common.

○ **Obsessive-compulsive disorders (OCD) generally begin before what age?**

25 years.

○ **What gender does obsessive-compulsive disorders predominate?**

Men.

○ **What are some common obsessions?**

Dirt and contamination, order and symmetry, religion and philosophy, daily decisions. Unfortunately, compulsion does not relieve the anxiety of the obsession. Serotonin reuptake inhibitors and exposure therapy can be helpful.

○ **Have medications been effective in treating OCD?**

No.

O **Is there a familial relationship in patients with paranoid personality disorder?**

There seems to be a relationship with family members who have a history of schizophrenia and/or delusional disorders.

O **A patient who is unable to express his anger, has few close friends, is indifferent to praise from others, is absentminded, and is emotionally cold and aloof probably has which kind of personality disorder?**

Schizoidia.

O **Are first-degree relatives of schizophrenics more likely to have schizoidia or schizophrenia?**

Schizoidia, at a ratio of 3:1.

O **What is a differentiating characteristic of schizoid when compared to schizophrenia?**

Schizoid patients do not have a need or behavior that dangers or involves others, while schizophrenia does.

O **Tom is a 14-year-old adolescent who has been exhibiting behavior that is unusual, along with odd beliefs and feels that he possesses magical abilities. What is the most likely diagnosis for Tom?**

Schizotypal personality disorder.

O **What are some more common disorders in patients with schizotypal disorders?**

Anxiety and substance abuse are common problems.

O **Which class of medications can be helpful in managing a patient with schizotypal disorder?**

Antipsychotics.

• • • PSYCHOSES • • •

O **Can patients with delusional disorder have hallucinations?**

Yes, tactile and olfactory hallucinations can be present in these patients.

O **What are some types of delusions?**

Erotomanic, grandiose, jealous, persecutory, somatic, and mixed.

O **What are some differential diagnoses with delusional disorder?**

Schizophrenia, schizoaffective, mood disorders, psychoses, and substance abuse.

O **Which classes of drugs are used to help control delusions?**

Antipsychotics.

O **What percentage of melancholic episodes are associated with hallucinations and/or delusions?**

20%.

○ **Cite an example for each of the following perceptual disturbances: illusion, complete auditory hallucination, functional hallucination, and extracampine hallucination:**

Illusion: A kitten is perceived as a dragon. (*The patient misinterprets reality.*)

Complete auditory hallucination: The patient claims to hear people talking when no one is around. (*Clear voices are reportedly heard. They are perceived as being external to the patient.*)

Functional hallucination: The patient hears voices only when cars honk their horns. (*Hallucinations occur only after sensory stimulus in the same category as the hallucination.*)

Extracampine hallucination: The patient can see people waving from the top of the Eiffel Tower, even though she is in Chicago. (*Hallucinations are external to the patient's normal range of senses.*)

○ **What is the difference between schizophrenia and schizophreniform disorder?**

Schizophreniform disorder implies the same signs and symptoms as schizophrenia, yet these symptoms have been present for less than 6 months. The impaired functioning in schizophreniform disorder is not consistent. Schizophreniform disorder is generally a provisional diagnosis with schizophrenia following.

○ **What are some characteristics of schizophrenia?**

Delusional disorder, hallucinations (usually auditory), disorganized thinking, loosening of associations, disheveled appearance, and the inability to realize thoughts and behavior are abnormal.

○ **What are the five first schizophrenia rank symptoms according to Schneider?**

1. Experiences of influence
2. Thought broadcasting
3. Experiences of alienation
4. Complete auditory hallucinations
5. Delusional perceptions

First-rank symptoms occur in 60% to 75% of schizophrenics. They also develop in patients with affective disorder, more commonly during manic stages.

○ **What are the five criteria for diagnosing schizophrenia?**

1. Psychosis
2. Emotional blunting
3. Absence of affective features or episodes
4. Clear consciousness
5. Absence of coarse brain disease, systemic illness, and drug abuse

○ **What percentage of patients with schizophrenia become chronically ill?**

60% to 80%. Men are at a greater risk for chronic illness.

○ **The onset of schizophrenia generally occurs by what age?**

80% of schizophrenics develop the disease before their early twenties. The disease is very rare after age 40.

○ **What are the five causes of schizophrenia?**

1. Viral infection in the CNS
2. Problem during pregnancy that affects the neuronal development
3. Head injury
4. Seizure disorder
5. Street drugs

○ **What psychiatric problems are associated with violence?**

Acute schizophrenia, paranoid ideation, catatonic excitation, mania, borderline and antisocial personality disorders, delusional depression, posttraumatic stress disorder, and decompensating obsessive-compulsive disorder.

○ **What is the average age of onset for schizophrenia?**

Men: 18 to 25 years
Women: 25 to 35 years

○ **What are the ages that are considered late and very late for the onset of schizophrenia?**

Late: after age 45
Very late: after age 65

○ **What percentage of schizophrenics is successful at suicide?**

10% to 13%.

○ **What are some secondary reasons for acute psychosis?**

Viral and bacterial infections, CNS infections, parasites, medications, anticholinergics drugs, hallucinogens, and over-the-counter stimulants.

○ **What are some hallmark signs and symptoms of schizophrenia?**

Delusions, hallucinations, disorganized speech and thoughts, and negative symptoms (deficits of normal function but not psychotic).

○ **What class of medications are the first-line treatment of schizophrenia?**

Antipsychotics.

○ **What are the five criteria for brief reactive psychosis?**

1. Precipitating stressful event
2. Rapid onset of the psychosis
3. Affective lability and mood intensity
4. Symptoms that match the stressful event
5. Resolution of symptoms once the stressor is removed, generally within 2 weeks

○   **What brain lesions sites are most commonly associated with psychosis?**

The temporolimbic system, caudate nucleus, and frontal lobes.

○   **List some life-threatening causes of acute psychosis:**

WHHHIMP:

Wernicke encephalopathy

Hypoxia

Hypoglycemia

Hypertensive encephalopathy

Intracerebral hemorrhage

Meningitis/encephalitis

Poisoning

○   **What signs and symptoms suggest an organic source for psychosis?**

Acute onset, disorientation, visual or tactile hallucinations, age under 10 or over 60 years, and any evidence suggesting overdose or acute ingestion, such as abnormal vital signs, pupil size and reactivity, or nystagmus.

○   **When are women at the greatest risk for psychiatric illness?**

The first few weeks postpartum. A psychiatric illness most often occurs in patients who are primiparous, have poor social support, or have a history of depression.

○   **When does postpartum psychosis begin?**

Within a week to 10 days following childbirth. A second, smaller peak occurs 5 to 7 months later, correlating with the first menses postpartum. The risk of psychosis is lowest during pregnancy.

• • • SOMATOFORM DISORDER • • •

○   **A 30-year-old woman complains of calf pain, headache, shooting pain when flexing her right wrist, random epigastric pain, bloating, and irregular menses, all of which cannot be explained after medical examination. What is the diagnosis?**

Somatization disorder, many unexplained medical symptoms involving multiple systems. In order to diagnose a patient with somatization disorder, one must have four or more unexplained pain symptoms. Symptoms generally begin in childhood and are fully developed by age 30. This is more common in women than in men.

○   **What percentage of primary care patients exhibits some form of somatizations in clinic visits?**

25%.

○   **What is a classic type of patient that presents with somatoform disorder?**

Young, unmarried, non-white woman from a rural area and who is uneducated.

○ **What is the treatment of somatoform disorder?**

It is extremely difficult. First, you have to detect the disorder and then convince the patient that they have this problem. Second is to have the patient exhibit more than two to three office visits that are legitimate problems. Make sure to examine all symptoms and orders tests as needed, and lastly prescribe any medications that may help the said illness and monitor for improvement.

● ● ● OTHER BEHAVIORAL DISORDERS ● ● ●

○ **What are some criteria to meet in a acute stress disorder (ASD)?**

Primary—Patient has to be witness to a traumatic event or involved. The event has to involve the patient's fear or helplessness.

Secondary—While during this event, the patient has a sense of detachment, will be in a daze and not able to function normally, and have a detachment from memory about the event. This may also cause the patient to have recall of the event, flashbacks, and reminders of the trauma. This experience will create a significant impairment for the patient.

○ **If a patient has an ASD from an event, what is he/she likely to develop?**

Up to 80% of these patients will later be diagnosed with PTSD.

○ **What are the three categories of child maltreatment?**

Child neglect, physical abuse, and sexual abuse.

○ **How many children die each year as a result of abuse?**

1500.

○ **What are some parental factors that lend to child abuse?**

Lower parental education, mental illness, alcoholism, and substance abuse.

○ **In what percentage of child sexual abuse cases is the abuser known by the child?**

90%. In 50% of such cases, the mother is also abused.

○ **In addition to the history, physical examination, laboratory tests, and collection of physical evidence, what needs to be done in cases of child sexual abuse?**

File a report with child protective services and law enforcement agencies. Provide emotional support to the child and family. Give a return appointment for follow-up of STD cultures and testing for pregnancy, HIV, or syphilis as indicated. Assure follow-up for psychological counseling by connecting the child/family to the appropriate services in your area.

○ **Is violence more likely between family members or nonfamily members?**

Family members: 20% to 50% of the murders in the United States are committed by members of the victims' families. Spouse abuse is as high as 16% in the United States.

○ **What is the epidemiology of domestic violence?**

95% of the victims are women. An estimated 4 million women are battered each year. Domestic abuse is the number one cause of injuries to women. More than half of all women murdered in the United States are killed by their intimate partner.

○ **What are the clinical clues for domestic violence?**

Any evidence of injury during pregnancy or late entry into prenatal care. Injuries presenting after significant delay or in various stages of healing; especially to the head, neck, breasts, abdomen, or areas suggesting a defensive posture, such as bruises on the forearms. Vague complaints or unusual injuries, such as bites, scratches, burns, or rope marks.

○ **What is the standard of care for victims of domestic violence currently recommended by JCAHO, the AMA, and the CDC?**
  • Establish a confidential system to identify DV victims
  • Document the abuse
  • Collect physical evidence
  • Evaluate safety issues and potential for lethality or suicide
  • Formulate a safety plan with the victim
  • Advise the victim of all his/her options and resources
  • Refer for counseling and other services, including legal assistance
  • Coordinate with law enforcement
  • Transport to a shelter if desired or needed
  • Follow-up with a domestic violence advocate

○ **What are the prodromes of violent behavior?**

Anxiety, defensiveness, volatility, and physical aggression.

○ **What are the only reliable indicators of a potentially violent patient?**

Male gender, history of violence, and history of substance abuse. Cultural, educational, economic, and language barriers to effective patient/staff communication can increase the patient's frustration and lower his or her threshold for violence as can trivialization of the patient or the family's concerns.

○ **Bereavement generally lasts how long?**

6 months. Full melancholic syndrome, hallucinations, and suicidal ideation are not common in bereavement.

○ **When do you medically treat uncomplicated bereavement?**

When the symptoms mimic depression and last for more than 13 months. This would be the expected time that uncomplicated bereavement should subside.

○ **Who is more successful at suicide, men or women?**

Men (a 3:1 men-to-women ratio). However, women attempt suicide three times as often as men.

○ **True/False: Fantasies frequently precede suicidal acts:**

True.

○ **What percentage of patients with melancholia attempt suicide?**

15%.

○ **What is the number one cause of death for African American men between the ages of 10 and 24 years?**

Firearm injury. The overall homicide rate for young men in the United States is more than seven times that of the next developed country.

○ **Do intentional or unintentional causes account for more firearm-related deaths?**

Intentional causes account for 94% of firearm deaths, suicide for 48%, and homicide for 46%. Unintentional firearm injuries account for about 4%. Only 1% of firearm deaths occur as a result of legal intervention. The number of firearm-related fatalities has more than doubled in the last 30 years.

○ **What are risk factors for homicide?**

Most homicide victims are killed by someone they know, someone of the same race, and usually during an argument or fight. Drugs and alcohol are important cofactors as is the presence of a handgun.

○ **What are the relative risks for suicide and homicide if a gun is kept in the home?**

Suicide is five times more likely. Homicide is three times more likely. The victim is 43% more likely to be a member of the family than an intruder. In the case of domestic violence, a gun at home increases the risk of homicide 20-fold.

● ● ● SUBSTANCE USE DISORDERS ● ● ●

○ **What is the prevalence of alcoholism in the United States?**

10% to 15% is the lifetime prevalence, and 10% of men and 3.5% of women are alcoholic.

○ **What age range has the highest prevalence of drinking problems?**

18 to 29 year olds have the greatest prevalence.

○ **What laboratory changes are suggestive of alcoholism?**

Look for an increase in ALT, AST, alkaline phosphatase, amylase, bilirubin, cholesterol, GGT, LDH, MCV, prothrombin time, triglycerides, and uric acid and a decrease in BUN, calcium, coagulopathy, hematocrit, magnesium, phosphorus, platelet count, and protein.

○ **Describe the symptoms of alcohol withdrawal and their temporal relations:**

Autonomic hyperactivity: Tachycardia, hypertension, tremors, anxiety, and agitation occur 6 to 8 hours after patient's last drink

Hallucinations: Auditory, visual, and tactile occur 24 hours after patient's last drink.

Global confusion: Occurs 1 to 3 days after patient's last drink.

○ **What is the difference in the treatment methods between alcohol withdrawal compared to sedative hypnotic withdrawal?**

Alcohol withdrawal is treated with benzodiazepine, carbamazepine, or paraldehyde. Sedative hypnotic withdrawal is treated with the substitution of a long-acting barbiturate.

○ **What is the most effective long-term treatment program for alcoholism?**

Alcoholics Anonymous.

○ **What should you do when handling intoxicated, violent, psychotic, or threatening patients?**

Conduct careful histories and physicals with attention to mental status. Look for evidence of trauma, toxic ingestion, or metabolic derangement. Historical sources (e.g., family, paramedics, mental health workers, police, or medical records) may need to be accessed. Patients may need to be physically or chemically restrained in order to obtain an adequate examination and to ensure the safety of the patient and hospital staff.

○ **What is the most common mental illness in large cities?**

Substance abuse. Substance abuse is prevalent in rural communities as well but the addiction percentages are lower. Incidentally, opiates are predominantly a city drug, while marijuana, alcohol, and amphetamines are found in both the rural and urban settings.

○ **A patient presents with tearing eyes, a runny nose, tachycardia, hair on end, abdominal pains, nausea, vomiting, diarrhea, insomnia, pupillary dilation, and leukocytosis. What is the diagnosis?**

Opiate and/or opioid withdrawal. Treat with methadone or Dolophine. Clonidine may blunt some of the side effects.

○ **Wild and abundant dreams may result from the withdrawal of what drugs?**

Antidepressants. Other side effects of withdrawal are anxiety, akathisia, bradykinesia, mania, and malaise.

○ **What percentage of deaths has been associated with tobacco use?**

25%.

○ **What are some of the more common diseases associated with tobacco use?**

Coronary heart disease, oral cancers, dental disease, emphysema, lung cancer, and low birth weight in pregnant women.

○ **What are the components of the multiaxial diagnostic system?**

Axis I: Symptoms and syndromes comprising a mental disorder, including substance abuse/addiction
Axis II: Personality and developmental disorders underlying the axis I diagnosis
Axis III: Physical medical problems/conditions that may or may not contribute to the axis I diagnosis
Axis IV: Psychosocial factors
Axis V: Adaptive ability/disability

○ **What is the most common cause of catatonia?**

Affective disorder.

○ **What is a previously healthy patient most likely suffering from when he becomes suddenly and intensely excited, goes into a delirious mania, develops catatonic features, and a high fever.**

Lethal catatonia. Such patients have a 50% death rate without treatment. Treat these patients with ECT.

○ **How is lethal catatonia differentiated from neuroleptic malignant syndrome?**

By the timing of the hyperthermia. In lethal catatonia, severe hyperthermia occurs during the excitement phase before catatonic features develop. In neuroleptic malignant syndrome, hyperthermia develops later in the course of the disease with the onset of stupor.

○ **In infancy, simple repetitive reactions like nail-biting, thumb-sucking, masturbation, or temper tantrums are manifestations of what psychological reaction?**

Adjustment reactions. These are responses to separation from the caregiver and are often associated with developmental delay.

○ **What is the prevalence of conduct disorder?**

10%. It is more common in boys and is hereditary.

○ **Children with conduct disorders will probably develop what adult disorder?**

Antisocial personality disorder. About 40% will have some pathology as adults.

○ **What is conversion disorder?**

An internal psychological conflict that manifests itself through somatic symptoms. Voluntary motor or sensory functions are affected. Examples include weakness, imbalance, dysphagia, and changes in vision, hearing, or sensation. These symptoms are not feigned or intentionally produced. They are also not fully explained by medical conditions.

○ **What are the five Kübler-Ross stages of dying?**

1. Denial
2. Anger
3. Bargaining
4. Depression
5. Acceptance

Patients may undergo either all or only a few of these stages.

○ **What psychiatric disease is the most hereditary?**

Idiopathic enuresis. If one parent has enuresis, there is a 44% chance that the child will also have the disease. If both parents have it, the likelihood increases to 77%.

○ **What is an extreme case of factitious disorder?**

Munchausen syndrome. These patients may actually try to cause harm to themselves (e.g., by injecting feces into their veins) and are very accepting/seeking of invasive procedures. Munchausen by proxy is another example. In this disease, the patient seeks medical care for another, usually a child.

○ **Give examples of the following thought disorders: perseveration, nonsequiturs, derailment, tangential speech, neologism, private word usage, and verbigeration:**

Perseveration—"I've been wondering if the mechanical mechanisms of this machine are mechanically sound. Mechanically speaking, I must understand the mechanisms." (*A repetition of certain words or phrases is found in the natural flow of speech.*)

Nonsequiturs—Q: "Are you nervous about the upcoming boards?" A: "Why no, the king of France is an excellent king." (*The patient's answers are unrelated to the questions asked.*)

Derailment—"I first became interested in the study of medicine after mom bought me a toy ambulance. Toys can be very dangerous, especially if they are very small and can be swallowed. I've been having difficulty swallowing lately." (*The patient suddenly switches lines of thought, though the second follows the first.*)

Tangential speech—A: "Those are nice clothes you're wearing today." B: "Of course I'm wearing clothes today." A: "I mean, I like the outfit you have on." B: "I think everyone should wear clothes, except on Friday, because Friday is casual day at my office." (*Conversations are on the right subject matter; however, the responses are inappropriate to the previous questions or comments.*)

Neologism—"I'm going to explaphrase (*explain by paraphrasing*) the meaning of agnonoctaudiophobia (*things that go bump in the night*)." (*Neologisms are meaningless combinations of two or more words to invent a new word.*)

Private word usage—"I can't believe the loquacious way he is formicating those tripods." (*Words and or phrases used in unique ways.*)

Verbigeration—"I have been studying, have been studying, have been studying, for hours for hours hours hours." (*The patient repeats words, especially at the end of thoughts, thoughts, thoughts, thoughts.*)

○ **Matching:**

1. Hypomania	a. 1 or more hypomanias plus 1 or more major depressive symptoms
2. Melancholia	b. A mild manic episode
3. Bipolar II	c. Deep depression and vegetative characteristics
	d. Manic episodes only
4. Unipolar mania	e. Many mild episodes of hypomania and depression
5. Cyclothymia	

Answers: (1) b, (2) c, (3) a, (4) d, and (5) e.

○ **A patient is brought in because she believes butterflies are landing all around her. The butterflies talk to her and tell her to love everyone. She denies suicidal ideation and any desire to harm herself or others. She has no record of harming people in the past. Can this person be institutionalized against her will?**

No. Unless the patient is a danger to herself or others, she cannot be confined to an institution despite questionable mental status.

○ **What is the difference between a malingering and a factitious disorder?**

A malingerer's incentive is external, such as workman's compensation. The goal of someone with a factitious disorder is to enter into the sick role. Both involve feigning illness.

○ **According to Holmes and Rahe, what are life's top 10 most stressful events?**

1. Death of spouse or child
2. Divorce
3. Separation
4. Institutional detention
5. Death of close family member
6. Major personal injury or illness
7. Marriage
8. Job loss
9. Marital reconciliation
10. Retirement

● ● ● REFERENCES ● ● ●

Brunton Laurence L, L J. *Goodman and Gilman's The Pharmacological Basis of Therapeutics.* 11th ed. New York, NY: McGraw-Hill; 2006.

Ebert ML, Nurcombe B, Leckman JF. *Current Diagnosis and Treatment, Psychiatry.* 2nd ed. New York, NY: McGraw-Hill; 2008.

Fauci Anthony S., B. E. (2008, 7 1). Harrisons Online. New York, NY.

McPhee Stephen J, PM. *Current Medical Diagnosis and Treatment 2009.* New York, NY: McGraw-Hill; 2009.

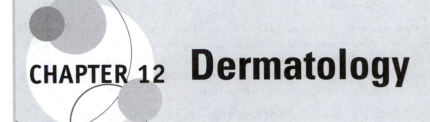

CHAPTER 12 Dermatology

Kimberly K. Dempsey, MPA, PA-C

● ● ● ECZEMATOUS ERUPTIONS ● ● ●

○ **A 5-year-old girl presents with a 3 cm, hyperpigmented, scaling plaque located at the umbilicus. She also has smaller similar lesions on both ear lobes at the site of her ear piercings. Her mother states that this is extremely pruritic. What does this represent?**

This reaction is consistent with an allergic contact dermatitis to nickel. Buttons, snaps, and other clothing closures all contain nickel. Costume jewelry also contains nickel. Nickel is a common sensitizing agent that causes an eczema-like reaction at sites of contact. Avoidance of metal is crucial in treatment and prevention. Occlusive techniques such as clear nail polish and duct tape provide minimal improvement. Avoidance and treatment with an appropriate topical steroid and oral antihistamine for itch relief is appropriate treatment.

○ **What is the appropriate treatment of contact dermatitis caused by poison ivy?**

Wash all clothing that may have come into contact with the oils from the poison ivy plant. Topical treatment with a class I–III topical steroid is effective for limited or early lesions. Oral steroids are indicated for severe cases. Prednisone beginning at 60 mg (adults), tapering by 10 mg over a 2-week period. The pediatric dosing is 2 mg/kg PO qd as an initial dose, tapering over 2 weeks. Oral antihistamines such as Benadryl or hydroxyzine may provide relief from pruritus.

○ **A 17-year-old female patient has a rash on her elbows and knees. Upon examination, you find several well-demarcated erythematous plaques covered with silvery scales that exhibit pinpoint bleeding when removed. These lesions are located on her extensor surfaces. Examination of her nails reveals pitting. What is her diagnosis?**

Psoriasis. This is a chronic disorder with bimodal peaks in incidence of 22.5 years and 55 years. Early onset is indicative of a more severe and long-lasting disease. There may be associated arthritis; otherwise, the disease is limited to the skin and nails. *Remember*: "Silvery scales and pitting nails."

○ **A 13-year-old patient presents with erythema and yellow scaly plaques in his eyebrows, eyelids, and nasolabial folds. What is the most likely diagnosis?**

This patient most likely has seborrheic dermatitis. Infantile and adolescent seborrheic dermatitis often improves with age. There is frequently a hereditary component. It occurs in areas where there is a concentration of sebaceous glands.

○ **What are the diagnostic criteria for atopic dermatitis?**

Essential clinical features include pruritus and eczematous changes in a predictable distribution. There is a specific distribution by age group. Infants may have involvement of the face and extension to the trunk, especially the extensor surfaces. Children from the age of 2 to puberty usually have involvement of the extremities, particularly the wrists, ankles, hands, feet, and popliteal and antecubital fossae. Beginning at puberty, the distribution changes to include the flexural creases, face, neck, and the dorsum of the hands and feet.

Supporting features of atopic dermatitis include early age of onset, family history of atopy, and xerosis.

○ **What is the treatment for atopic dermatitis?**

Management of atopic dermatitis includes limiting bathing to 10 minutes daily with soap-free cleansers. In addition, liberal use of thick emollients especially right after bathing will help maintain skin hydration. Avoidance of irritant or allergens is also crucial to help control atopic dermatitis. Topical steroids are the first-line pharmacological treatment for atopic dermatitis. Pruritus can also be relieved with the use of oral antihistamines.

○ **A mother brings her 6-month-old daughter in for a diaper rash that has been unresponsive to over-the-counter diaper creams. On physical examination, you find a well-demarcated beefy red rash with pinpoint satellite papules. What is the most common causative organism?**

Candida albicans commonly occurs in infants. The moist occlusive diaper provides an optimal environment for proliferation of this organism. Systemic antibiotics can also contribute to proliferation.

○ **Which chronic disorder with acute exacerbations is characterized by deep-seated vesicles located on the palms, soles, and lateral aspects of the fingers and intense pruritus?**

Dyshidrotic eczema. Exacerbations are treated with moderate to potent topical steroids. Oral antihistamines help with pruritus.

○ **What is lichen simplex chronicus and how is it treated?**

This is also called circumscribed neurodermatitis, which is a self-perpetuated skin disorder causing the skin to turn into dry, leathery, lichenified patches most commonly seen on the nape of the neck, wrists, forearms, and lower legs and perineal area. The best treatment for this disorder is to use flurandrenolide tape, which will prevent the patient from scratching while healing the dermatitis. Also, the use of oral antihistamines to relieve itching can be beneficial.

• • • PAPULOSQUAMOUS DISEASES • • •

○ **What type of reaction is erythema multiforme and what are its common causes?**

Erythema multiforme is a hypersensitivity reaction. There are numerous possible inciting agents. Some of the most common are:

- **infection,** especially herpes simplex, *Mycoplasma*
- **drugs** such as sulfonamides, NSAIDS, phenytoin, barbiturates, and salicylates
- **malignancy**
- **idiopathic**

○ **What is the most common location of erythema nodosum?**

The most common site for erythema nodosum is the shin. These can also be found on the knees and extensor surfaces of the forearms. Skin findings are deep-red tender nodules. Erythema nodosum is a hypersensitivity reaction to a variety of stimuli and its causes include infectious organisms, drugs, malignancies, and connective tissue diseases. Often the cause is idiopathic.

○ **What is the Koebner phenomenon?**

The development of plaques/lesions in areas where trauma has occurred. Just a scratch can trigger the development of a plaque. This is common in numerous conditions such as psoriasis, lichen planus, molluscum contagiosum, and verrucae.

○ **A 17-year-old male patient complains of spreading spots. They began several months ago on his upper back and have spread to involve the upper chest and upper arms. There are no associated symptoms; he is just concerned that he is becoming "spotted." On physical examination, you see small, circular, tan macules with fine scaling. What is the presumptive diagnosis and how would you confirm your diagnosis?**

This patient most likely has tinea versicolor, which is caused by the lipophilic yeast *Malassezia furfur*. This infection is most common during adolescence and early adulthood when sebaceous gland activity is at its peak. The easiest way to confirm the diagnosis is to perform a KOH Prep with 10% to 20% KOH. Visualization of hyphae (usually shortened) and spores is confirmatory; this is the classic "spaghetti and meatball" appearance.

○ **What are the treatment alternatives and appropriate patient education for the above patient?**

Treatment options include antifungal shampoo such as selenium sulfide or ketoconazole 2% left on for 10 minutes before washing. This can be done daily for up to 2 weeks. Topical imidazoles such as ketoconazole, econazole, and oxiconazole can be applied twice daily for 2 weeks. For severe, recurrent or intractable cases PO ketoconazole 400 mg can be used.

○ **Urticaria that results within seconds of firm stroking of the skin is:**

Dermatographism. This is a very common physical urticaria. Pressure urticaria, swelling resulting from local pressure, is a variant of dermatographism.

○ **A 20-year-old female patient complains of a spreading rash. She states it started with a dry scaling patch on the abdomen that was larger than the current lesions. Now she has smaller dry scaling patches located on her chest and pack. She denies any associated symptoms. What is the presumptive diagnosis?**

The characteristic rash of pityriasis rosea begins with a "herald patch," which is usually 2 to 5 cm. Within a week or two, smaller lesions distributed over the torso and proximal extremities develop along the cleavage lines ("Christmas tree" distribution). These are scattered scaling patches that may be asymptomatic or mildly pruritic. Treatment is symptomatic since this resolves spontaneously in 6 to 12 weeks. Oral antihistamines help with pruritus.

○ **What rash is classically associated with a "herald patch"?**

Pityriasis rosea. Most cases begin with a single large, oval patch (herald patch). Then, there is a secondary eruption of small oval patches with a collarette of scale appear on the trunk parallel to the lines of cleavage, the "Christmas tree" distribution. A history of mild pharyngitis and malaise may precede the rash.

○ **A 14-year-old adolescent presents to the emergency department with 103.1°F fever and dysphagia. He appeared ill and had small vesicles on the nasal and oral mucosa. An erythematous rash on his chest coalesced on the trunk with many small vesicles, some forming bullae. Vesicles were also present on the penis and scrotum. What is the likely diagnosis?**

Stevens-Johnson syndrome (SJS)/toxic epidermal necrolysis (TEN) are considered to be variants of the same disorder. SJS was formerly referred to as erythema multiforme major. Patients may initially present with SJS and evolve into TEN depending on the degree of epidermal detachment. Features of each include targetoid lesions that can develop into bullae with prominent mucosal involvement. Sometimes the bullae may become confluent and detach leaving a denuded base. SJS is diagnosed when there is less than 10% epidermal detachment, SJS–TEN is diagnosed with 10 % to 30% epidermal detachment, and TEN when there is greater than 30% detachment.

○ **A 25-year-old male patient presents with a well-defined oval violaceous lesion located in the groin. He states that it is pruritic and occurred approximately an hour after taking acetaminophen for a headache. He states this has happened before under similar circumstances. What is the likely diagnosis?**

Fixed drug eruption. Common inciting agents in fixed drug eruptions are antimicrobial agents, tetracyclines, metronidazole, anti-inflammatory agents, oral contraceptives, phenolphthalein, and yellow food coloring. The eruptions usually appear within 30 minutes to 8 hours after ingesting the offending agent. The lesions are well defined, usually round or oval, and dusky red to violaceous macules. Thes may become edematous with erosions or bullae.

○ **What drugs are most often implicated in toxic epidermal necrolysis (TEN)?**

Sulfonamides, penicillins, anticonvulsants, allopurinol, sulfonylureas, barbiturates, and NSAIDs.

○ **What is Nikolsky sign?**

A positive Nikolsky sign is when the gentle pressure on the skin causes the epidermis to separate and leave a raw, denuded base.

○ **A 77-year-old man presents to your clinic complaining of multiple fluid-filled blisters to the flexor surfaces of his forearms. He states that he has had itching to these areas for quite sometime but now this has occurred. On examination, you see multiple tense bullae to the flexor surfaces of the arms with an irritated erythematous base. What is the most likely diagnosis?**

Bullous pemphigoid. These are lesions that will have a life span of up to 5 to 6 years. The diagnosis is made by biopsy and immunofluorescence and treated with ultrapotent steroids.

● ● ● **ACNEIFORM LESIONS** ● ● ●

○ **What are the typical clinical manifestations of hidradenitis suppurativa?**

Typical skin lesions include open comedones, particularly the double comedones, and tender abscesses that may drain purulent or seropurulent material. Sinus tracts may also form. These lesions are most common in the axillae, anogenital region, and under the breast.

○ **What is the best treatment for the comedonal lesions (white heads and black heads) of acne vulgaris?**

Topical retinoids are the treatment of choice for comedonal acne. Topical benzoyl peroxide and salicylic acid preparations have a mild comedolytic effect.

○ **What are the side effects of tetracycline antibiotics commonly used to treat inflammatory acne?**

Side effects include dental staining in children younger than 9 years, GI upset, photosensitivity, pseudotumor cerebri, and vulvovaginal candidiasis. Minocycline has the added side effects of blue-gray skin pigmentation of the skin or mucosa, lupus-like reactions, and vertigo.

○ **Describe the clinical manifestation of acne rosacea:**

Early manifestations include facial flushing in response to heat, spicy foods, alcohol, warm drinks, and sun exposure. Tiny papules and pustules may also be present early. Later manifestations can include telangiectasias, sebaceous hyperplasia, and rhinophyma. Ocular symptoms, such as blepharitis, conjunctivitis, and episcleritis, may occur. Distribution is primarily on bilateral cheeks. There are no comedones present.

○ **Describe the different forms of folliculitis:**

Folliculitis depends on the source of the infection. The most common cause is staphylococcal bacteria and is more common in diabetic patients. Other causes include "hot tub" folliculitis, which is caused by *Pseudomonas* and produces follicular pustules, and nonbacterial folliculitis, which can be caused by friction and oils.

• • • INSECTS/PARASITES • • •

○ **A 12-year-old female patient complains of intense generalized itching; it worsens at night. On physical examination, she has erythematous papules on her hands and feet including the palms or soles. She also has papules and nodules around the umbilicus and in the genital area. Close examination reveals a linear lesion in the webspace on her hands. What is the presumptive diagnosis and how would you confirm your suspicion?**

Scabies. Scabies are due to the mite *Sarcoptes scabiei* var. *hominis*. To confirm your diagnosis, an intact burrow or papule should be scraped and the scraping should be placed on a glass slide with mineral oil. Visualization of a mite, eggs, or feces is diagnostic for scabies.

○ **What is the appropriate treatment for the patient described in the previous question?**

Appropriate treatment is application of 5% permethrin cream applied from the neck to toes and left on overnight (8 hours) and then washed off. All people who live in the same residence should be treated at the same time. After treatment, carpets and upholstered furniture should be vacuumed and sheets and clothing should be washed in hot soapy water. This treatment should be repeated in 1 week to kill any mites that have hatched in the interim. Oral antihistamines can be prescribed to ameliorate pruritus. Very frequently, the patient has a postscabetic dermatitis that can be treated with appropriate topical steroids.

○ **What is the drug of choice for pediculosis capitis (head lice)?**

1% permethrin (which is available OTC).

○ **What is the treatment of choice for scabies and how should it be used?**

5% permethrin cream applied overnight to all skin surfaces from the neck down. Special attention should be given to webspaces and skin under the nails. Treatment should be repeated in 1 week.

○ **What are two potential skin manifestations that can be caused by a brown recluse spider?**

Local pain and cellulitis, which can progress to an area of necrosis that spreads.

● ● ● NEOPLASMS ● ● ●

○ **A 62-year-old male tennis player with androgenetic alopecia presents with small scattered areas of skin-colored hyperkeratotic scale. When scraped, they are tender. The texture is that of sandpaper when palpated. What does this most likely represent?**

This presentation is consistent with actinic keratosis. These are more common in middle-aged men, especially those who spend a great deal of time outdoors. These lesions are often easier to feel than to see. AKs are isolated or scattered discrete lesions distributed in sun-exposed areas. They can progress to squamous cell carcinoma.

○ **Brown plaques with a warty "stuck on" appearance that erupt after the age of 30 and that have no malignant potential are consistent with:**

Seborrheic keratosis.

○ **A 50-year-old man present with two pearly papules: one on the nostril and another on the nasolabial fold. These papules are smooth and dome shaped with some overlying telangiectasias. Your patient states that these have been growing slowly. What do these papules most likely represent?**

Basal cell carcinoma (BCC) is the most common cutaneous malignancy. These lesions most likely represent the most common variant of BCC, nodular basal cell carcinoma. The papules may also display a raised, rolled border and may be red or skin colored. Later stages may also display central ulceration, bleeding, and crusting. Other types of BCC include ulcerating BCC, sclerosing BCC, superficial multicentric BCC, and pigmented BCC.

○ **Nevi should be examined for what characteristics when evaluating for atypia?**

Asymmetry: one-half is unlike the other half

Border irregularity: irregular, scalloped, or poorly defined borders

Color variation: variations in color present (tan, brown, black, white, red)

Diameter: >6 mm in acquired after the age of 1 year

Evolution: mole that looks different than the rest or is changing

○ **What are the risk factors for melanoma?**

- Fair complexion
- History of sunburns
- More than 50 moles
- Atypical moles
- Family history of melanoma

○ **A periungual extension of brown-black pigmentation from longitudinal melanonychia onto the proximal nail fold is an indicator of?**

This is consistent with a Hutchinson sign, which is an indicator of subungual melanoma. However, it is not pathognomonic. Diagnosis is made histologically.

○ **What are the most common locations of melanomas in African Americans? In Caucasian Americans?**

African Americans: palms, soles, nails, and mucous membranes

Caucasian Americans: back and lower legs

○ **What are the clinical characteristics of dysplastic nevi?**

They may be large (>6 mm), have variations of color, be asymmetric, and/or have irregular borders.

• • • HAIR AND NAILS • • •

○ **A patient presents with the complaint of losing her hair. On physical examination, you note that there is a smooth patch of loss of hair and also note the presence of small "exclamation hairs." What is the likely diagnosis?**

Alopecia areata. The patient could develop more extensive patches that will extend to the entire scalp or body. In some cases, this may be associated with Hashimoto thyroiditis, Addison disease, pernicious anemia, and vitiligo.

○ **How is onychomycosis diagnosed and what is the appropriate treatment?**

Clinical diagnosis must be confirmed by laboratory examination. The preferred method of confirmation can be achieved by isolation of fungus on culture medium. Fungal culture allows for confirmation of the species of fungus. KOH examination of subungual debris or nail plate can be used to confirm the presence of hyphae.

Approved treatment regimens are

- Terbinafine 250 mg/day for 6 weeks (fingernails) and 12 weeks (toenails)
- Itraconazole 200 mg/day for 6 weeks (fingernails) and 12 weeks (toenails)

Patients should be advised that nails do not appear completely normal after treatment due to slow growth of the nails. However, new growth should appear as normal.

○ **A patient presents with red, tender, and indurated lateral nailfold with purulent drainage on his ring finger. What is the diagnosis?**

Paronychia is inflammation surrounding the nail. Acute paronychia is painful, erythematous, and frequently has purulent drainage. The common causative organism is *Staphylococcus aureus*; however, bacterial cultures should be performed to confirm and rule out resistant organisms.

○ **What are Beau lines?**

Transverse grooves in the nailbed. Single nail involvement usually indicates a traumatic inciting event. Multiple nail involvement usually indicates trauma, dermatologic disorder, or systemic illness.

○ **A 6-year-old African American boy presents with diffuse patchy scaling in the scalp with areas of black dot alopecia. What is the presumptive diagnosis and how is it treated?**

Tinea capitis is extremely common in school-aged children especially those from the inner city. There is usually posterior cervical lymphadenopathy associated with this infection. Diagnosis is confirmed with a fungal culture. Only 10% of tinea fluoresces with Wood lamp examination making it less than useful in diagnosing. The gold standard for treatment is griseofulvin (15 mg/kg/day for 6–8 weeks) and an antifungal shampoo (ketoconazole 2% or selenium sulfide 2.5%) two to three times a week. The shampoo should be allowed to sit on the scalp for 10 minutes before washing out.

• • • VIRAL DISORDERS • • •

○ **Describe the treatment options for a woman with condyloma acuminatum:**

Genital warts can be treated with a couple of therapies. Podophyllin resin in tincture of benzoin is commonly used. Other therapies include cryotherapy, CO_2 laser therapy, podofilox, or imiquimod cream.

○   **A 5-year-old child develops a rash that starts on the face and quickly spreads to the trunk. The lesions begin as small vesicles on a red base. After a couple of days the lesions crust over, but new ones are still forming. This is the characteristic rash of:**

Chicken pox, varicella zoster virus, is transmitted by airborne droplets and is highly contagious. Patients are contagious 48 hours before the characteristic rash appears. This continues until all lesions are crusted over. Chicken pox used to be a common childhood illness until the vaccination became routine.

○   **A 4-year-old boy who recently had a few days of bright red cheeks now has a lacy appearing rash on both upper extremities. There are no associated symptoms. What is the most likely cause?**

This represents erythema infectiosum or fifth disease. The causative organism is Parvovirus B19.

This viral exanthem has three overlapping phases. First is the "slapped cheek" phase, which is characterized by fiery red facial erythema. The second phase is the exanthem, which affects the trunk and extremities. It is characterized by a lacy or reticulated rash. Third is the recurrent phase, which usually fades but recurs on exposure to sunlight and warmth or with physical exercise.

○   **A mother brings her 14-year-old boy to you a week after you prescribed ampicillin for his pharyngitis. Mom says he developed a rash over his torso, arms, legs, and even the palms of his hands. Upon examination, the patient has an erythematous, macular, and papular rash. What might the adolescent have other than pharyngitis?**

Infectious mononucleosis. In almost 95% of patients with Epstein–Barr viruses that are treated with ampicillin, a rash will develop. The rash and subsequent desquamation will last about a week.

○   **A 72-year-old woman has a painful red rash with vesicles on erythematous bases in a bandlike distribution on the right side of her lower back, which spreads down and out toward her hip. What is your diagnosis?**

Shingles or herpes zoster disease. This is due to the reactivation of a dormant varicella zoster virus in the sensory root ganglia of a patient with a history of chicken pox. The rash is in the distribution of the dermatome, in this case L5. It is most common in those older than 50 years or in patients who are immunocompromised.

○   **A patient with shingles extending to the tip of his nose is at risk for what?**

Vesicles at the tip of the nose is Hutchinson sign. This indicates that the varicella zoster virus resides in the nasociliary branch of the ophthalmic nerve. Complications include ocular inflammation and corneal denervation. This is a medical emergency and needs immediate referral.

○   **What is the causative organism of verruca vulgaris and what are its appropriate treatment options?**

Verruca vulgaris is caused by the human papilloma virus (HPV). Treatment options range from watchful waiting, OTC salicylic acid preparations, manual paring, cryotherapy, topical imiquimod cream, and injection therapy with candida antigens. Pulsed dye laser has also been useful but can cause scarring.

○   **An otherwise healthy 8-month-old female infant runs a high fever (105°F). Just as the fever subsides, a rash of pale pink oval macules appear on the trunk. These quickly become confluent. Within 48 hours, the rash subsides. What is the most likely diagnosis?**

Roseola (exanthem subitum) is a viral disorder that affects children between the ages of 6 months and 4 years. The causative organism is HHV-6 and HHV-7. The prodrome is a high fever between 104 and 106°F in an otherwise well child. Just as the fever subsides, the rash appears. The rash consists of numerous pale pink oval macules on the trunk and neck that become confluent. Within 48 hours, the rash subsides without scaling or peeling.

○ **A patient with AIDS presents with a grayish-white "corduroy-like" plaque on the lateral borders of her tongue that does not scrape off. What is the presumptive diagnosis?**

Oral hairy leukoplakia, which is caused by EBV infection of the oropharynx.

○ **What are the goals of management of herpes zoster?**

Reduce viral shedding, promote healing of lesions, prevent secondary infection, minimize pain, and prevent or minimize postherpetic neuralgia.

○ **What are Koplik spots and with which viral exanthem are they associated?**

Koplik spots are gray-white papules on the buccal mucosa. They are pathognomonic for rubeola (measles). Other symptoms of rubeola include the three Cs: cough, coryza, and conjunctivitis.

● ● ● BACTERIAL INFECTIONS ● ● ●

○ **What is a carbuncle?**

A carbuncle consists of multiple deep loculated dermal and subcutaneous abscesses. There may be multiple openings that drain pus. They are extremely painful. Carbuncles occur mainly in hair-bearing areas and sites of friction and sweating. Risk factors for development include obesity, immunosuppression, hyper-IgE, chronic granulomatous disease, and malnutrition.

○ **Differentiate between ecthyma and impetigo:**

Impetigo is a superficial bacterial infection of the skin most commonly caused by *S. aureus* or group A *Streptococcus*. Classic skin findings include small erosions and golden-yellow crusting. Common distribution is on the nose and lip or as secondary infection of various dermatoses. Ecthyma is a deep erosion or ulcer with a thick crust most commonly caused by *S. aureus* or group A *Streptococcus*. Lesions are more common on distal extremities.

○ **Differentiate between erysipelas and cellulitis:**

Erysipelas and cellulitis are both red, hot, tender areas of skin. Erysipelas, however, is well demarcated, with sharp, raised advancing borders and is more superficial and commonly has lymphatic involvement. Cellulitis has more indiscreet margins and no lymph involvement. The most common pathogen of both the disorders is Group A *Streptococcus*.

○ **A mother brings her 4-year-old girl to you because she has a terrible rash. The child's face has patches of shallow erosions covered in a thick, honey-colored crust. Just 2 days ago, these lesions were small red papules. What is your diagnosis?**

Impetigo. This is most common in children and usually occurs on exposed areas of skin. Most limited cases can be treated with topical mupirocin antibiotic ointment. However, extensive disease should be treated with systemic antibiotics. For staphylococcal, use dicloxacillin, cephalexin, or amoxicillin plus clavulanic acid. For streptococcal, use Benzathine penicillin, penicillin V, or cephalexin. For penicillin-allergic patients, use erythromycin, clarithromycin, or azithromycin.

○ **Which organism is probably responsible for the infection described in the previous question?**

Most impetigo cases are caused by *Staphylococcus aureus*. β-Hemolytic *Streptococcus* is the second most common infecting agent. It can also be coinfecting with *Staphylococcus aureus*.

○ **What is the appropriate treatment for a cyst/abscess that occurs just above the gluteal fold in the sacrococcygeal region?**

Appropriate treatment for a pilonidal cyst is incision and drainage (I&D) of the cyst. The incision should extend to the subcutaneous tissue with removal of all hair and debris. The wound should be packed. No antibiotics are necessary unless there is an associated cellulitis. Follow-up with a surgeon shortly after I&D is recommended since the recurrence rate is high.

○ **What age group does staphylococcal scalded skin syndrome (SSSS) usually affect?**

SSSS most often occurs in neonates and young children (<5 years).

○ **What is the treatment for SSSS?**

Oral or IV penicillinase-resistant penicillin, first- or second-generation cephalosporins, or clindamycin are appropriate. Modification may be made after sensitivities are determined. In patients with severe infection, hospitalization is required often times in burn units with special attention given to fluid and electrolyte management, pain management, and infection control.

○ **A 2-year-old girl has significant perianal erythema and small discrete red papules in the gluteal area. She has also been constipated because she is withholding her bowel movements due to pain. What is the presumptive diagnosis?**

Perianal staphylococcal/streptococcal infection. The diagnosis can be confirmed with a bacterial culture. This usually responds well to topical mupirocin ointment. Oral penicillin V (or erythromycin in allergic patients) can also be used.

○ **What is the inciting event for the development of decubitus ulcers?**

Decubitus ulcers result from ischemia caused by prolonged exposure to pressure.

○ **Describe the presentation of SSSS:**

It is most common in children younger than 5 years of age, particularly in those younger than 3 years. It may begin as a conjunctivitis, or local infection of nares, mouth, or umbilicus; but often no clinical infection is apparent. Initially, the lesions consist of diffuse ill-defined erythema or a scarlatiniform rash. This quickly progresses to with deepening erythema and the onset of tenderness. Bullae may be present especially in infants. Within 24 to 48 hours, the lesions become more widespread. Later, the skin peels off with gentle pressure (Nikolsky sign). During the healing phase, desquamation occurs. Because SSSS does not have mucosal involvement, it can be differentiated from TEN.

● ● ● OTHER DERMATOLOGIC DISORDERS ● ● ●

○ **Upon routine examination, a 76-year-old female patient is found to have thickening and brown hyperpigmentation of the skin on the neck and axillae. This finding can be a marker for what disorders?**

Acanthosis nigricans is most commonly associated with obesity and insulin resistance. However, endocrine disorders, drug administration, and malignancy should also be considered. It is the velvety brown hyperpigmentation and thickening of intertriginous areas. It is most common around the neck and in the axillae. Overweight and obese patients should be worked up for insulin resistance. However, acanthosis nigricans can also be associated with malignancy, particularly of the gastrointestinal and genitourinary systems.

○ **A port-wine stain (PWS) in the distribution of the first branch of the trigeminal nerve (V1) is characteristic of what disorder?**

Sturge-Weber syndrome (SWS) is a neuroectodermal disorder with a characteristic PWS in a V1 distribution. Other branches of the trigeminal nerve (V2 and V3) can also be involved. There is also a central nervous system (CNS) component of SWS. The most common CNS manifestation is seizures. Glaucoma is also a frequent manifestation of SWS. It may be present at birth or any time before the fourth decade.

○ **Transient erythematous well-circumscribed wheals that are intensely pruritic are characteristic of:**

Urticaria; these are representative of a type I hypersensitivity reaction.

○ **Xanthomas are associated with which metabolic disorder?**

Familial hyperlipidemia. Xanthomas are yellow-brown or orange plaques, papules, or infiltrations in tendons. They are most common on the extensor surfaces of the extremities. Eruptive xanthomas are most common on the buttocks, elbows, or knees.

○ **A 5-year-old African American boy presents with a sharply demarcated annular macule with complete loss of pigment on his right knee. He also has a well-defined hypopigmented macule located on his right temporal area. There is no scaling or erythema noted. What disorder does this most likely represent?**

This patient most likely has vitiligo. Vitiligo is thought to be an autoimmune disorder that affects melanocytes. There may be areas of involvement in differing stages with a range of macules slightly lighter than normal pigmentation to complete loss of pigment.

○ **What examination technique is helpful in identifying vitiligo lesions in lighter skin types and in sun-protected areas where contrast may not be as obvious?**

Wood lamp examination in a completely darkened room without windows will show accentuation of vitiligo lesions.

○ **A patient presents with a red pedunculated papule that has a collarette of scale. She states that it appeared less than a week ago and has been growing rapidly. She reports that it bleeds profusely in response to minor trauma. What is the probable diagnosis and treatment?**

This most likely represents a pyogenic granuloma. This is an acquired vascular lesion that often forms in response to trauma, such as an insect bite or scratch. Treatment for pyogenic granuloma includes shave excision followed by electrodessication to achieve hemostasis and prevent reoccurrence.

○ **What are the diagnostic criteria for Kawasaki disease?**

Fever for 5 days or more with at least four of the following:

- Bilateral injected conjunctiva
- Red fissured crusted lips, hyperemia of oropharynx, and red strawberry tongue
- Erythema and/or edema of the extremities
- Skin manifestations (diffuse macular and papular, erythematous eruption, diffuse urticarial rash, or scarlet fever-like rash)
- Cervical lymphadenopathy

○ **What is the treatment for Kawasaki disease?**

Treatment is directed toward reducing inflammation and preventing damage to the arterial wall. Standard treatment regimen includes intravenous immunoglobulin (IVIG) and aspirin. Rapid diagnosis is crucial because treatment should be started within the first 10 days of the illness.

○ **A 6-year-old boy presents with palpable purpura on bilateral lower extremities. He also complains of pain and mild swelling in his ankles and knees. Today, he is experiencing some abdominal discomfort as well. He is recuperating from streptococcal pharyngitis. What is his most likely diagnosis?**

Henoch-Schönlein purpura (HSP) is a vasculitic disorder that primarily affects children between the ages of 2 and 11 years. Classic presentation includes palpable purpura in dependent areas, arthritis, abdominal pain, and glomerulonephritis. There are many possible etiologies including group A β-hemolytic streptococci, viruses, immunizations, and drugs.

○ **What are the diagnostic criteria for neurofibromatosis type 1 (NF1)?**

Café-au-lait macules: six or more measuring ≥0.5 cm before puberty (≥1.5 cm in adults)

Axillary and/or inguinal freckling

Fibroma: 2+ dermal neurofibromas

Eye: 2+ Lisch nodules

Skeletal dysplasia

Pedigree: first-degree relative with NF1

Optic

Tumors: optic nerve glioma

○ **Small, follicular-based, hyperkeratotic papules located on the outer aspects of the upper arms and thighs are consistent with what chronic condition?**

Keratosis pilaris is a chronic disorder seen in early childhood through adulthood. Usually there is improvement as the patient progresses into adulthood. Treatment consists of keratolytic agents, which may help smooth the affected skin.

○ **What side effects are associated with topical corticosteroids?**

Atrophy, striae, telangiectasia, erythema, and hypopigmentation of the skin are common side effects. Topical corticosteroids used on the eyelid can cause cataracts and glaucoma. Systemic side effects include hypothalamic-pituitary-adrenal axis suppression.

○ **A 5-year-old boy presents with small discrete erythematous papules in a perioral and nasolabial distribution. What is the diagnosis and proper treatment?**

This is consistent with perioral dermatitis. The etiology is unknown. Proper treatment is with topical antibiotics such as erythromycin, clindamycin, and metronidazole. In more severe cases, oral erythromycin or tetracyclines (in patients older than 8 years) are required. Recurrence is common.

○ **What is the reaction when perioral dermatitis is treated with a topical steroid?**

A granulomatous perioral dermatitis results from treatment with a topical steroid. The patient must be weaned off of the topical steroid and treated with an appropriate topical antibiotic to prevent a rebound flare.

○ **Name some of the more common etiologies that produce exanthems:**

The morbilliform exanthems can be caused by drugs as well as viral infections such as rubeola, rubella, erythema infectiosa, Epstein Barr, Coxsackie virus, HIV, and adenovirus. Bacterial forms can be caused by typhoid, rickettsia, syphilis, and meningococcemia. The scarlatina forms can be caused by scarlet fever, toxic shock, and Kawasaki disease.

○ **An 89-year-old bedridden nursing home patient is found to have a superficial ulceration involving only the epidermis located in the sacral region. What is the presumptive diagnosis?**

This most likely represents a stage II decubitus ulcer. Common sites for decubitus ulcers are the hip and buttock regions. Decubitus ulcers are classified in stages:

Stage I: intact skin with blanchable erythema

Stage II: partial thickness skin loss, involves epidermis and possibly the dermis

Stage III: full thickness skin loss involves subcutaneous tissue up to fascia

Stage IV: full thickness skin loss with damage to muscle, bone, tendon, or joint

• • • REFERENCES • • •

Paller AS, Mancinic AJ. *Hurwitz Clinical Pediatric Dermatology: A Textbook of Skin Disorders of Childhood and Adolescence.* 3rd ed. Elsevier Saunders; 2006.

Habif TP, Campbell JL, Chapman MS, Dinulos JG, Zug KA. *Skin Disease: Diagnosis and Treatment.* 2nd ed. Philadelphia, PA: Elsevier Mosby; 2005.

Wolff K, Johnson RA. *Fitzpatrick's Color Atlas and Synopsis of Clinical Dermatology.* 6th ed. New York, NY: McGraw-Hill; 2009.

Pryor JP, Todd B, Dryer M. *Clinician's Guide to Surgical Care.* Lange Series. New York, NY: McGraw-Hill; 2008.

CHAPTER 13 Hematology

Anthony Brenneman, MPAS, PA-C

● ● ● **ANEMIAS** ● ● ●

○ **What is the most common cause of hyperviscosity syndrome?**

Waldenstrom macroglobulinemia.

○ **In anemia, which way is the oxygen dissociation curve shifted?**

The right (affinity of hemoglobin for oxygen is decreased).

○ **What are the factors contributing to the pathophysiology of anemia of chronic disease?**

Decreased red cell life span (hyperactive reticuloendothelial system), hypoactive bone marrow, erythropoietin production inadequate for degree of anemia, and abnormal iron metabolism.

○ **What is the formula for calculating the proper volume of red cells to transfuse in an anemic patient?**

Desired hemoglobin (g/dL) = observed hemoglobin (g/dL) × weight (kg) × 3.

○ **What should be considered in a patient who presents in a coma and with anemia and rouleaux formation in the peripheral blood smear?**

Primary macroglobulinemia (hyperviscosity syndrome).

○ **A 20-year-old male patient presents with pancytopenia. On smear you note anemia associated with decreased reticulocytes and the morphology is unremarkable. Neutrophils and platelets are reduced in number and no immature or abnormal forms are seen. Bone marrow biopsy and aspirate is hypocellular. What is your most likely diagnosis?**

Aplastic anemia.

○ **The primary cause of aplastic anemia is:**

Unknown.

○ **Aplastic anemia is characterized by two peaks in frequency of disease appearance. At what ages are these peaks?**

Ages 15 to 25 years and 65 to 69 years.

○ **What diagnosis should be considered in a patient who presents with macrocytic anemia, macro-ovalocytes, and hypersegmented neutrophils on peripheral blood smear, along with a serum vitamin B12 level of <100 pg/mL?**

Vitamin B12 deficiency.

○ **A 36-year-old female patient presents to your clinic with anemia. In her history, you learn that she is a strict vegan (a strict vegetarian that avoids all animal products). What is at the top of your differential?**

Vitamin B12 deficiency.

○ **What are the common signs and symptoms of Vitamin B12 deficiency?**

- Decreased vibration and position sense is common early in the disease; later paresthesias, balance disorders, and impaired cerebral function develop
- Patients are usually pale and mildly icteric

○ **Treatment for pernicious anemia after initial replacement is provided by:**

Intramuscular injections of 100 μg of vitamin B12 monthly for life.

○ **What diagnosis should be considered in a patient who presents with macrocytic anemia, macro-ovalocytes, and hypersegmented neutrophils on peripheral blood smear, along with a serum vitamin B12 level of 298 (normal range 203–339)?**

Folate deficiency.

○ **A 21-year-old woman presents to your office looking pale, fatigued, and thin. She states that she has been trying to lose weight despite being underweight by today's measurement. When discussing her oral intake you learn that she almost never eats any fresh fruits or vegetables. What is the likely diagnosis?**

Folate deficiency.

○ **The best way to differentiate between vitamin B12 deficiency and folate deficiency is by which laboratory tests?**

A normal vitamin B12 and a low serum folate level.

○ **What does treatment for folate deficiency consists?**

Folic acid 1 mg/day orally with response seen within 5 to 7 days and resolution of all symptoms within 2 months.

○ **Why are red cell transfusions rarely required to treat iron deficiency anemia?**

Nucleated red blood cells and reticulocytes appear in the blood stream within 72 hours after starting oral iron replacement.

○ **What is the progression of biochemical and hematological events in iron deficiency anemia?**

Decreased serum ferritin, then decreased serum iron and total iron binding capacity, followed by a fall in MCV and MCH, and a rise in RDW. Thrombocytosis may occur.

○ **A serum ferritin level less than 12 μg/L is notable for what diagnosis?**

Iron deficiency anemia.

○ **What are common causes of iron deficiency anemia?**

Dietary deficiency, decreased absorption, pregnancy, and blood loss.

○ **A 24-year-old woman who changed her dietary intake within the past 6 months to vegan complains of fatigue and tachycardia over the last 2 to 3 months. Recently, she has also developed palpitations and tachypnea on exertion. Her history is notable for heavy menstrual cycles. What laboratory test should you obtain?**

Serum ferritin to evaluate for iron deficiency anemia.

○ **Early laboratory findings on blood smear looking for iron deficiency will include:**

Anisocytosis.

○ **Later laboratory findings in iron deficiency include:**

Normochromic, normocytic anemia.

○ **What is the most common human enzyme defect?**

Glucose-6-phosphate dehydrogenase (G-6-PD) deficiency.

○ **Clinical manifestations of individuals who inherit the common (polymorphic) forms of G-6-PD deficiency include:**

No manifestations.

○ **Usually the anemia of G-6-PD is episodic and associated with stress most commonly from:**

Drug administration, infection, and in some cases fava beans.

○ **What is the best therapy for a person with G-6-PD?**

None, unless a hemolytic episode occurs. The use of transfusions is recommended in patients with brisk hemolysis along with good urine output. Avoiding drugs that might cause hemolysis should be considered but the drugs must not be avoided if the benefit outweighs the risk for the patient. In many cases patients with G-6-PD can tolerate many medications that previously were thought to be avoided.

○ **What syndrome is suggested in a child who is 6 months to 4 years old with an antecedent URI, fever, acute renal failure, microangiopathic hemolytic anemia (MAHA), and thrombocytopenia?**

Hemolytic uremic syndrome.

○ **What malignancy is most frequently associated with MAHA?**

Gastric adenocarcinoma.

○ **What is the most common worldwide cause of hemolytic anemia?**

Malaria.

○ **Hemolytic uremic syndrome (HUS) is associated with several etiologies that are grouped into two major classifications. It is important to recognize the differences because the clinical course and prognosis differ for each group. The two major groups are:**

1. Diarrhea-associated HUS (D+HUS) 2. non–diarrhea-associated HUS (D-HUS).

○ **What is the most common cause of hemolytic uremic syndrome in the United States?**

Diarrhea-associated HUS (D+HUS) from ingestion of *E. coli* 0157:H7.

○ **In a Coombs-positive hemolytic anemia patient, what should the differential include?**

Autoimmune, drugs, infection, lymphoproliferative disease, and Rh or ABO incompatibility.

○ **What is the most common hemoglobin variant?**

Hemoglobin S (valine substituted for glutamic acid in the sixth position on the β-chain).

○ **Which clinical crises are seen in patients with sickle cell disease?**

- Vasoocclusive (thrombotic, painful) crisis
- Aplastic crisis
- Sequestration crisis
- Hemolytic crisis

○ **Which is the most common type of sickle cell crisis?**

Vasoocclusive and is the hallmark of sickle cell crisis. It can occur almost daily to once per year.

○ **What percentage of patients with sickle cell disease have gallstones?**

50% to 70% of adults have bilirubin gallstones and these may be found in children as young as 6 years.

○ **Current therapeutic recommendations for a patient in sickle cell crisis may include:**

- Hydration
- Analgesia (if pain is associated)
- Oxygen (only beneficial if patient is hypoxic)
- Cardiac monitoring (if patient has history of cardiac disease or is having chest pain)

○ **What is the most commonly encountered sickle hemoglobin variant?**

Sickle cell trait.

○ **What is appropriate preventive immunization for a child with the sickle cell trait?**

Pneumococcal conjugate and polysaccharide vaccine should be administered to all children who have sickle cell disease. Other routine immunizations, including yearly vaccination against influenza, should be provided.

○ **What is the difference between sickle cell anemia and sickle cell trait?**

Sickle cell anemia is the homozygous form of the disease while sickle cell trait is the heterozygous form. People with the sickle trait are generally not anemic, are asymptomatic, and have a normal life span compared to those with the disease.

○ **How does a patient older than 12 months present with sickle cell disease?**

By age 1 year, a severe hemolytic anemia may be present. The child will present with pallor, fatigue, and jaundice, and will be predisposed to developing gallstones. They may have splenomegaly due to sequestration and are at great risk for infection with encapsulated bacteria.

○ **A cure for β-thalassemia major is possible with what treatment?**

Allogeneic bone marrow transplant.

○ **Increased levels of hemoglobin A2 are found in what condition?**

Thalassemia trait.

○ **RBC basophilic stippling occurs with what two disorders?**

Thalassemia and lead poisoning.

○ **Hemosiderosis from chronic transfusion therapy for thalassemia can be successfully treated with:**

Deferoxamine.

○ **Thalassemias are characterized by:**

Microcytosis, family history, acanthocytes, and target cells.

○ **Thalassemias are classified into clinical categories based on outcomes. Identify the category and the outcome for each level:**

1. Trait—without significant long-term clinical outcome
2. Intermedia—red blood cell transfusion requirements or other moderate clinical impact
3. Major—disorder is life-threatening

○ **In people with high transfusion requiring thalassemias, what is one of the primary laboratory values to monitor, along with primary therapy to apply?**

Serum iron levels and iron chelation, using deferoxamine infusion.

• • • COAGULATION DISORDERS • • •

○ **What common drugs have been implicated to acquired bleeding disorders?**

Ethanol, ASA, NSAIDs, warfarin, and antibiotics.

○ **Mucocutaneous bleeding, including petechiae, ecchymoses, epistaxis, GI, GU, and menorrhagia, indicate what coagulation abnormalities?**

Qualitative or quantitative platelet disorders.

○ **Delayed bleeding and bleeding into joints or potential spaces, such as the retroperitoneum, suggest what type of bleeding disorder?**

Coagulation factor deficiency (such as in hemophilia).

○ **What is primary hemostasis?**

The platelet interaction with the vascular subendothelium that results in the formation of a platelet plug at the site of injury.

○ **What four components are required for primary hemostasis?**

1. Normal vascular subendothelium (collagen)

2. Functional platelets

3. Normal von Willebrand factor (connects the platelet to the endothelium via glycoprotein Ib)

4. Normal fibrinogen (connects platelets to each other via glycoprotein IIB-IIIA)

○ **What is the end product of secondary hemostasis (coagulation cascade)?**

Cross-linked fibrin.

○ **What is the principal physiologic activator of the fibrinolytic system?**

Tissue plasminogen activator (tPA). Endothelial cells release tPA, which converts plasminogen, adsorbed in the fibrin clot, to plasmin. Plasmin degrades fibrinogen and fibrin monomer into fibrin degradation products (FDPs, once called fibrin split products) and cross-linked fibrin into D-dimers.

○ **How can an overdose of warfarin be treated? What are the advantages and disadvantages of each treatment?**

Fresh frozen plasma (FFP) or vitamin K. However, if there are no signs of bleeding, temporary discontinuation may be all that is necessary. Treatment depends on the severity of symptoms, not the degree of prolongation of the prothrombin time (PT).

FFP:

advantages: rapid repletion of coagulation factors and control of hemorrhage.

disadvantages: volume overload, possible viral transmission.

Vitamin K-advantages: ease of administration.

disadvantages: possible anaphylaxis when given IV; delayed onset of 12 to 24 hours; effects may last up to 2 weeks, making anticoagulation of the patient difficult or impossible.

○ **Which four hemostatic alterations are seen in patients with liver disease?**

1. Decreased protein synthesis leading to coagulation factor deficiency
2. Thrombocytopenia
3. Increased fibrinolysis
4. Vitamin K deficiency

○ **What five treatments are available to bleeding patients with liver disease?**

1. Transfusion with Packed RBCs (maintains hemodynamic stability)
2. Vitamin K
3. Fresh frozen plasma
4. Platelet transfusion
5. DDAVP (desmopressin)

○ **What hemostasis test is often prolonged in uremic patients?**

Bleeding time.

○ **What treatment options are available to patients with renal failure and coagulopathy?**

- Dialysis
- Optimize hematocrit (by recombinant human erythropoietin or transfusion with PRBCs)
- Desmopressin
- Conjugated estrogens

Cryoprecipitate and platelet transfusions if hemorrhage is life-threatening.

○ **What factors are deficient in classic hemophilia, Christmas disease (hemophilia b), and von Willebrand disease, respectively?**

- Classic hemophilia: Factor VIII
- Christmas disease: Factor IX
- von Willebrand disease: Factor VIIIc and von Willebrand cofactor

○ **Vitamin K-dependent factors of the clotting cascade include:**

X, IX, VII, and II. Remember 1972.

○ **What are the clinical complications of Disseminated intravascular coagulation (DIC)?**

Bleeding, thrombosis, purpura fulminans, and multiorgan failure.

○ **Which three laboratory studies are most helpful in diagnosing DIC?**

1. Prothrombin time (prolonged)
2. Platelet count (usually low)
3. Fibrinogen level (low)

○ **There is a simultaneous activation of coagulation and fibrinolysis in what pathologic condition?**
Disseminated intravascular coagulation.

○ **What are some common ischemic complications of DIC?**
Renal failure, seizures, coma, pulmonary infarction, and hemorrhagic necrosis of the skin.

○ **What is the most important aspect of treating DIC?**
Attempting to correct the underlying disorder (usually septic shock).

○ **A classic hemophiliac (hemophilia A) suffers a major head injury. What treatment should be given?**
Give factor VIII.

○ **What pathway involves factors VIII and IX?**
Intrinsic pathway.

○ **What effect does deficiency of factors VIII and IX have on PT and on PTT?**
Deficiency leads to an increase in PTT.

○ **What agent can be used to treat mild hemophilia A and von Willebrand disease type 1?**
1-Deamino-8-D-arginine vasopressin (DDAVP) induces a rapid rise in factor VIII levels.

○ **What are the most common sites for bleeding in patients with hemophilia?**
Joints, muscles, and subcutaneous tissue.

○ **What is the only coagulation factor not synthesized by hepatocytes?**
Factor VIII.

○ **What is the leading cause of death in hemophiliacs who received treatments prior to 1985?**
AIDS.

○ **Hemophilia B is symptomatic in what patient populations?**
Men; disease is X-linked.

○ **Patients with hemophilia B who are treated episodically early in childhood will develop what complications?**
Severe arthritis and limited range of motion in affected joints.

○ **What is the mainstay of therapy for patients with factor XI disorders?**
Fresh frozen plasma.

○ **For patients with factor XI disorders that need a surgical procedure or are bleeding into mucosal surfaces, what therapy is regarded as mandatory for treatment?**

Aminocaproic acid.

○ **In the thrombocytopenic patient, one unit of platelets will raise the platelet count by about how much?**

One unit raises the platelet count by about 10,000/mm^3.

○ **Below what platelet count is spontaneous hemorrhage likely to occur?**

<10,000/mm^3.

○ **What patients with thrombocytopenia are unlikely to respond to platelet infusions?**

Those with antiplatelet antibodies (ITP or hypersplenism).

○ **What are the three major categories for the occurrence of thrombocytopenia?**

Decreased production of platelets, increased destruction of platelets, and sequestration.

○ **Idiopathic thrombocytopenic purpura (ITP) disease course is different in children than in adults. How do the two differ?**

In children, it is usually an acute disease often following an infection and is usually self-limited, while in adults it tends to take a more chronic disease course.

○ **Idiopathic thrombocytopenic purpura (ITP) is considered a secondary process when it is associated with an underlying autoimmune process. What are three common causes of ITP as a secondary process?**

Systemic lupus erythematosus, and infections such as HIV and hepatitis C.

○ **Idiopathic thrombocytopenic purpura (ITP) is characterized by mucocutaneous bleeding and what on peripheral blood smear?**

Often a very low platelet count and otherwise a normal peripheral blood smear.

○ **What is the characteristic bone marrow finding in idiopathic thrombocytopenic purpura (ITP)?**

Increased or normal megakaryocytes.

○ **A patient is diagnosed with ITP. The patient has purpura noted on the extremities and a platelet count of 54 × 10^9/L, what is the most appropriate treatment for the individual?**

Observation.

○ **What are the potential treatment modalities for ITP?**

Gamma globulins (IVIG), steroids, splenectomy, anti-(RH) D, danazol, and antineoplastic drugs. However, the treatment modality should be tailored according to the patient's condition as well as depending on bleeding issues; most patients require only observation of platelet counts, activity level of, and bleeding frequency.

○ **How do gamma globulin and steroids work in the treatment of ITP?**

These block the uptake of antibody-coated platelets by splenic macrophages.

○ **Under what circumstances is a bone marrow aspirate appropriate in the diagnosis and treatment of ITP?**

If the patient is younger than 60 years, a bone marrow aspirate should be performed to rule out leukemia.

○ **What is the classic pentad of thrombotic thrombocytopenic purpura (TTP)?**

1. Fever
2. Thrombocytopenia
3. Neurologic symptoms
4. Renal insufficiency
5. Microangiopathic hemolytic anemia (MAHA)

○ **What is the most common precipitating event for thrombotic thrombocytopenic purpura?**

Pregnancy.

○ **What is the recommended treatment for acquired thrombotic thrombocytopenic purpura (TTP)?**

Daily plasma exchange until several days after remission is obtained, denoted by normalization of platelet counts and LDH combined with clinical resolution of tissue ischemia and thrombosis.

○ **What are some signs and symptoms of thrombotic thrombocytopenic purpura (TTP)?**

Thrombocytopenia, purpura, and microangiopathic hemolytic anemia. Patient with TTP presents with fever, fluctuating neurologic signs, and renal complications. If the disease goes untreated, it is almost uniformly fatal. Therapy includes steroids, splenectomy, plasmapheresis and exchange, and antiplatelet agents, such as dipyridamole and aspirin.

○ **What is the most common clinical presentation of TTP (thrombotic thrombocytopenic purpura)?**

The most common clinical findings are thrombocytopenia and MAHA; however, most people present with neurologic symptoms including headache, confusion, cranial nerve palsies, coma, and seizures and through history purpura and other findings related to thrombocytopenia are noted.

○ **What is the most common inherited bleeding disorder?**

von Willebrand disease.

○ **What is the currently approved mode of therapy for bleeding in patients with von Willebrand disease? What is the dose?**

DDAVP, 0.3 μg/kg IV or subcutaneously every 12 hours for three to four doses.

○ **There are several types of von Willebrand disease; of these, which type is the most common?**

von Willebrand disease type 1 accounts for 70% of clinically significant vWD.

○ **What is the most common clinical symptom with von Willebrand disease type 1?**

Mucocutaneous bleeding. Other common findings are epistaxis, easy bruising, and hematoma.

○ **What is von Willebrand disease?**

An autosomal dominant disorder of platelet function. It causes bleeding from mucous membranes, menorrhagia, and increased bleeding from wounds. Patients with von Willebrand disease have less (or dysfunctional) von Willebrand factor.

von Willebrand factor is a plasma protein secreted by endothelial cells and serves two functions: (1) It is required for platelets to adhere to collagen at the site of vascular injury, which is the initial step in forming a hemostatic plug. (2) It forms complexes in plasma with factor VIII, which are required to maintain normal factor VIII levels.

• • • MALIGNANCIES • • •

○ **What are some signs and symptoms of leukemia?**

Fever, fatigue and lethargy, petechia, bleeding, purpura, lymphadenopathy, hepatosplenomegaly, bone and joint pain, and pallor.

○ **What are some metabolic complications of leukemia?**

Hypercalcemia, hyperuricemia, and syndrome of inappropriate antidiuretic hormone.

○ **How is hyperleukocytosis treated?**

IV hydration, alkalinization, allopurinol, and antileukemic therapy.

○ **What percent of children with acute lymphoblastic leukemia (ALL) are cured by conventional chemotherapy?**

70%.

○ **What is the most common malignancy for individuals younger than 15 years of age?**

Acute lymphoblastic leukemia. It accounts for 23% of all cancers and 76% of all leukemia's within this age group.

○ **What is the most common clinical presenting symptom for acute lymphoblastic leukemia?**

Fever presents in approximately half of all patients with ALL. Other frequent findings are pallor, petechiae, and ecchymosis.

○ **The most common sites of extramedullary involvement for patients with ALL are:**

Liver, spleen, and lymph nodes.

○ **Patients with ALL, considered at high risk for relapse following conventional chemotherapy, are considered for BMT. What patients are included in this group?**
- Congenital or infants (<1 year) with ALL
- Chromosomal translocation t (4,11), t (9,22)-Philadelphia, t (8,14)
- FAB L-3 morphology (Burkitt)
- WBC > 100,000
- Patients taking more than 1 month to achieve remission
- Patients who relapse while on chemotherapy
- Patients with more than one extramedullary site of relapse without a marrow relapse
- Patients with second and subsequent remissions

○ **What do ALL and AML stand for?**

Acute lymphoblastic leukemia and acute myelogenous leukemia.

○ **At what ages is ALL most common?**

ALL peaks between ages 2 and 4 years. Incidence again rises in the sixth decade and reaches a second, smaller peak in the elderly.

Acute lymphoblastic leukemia (poor prognostic factors):

Lymphoblast high	**B**lood cells > 50,000
Younger than 1 year	**L**ymph node enlarged
Male	**A**nterior mediastinum masses
Philadelphia marker	**S**pleen enlarged
Hgb > 10_	**T**-cells
Older than 10 years	**I**nduction > 4 weeks
	Chromosome < 46

○ **AML accounts for what percentage of adult leukemias?**

80%.

○ **What is the most common gene rearrangement in chronic myelogenous leukemia (CML)?**

Translocation of abl 9 and bcr 22 commonly written t(9:22) or more commonly called the Philadelphia chromosome.

○ **What are common presenting symptoms in a patient with CML?**

Easy fatigability, loss of sense of well-being, decreased tolerance to exertion, anorexia, abdominal discomfort, and early satiety (related to splenic enlargement), weight loss, and excessive sweating.

○ **The most common cytogenetic finding on blood smear of a patient diagnosed with CML is:**

Philadelphia chromosome found in 90% of cases.

○ **The Ph+ chromosome rearrangement in CML is a positive long-term survival finding. In what disease is Ph+ chromosome rearrangement a poor prognostic finding with decreased median survival rate and early relapse?**

Acute lymphocytic leukemia.

○ **What are early signs/findings for acute myelogenous leukemia?**

Easy bruising, petechiae, epistaxis, gingival bleeding, conjunctival hemorrhages, and prolonged bleeding from skin injuries reflect thrombocytopenia.

○ **Most signs and symptoms of AML are related to what clinical feature?**

Anemia.

○ **What is the greatest risk factor in achieving a long-term remission in a patient diagnosed with AML?**

Age, remission rates approach 90% in children, 70% in young adults, 50% in middle age, and 25% in old age.

○ **Non-Hodgkins lymphoma most often presents with what clinical finding?**

Painless lymphadenopathy.

○ **A patient on chemotherapy for his Burkitt lymphoma is found to be hyperkalemic, hypocalcemic, hyperphosphatemic, and hyperuricemic. What is the presumptive diagnosis?**

Tumor lysis syndrome.

○ **What is the malignant cell in Hodgkin disease?**

The Reed-Sternberg cell.

○ **What are the peak age groups for Hodgkin disease?**

15 to 34 years and over 60 years.

○ **What are the signs and symptoms of Hodgkin disease?**

Painless supraclavicular or cervical lymphadenopathy, hepatomegaly, splenomegaly, unexplained fever, and night sweats.

○ **What are the indications for lymph node biopsy?**

The indications for lymph node biopsy are imprecise. The decision to biopsy may be made early in a patient's evaluation or delayed for up to 2 weeks. Prompt biopsy should occur if the patient's history and physical findings suggest a malignancy; examples include a solitary, hard, nontender cervical node in an older patient who is a chronic user of tobacco, supraclavicular adenopathy, and solitary or generalized adenopathy that is firm, movable, and suggestive of lymphoma.

○ **How are childhood cases of non-Hodgkin lymphomas different from adult cases?**

They grow rapidly, are rarely nodular, and are as likely to be T-cell lymphomas as B-cell lymphomas.

○ **What is the most common presentation of B-cell lymphomas?**

Lymphadenopathy and hepatosplenomegaly.

○ **What is the most common presentation of T-cell lymphomas?**

T cell lymphomas more likely present with cutaneous and bone marrow involvement.

○ **What condition should be suspected in a patient with multiple myeloma who presents with paraparesis, paraplegia, and urinary incontinence?**

Acute spinal cord compression. This condition occurs primarily with multiple myeloma and lymphoma; it is also encountered with carcinomas of the lung, breast, and prostate.

○ **Multiple myeloma is a malignancy of what cell line?**

Plasma cells.

○ **What are the most common presenting complaints with someone who will be diagnosed with multiple myeloma?**

Anemia, bone pain, and infection.

○ **What are common laboratory findings in a patient diagnosed with multiple myeloma?**

Hypercalcemia, proteinuria, elevated sedimentation rate, or abnormalities on serum protein electrophoresis.

○ **What is the hallmark laboratory finding in multiple myeloma?**

A paraprotein on serum protein electrophoresis (SPEP).

○ **What blood dyscrasias are currently being considered for treatment through BMT?**

Fanconi anemia, thalassemia major, sickle cell disease, Diamond-Blackfan syndrome, and congenital sideroblastic anemia.

○ **What is graft versus host disease (GVHD)?**

Engraftment of immunocompetent donor cells into an immunocompromised host, resulting in cell-mediated cytotoxic destruction of host cells if an immunologic incompatibility exists.

○ **When does acute GVHD present and what are the typical manifestations?**

Acute GVHD typically becomes apparent between weeks 2 and 4 as the patient begins to engraft, and is characterized by erythroderma, cholestatic hepatitis, and enteritis.

○ **What is the clinical definition of chronic GVHD (cGVHD)?**

Graft versus host disease lasting longer than 3 months posttransplant.

○ **How long is immunosuppressive treatment required for BMT recipients?**

Usually 6 to 12 months or until a state of tolerance is attained.

○ **What are the most common types of infections seen posttransplant engraftment (day 0–30)?**

Oral thrush, bacterial sepsis, catheter infections, fungal infections, pneumonia, and sinusitis.

○ **What are the most common types of infections seen in posttransplant postengraftment (day 30–100)?**

CMV and EBV infection, viral hepatitis, toxoplasmosis, diffuse interstitial pneumonia, and cystitis.

○ **What are the most common types of infections seen posttransplant postengraftment (day 100–365)?**

Varicella, herpes, CMV, toxoplasmosis, pneumocystis carinii pneumonia, viral hepatitis, and common bacterial infections.

○ **What components of whole blood are used for transfusion?**
- RBCs
- Platelets
- Plasma
- Cryoprecipitate

○ **How much will the infusion of 1 unit of PRBCs raise the hemoglobin and hematocrit in a 70-kg patient?**
Hemoglobin: 1 g/dL. Hematocrit: 4%.

○ **What are the three conditions under which the transfusion of PRBCs should be considered?**
1. Acute hemorrhage (blood loss > 1500 mL)
2. Surgical blood loss > 2 L
3. Chronic anemia (Hgb < 7–8 g/dL, symptomatic, or with underlying cardiopulmonary disease)

○ **What five factors indicate the need to type and cross-match blood in the emergency department?**
1. Evidence of shock from any cause
2. Known blood loss > 1000 mL
3. Gross GI bleeding
4. Hgb < 10; Hct < 30
5. Potential of surgery with further significant blood loss

○ **What are the main components of cryoprecipitate?**
- Factor XIII
- von Willebrand factor
- Fibrinogen
- Cold-insoluble plasma proteins

○ **What is the first step in treating all immediate transfusion reactions?**
Stop the transfusion.

○ **Since the advent of this testing method in blood products, viral infections are now considered negligible.**
Nucleic acid amplification testing (NAT)

○ **What is the current recommended emergency replacement therapy for massive hemorrhage?**
Type-specific, uncross-matched blood. Type O negative, although immediately lifesaving in certain situations, carries the risk of life-threatening transfusion reactions.

○ **In current practice, what blood components are routinely infused along with PRBCs in a patient receiving a massive transfusion?**
None. The practice of routinely using platelet transfusion and fresh frozen plasma is costly, dangerous, and unwarranted.

○ **What is the only crystalloid fluid compatible with PRBCs?**

Normal saline.

○ **What is the incompatibility risk of typed blood, screened blood, and fully cross-matched blood?**

The risk of incompatibility of ABO/Rh-compatible blood is 0.1% if the patient has never been transfused. The risk increases to 1.0% if the patient has had a previous transfusion. Adding a negative antibody screen decreases the risk to 0.06%. Fully cross-matched blood should carry a risk less than 0.05%.

○ **What is the most common blood group? What percentage of blood is Rh positive?**

The most common blood group is type O; 45% of whites, 49% of African Americans, 79% of Native Americans, and 40% of Orientals are blood type O. Approximately 85% of the population is Rh positive and 15% Rh negative.

○ **What are the indications for the administration of FFP?**

- Replacement of isolated factor deficiencies
- Reversal of coumadin effect
- Treatment of pathological hemorrhage in patients who have received massive transfusion
- Use in antithrombin III deficiency
- Treatment of immunodeficiencies

○ **What are the indications for cryoprecipitate administration?**

Treatment of congenital or acquired fibrinogen and factor VIII deficiencies. Cryoprecipitate can also be administered prophylactically for nonbleeding perioperative or peripartum patients with congenital fibrinogen deficiencies or for von Willebrand disease that is unresponsive to desmopressin (DDAVP).

○ **Is it necessary to administer ABO-specific platelets?**

The administration of ABO-specific platelets is not required because platelet concentrates contain few red blood cells. However, the administration of pooled platelet components of various ABO types can transfuse plasma-containing anti-A and/or anti-B, resulting in alloimmunization and a weakly positive direct antiglobulin test.

○ **What are the indications for platelet transfusion?**

Platelets should be administered to correct thrombocytopenia or platelet dysfunction (thrombocytopathy). Perioperative factors to consider for the transfusion of platelets for counts between 50 and 100×10^9/L are the type of surgery, anticipated and actual blood loss, extent of microvascular bleeding, presence of medications (e.g., aspirin), and disorders (e.g., uremia) known to affect platelet function and coagulation. The prophylactic administration of platelets is not recommended in patients with chronic thrombocytopenia caused by increased platelet destruction (e.g., idiopathic thrombocytopenic purpura).

○ **What is the potassium load with transfusion?**

It depends on the age of the blood. The potassium load steadily increases with time as extracellular potassium develops.

○ **What is the incidence of hemolytic transfusion reactions (HTR)?**

1 in 38,000 units. The HTR is potentially life-threatening and often regarded the most serious complication of transfusions.

○ **What are the types of HTRs and what is the pathophysiology of each one?**

HTRs are divided in to two types of reactions: (1) intravascular hemolysis and (2) extravascular hemolysis or delayed hemolytic reaction.

○ **What is the treatment for HTRs?**

The transfusion should be stopped immediately. Hypotension should be treated with fluids, inotropes, or other blood as appropriate. Renal output should be maintained with crystalloids, diuretics, or dopamine, as necessary. Component therapy should be used if DIC develops.

○ **What causes febrile reactions to blood and what are the incidences?**

The febrile reaction is the most common mild transfusion reaction and occurs in 1% to 3% of transfusions. It is caused by alloantibodies (leukoagglutinins) to white blood cell, platelet, or other donor plasma antigens. Fever is presumably caused by pyrogens liberated from lysed cells. It occurs more commonly in previously transfused patients.

○ **What is transfusion-related acute lung injury (TRALI)?**

TRALI is a form of noncardiogenic pulmonary edema, occurring within 2 to 4 hours after a transfusion. This reaction should be suspected in any patient who develops pulmonary edema after a transfusion in which volume overload is thought to be unlikely. Clinical signs of respiratory distress vary from mild dyspnea to severe hypoxia. It usually resolves within 48 hours in response to oxygen, mechanical ventilation, and other forms of supportive treatments.

○ **Petechia and bruising occur with platelet counts below what number? Internal hemorrhage occurs with count below what number?**

$<20,000/mm^3$ and $<10,000/mm^3$, respectively.

○ **What electrolyte abnormality is commonly associated with the transfusion of packed RBCs?**

Hypocalcemia secondary to citrate toxicity. Citrate, when rapidly infused, binds ionized calcium and therefore decreases the calcium level. Hyperkalemia may also develop, especially if the patient is in renal failure or if the blood products are old.

○ **Historically, what is the most common type of hepatitis transmitted through blood transfusions?**

Hepatitis C.

○ **What is the universal type of blood donor?**

Type Rh-negative blood with anti-A and anti-B titers of less than 1:200 in saline.

○ **What are the common presentations of a transfusion reaction?**

Myalgia, dyspnea, fever associated with hypocalcemia, hemolysis, allergic reactions, hyperkalemia, citrate toxicity, hypothermia, coagulopathies, and altered hemoglobin function.

○ **What is the most serious transfusion reaction?**

Hemolytic. Treat with aggressive fluid replacement and Lasix.

○ **What is the most common transfusion reaction?**

Fever.

○ **What is the most common cause of a coagulopathy in patients who require massive transfusions?**

Thrombocytopenia.

○ **What blood product is given when the coagulation abnormality is unknown?**

Fresh frozen plasma.

○ **In a nonacute noncardiac blood loss setting, what is the initial dose of blood given to children?**

10 mL/kg of packed RBCs.

○ **What pathway does the PT measure? What factor is unique to this pathway?**

Extrinsic pathway. Factor VII.

○ **What are the three major proteins that inhibit clotting?**

Antithrombin III, protein C, and protein S.

○ **The deficiency of antithrombin III, protein C, or protein S increases the risk of what?**

Venous thrombosis.

○ **Why should warfarin, as an <u>initial</u> treatment for venous thrombosis secondary to protein C deficiency, be avoided?**

It may, by inhibiting the synthesis of protein C, lead to paradoxical hypercoagulability. Always treat with heparin before warfarin.

○ **What are the signs and symptoms of splenic sequestration crisis?**

Pallor, weakness, lethargy, disorientation, shock, decreased level of consciousness, and enlarged spleen.

○ **What is the treatment of splenic sequestration crisis?**

Rapid infusion of saline and transfusion of red cells or whole blood.

○ **What are the major complications of hereditary spherocytosis?**

Hyperbilirubinemia in the newborn period, splenomegaly, and often gallstones.

○ **At what hematocrit level is the oxygen treatment capacity maximum?**

It occurs at a hematocrit of 30%.

○ **What does prothrombin time (PT) measure? How is it performed?**

PT measures the extrinsic and common pathways of the coagulation system. The time to clot formation is measured after the addition of thromboplastin. If the concentration of factors V, VII, IX, and X are significantly lower than usual, the PT may be prolonged.

○ **What does activated partial thromboplastin time (PTT) measure? How is it performed?**

PTT measures the intrinsic and common pathways of the coagulation cascade. After the blood sample is exposed to celite for activation and a reagent is added, the clot formation is measured. When factors II, V, VIII, IX, X, XI, XII, or fibrinogen are deficient, the PTT may be prolonged.

○ **What therapy should be initiated for a bleeding patient who is on warfarin and has a high PT?**

D/C warfarin, followed by a water soluble form of vitamin K. Prescribe SQ and consider a test dose. If the bleeding is severe or in a dangerous location (i.e., the brain), fresh frozen plasma containing active factors X, IX, VII, and II should be given. (*Remember*: 1972.)

● ● ● REFERENCES ● ● ●

Ambruso DR, Hays T, Goldenberg NA. Hematologic diseases. In: Hay WW Jr, Levin MJ, Sondheimer JM, eds. *Current Diagnosis and Treatment: Pediatrics.* 19th ed. New York, NY: McGraw-Hill; 2009:Ch 28.

Barrett KE, Barman SM, Boitano S, Brooks H. Circulating body fluids. In: Ganong WF, ed. *Review of Medical Physiology.*, 22nd ed. New York, NY: McGraw; 2005:Ch 27.

Beutler E. Disorders of iron metabolism. In: Lichtman MA, Beutler E, Kipps TJ, et al., eds. *Williams Hematology.* 7th ed. New York, NY: McGraw; 2006:Ch 40.

Beutler E. Disorders of red cells resulting from enzyme abnormalities. In: Lichtman MA, Beutler E, Kipps TJ, et al., eds. *Williams Hematology.* 7th ed. New York, NY: McGraw; 2006:Ch 45.

Cornett PA, Dea TO. Hematologic emergencies. In: Stone CK, Humphries RL, eds. *Current Diagnosis & Treatment: Emergency Medicine.*, New York, NY: McGraw; 2008:Ch 39.

Essentials of diagnosis, "vitamin B12 deficiency." Quick answers to medical diagnosis and therapy. http://www.accessmedicine.com/quickam.aspx.

Henry PH, Longo DL. Enlargement of lymph nodes and spleen. In: Fauci AS, Braunwald E, Kasper DL, et al., eds. Harrison's Principles of Internal Medicine. 17th ed. New York, NY: McGraw; 2008:Ch 60. http://www.accessmedicine.com/content.aspx?aID=2875326.

Kipps TJ. The hyperviscosity syndrome. In: Lichtman MA, Beutler E, Kipps TJ, et al., eds. Williams Hematology. 7th ed. New York, NY: McGraw; 2006:Ch 102.

Konkle BA. Bleeding and thrombosis. In: Fauci AS, Braunwald E, Kasper DL, et al., eds. *Harrison's Principles of Internal Medicine.* 17th ed. New York, NY: McGraw; 2008:Ch 59.

Konkle BA. Disorders of platelets and vessel wall. In: Fauci AS, Braunwald E, Kasper DL, et al., eds. *Harrisons Principles of Internal Medicine.* 17th ed. New York, NY: McGraw; 2008:Ch 109.

Lichtman MA, Shafer JA, Felgar RE, Wang N, eds. *Lichtman's Atlas of Hematology.* New York, NY: McGraw; 2007:Ch 22.

Linker CA. Blood Disorders. In: McPhee SJ, Papadakis MA, eds. Gonzales R, Zeiger R, online eds. *Current Medical Diagnosis and Treatment 2009.* New York, NY: McGraw; 2009:Ch 13.

Majerus PW, Tollefsen DM. Blood coagulation and anticoagulant, thrombolytic, and antiplatelet drugs. In: Burnton L, Lazo J, Parker K, eds. *Goodman and Gilman's Pharmacology, XI: Drugs Acting on the Blood and the Blood Forming Organs.* New York, NY: McGraw; 2006:Ch 54.

Morgan GE Jr, Mikhail MS, Murray MJ. Fluid management and transfusion. In: Morgan GE Jr, Mikhail MS, Murray MJ, eds. *Clinical Anesthesiology.* 4th ed. New York, NY: McGraw; 2006:Ch 29.

Prchal JT. Clinical manifestations and classification of erythrocyte disorders. In: Lichtman MA, Beutler E, Kipps TJ, et al., eds. *Williams Hematology.* 7th ed. New York, NY: McGraw; 2006:Ch 32.

Wittler MA, Hemphill RR. Acquired bleeding disorders. In: Tintinalli JE, Kelen GD, Stapczynski JS, eds., *Tintinalli's Emergency Medicine.*, New York, NY: McGraw; 2004:Ch 219.

Zeiger RF. McGraw-Hill's Diagnosaurus 2.0: http://www.accessmedicine.com/diag.aspx.

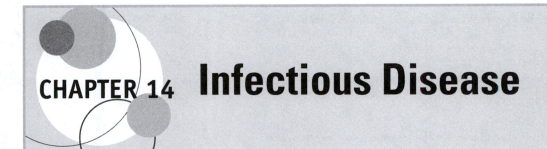

CHAPTER 14 # Infectious Disease

Daniel Thibodeau, MHP, PA-C

● ● ● FUNGAL DISEASE ● ● ●

○ **What are some of the clinical conditions that can present with candidiasis?**

Oral thrush, vaginitis, esophagitis, and mucocutaneous candida.

○ **What is the microscopic appearance of *Candida albicans*?**

Either as a singular oval budding yeast or as pseudohyphae (elongated).

○ **What types of patients are predisposed to develop disseminated candidiasis?**

Intravenous drug users and those with indwelling catheters and hyperalimentation, which can lead to right-sided endocarditis.

○ **How is candidiasis of the esophagus diagnosed?**

An air contrast barium swallow shows ulcerations with plaques. In contrast, herpes esophagitis produces punched out ulcerations with no plaques. Definitive diagnosis is made by upper GI endoscopy and fungal and viral cultures.

○ **Of the five antifungals listed, which drug would be the treatment of choice for each?**

1. Oral *candidiasis*
2. Esophageal
3. Vaginal
4. Mucocutaneous
5. Disseminated

1. Fluconazole
2. Fluconazole
3. Nystatin
4. Ketoconazole
5. Amphotericin B or fluconazole

○ **What is the method of contracting *Cryptococcus* in a human?**

Inhalation of contaminated soil, usually by bird droppings.

339

○ **Which species of *Cryptococcus* causes most human infections?**

C. neoformans.

○ **What would a chest X-ray reveal in a patient with early infection caused by *Cryptococcus*?**

A solitary nodule or a diffuse infiltrate.

○ **What is the drug(s) of choice for the treatment of *Cryptococcus*?**

Amphotericin B with fluconazole or flucytosine.

○ **Where is *histoplasmosis* more commonly found in the United States?**

Eastern and central United States, particularly in Mississippi, Ohio, and Missouri Valley areas.

○ **How does the *histoplasmosis* spore spread?**

Any activity that will cause the spores to move from their original site such as dry, windy conditions, demolition of old buildings, and barns where birds and bats have helped the spores proliferate.

○ **What test is used to accurately diagnose *histoplasmosis*?**

Cultures either from blood, marrow, tissue, or sputum via bronchoalveolar lavage.

○ **What is the drug of choice for the treatment of a *histoplasmosis* infection?**

Amphotericin B.

○ **What is the newer and more appropriate species for a pneumocystis infection in humans?**

Pneumocystis jiroveci. P. carinii infects only rats and not humans.

○ **What is the most common opportunistic infection in children and infants with HIV?**

Pneumocystis carinii pneumonia (PCP)

○ **What is the definitive diagnostic test for *pneumocystis* infection?**

Obtaining a respiratory tract specimen, either by tissue sample or aspiration of secretions.

○ **What is the drug of choice for the treatment of *pneumocystis* infection?**

Trimethoprim-sulfamethoxazole IV.

○ **What if the patient is sulfa allergic or cannot tolerate the medication?**

Alternate drug to use would be pentamidine.

○ **How is the diagnosis of pulmonary *zygomycosis* made?**

By biopsy.

○ **How does one diagnose invasive *aspergillosis*?**

By biopsy.

● ● ● BACTERIAL DISEASE ● ● ●

○ **How is botulism contracted, and what are the principal clinical features?**

It is contracted by consumption of contaminated foods, by injury from nonsterile objects (wound botulism), and in infants from intestinal colonization by *Clostridium botulinum* (lack of normal intestinal flora permit this colonization). The clinical features are that of a descending paralysis with complete ophthalmoplegia, bulbar, and somatic palsy.

○ **What is the best test to use to confirm a diagnosis of botulism?**

Stool and/or gastric aspirate for culture.

○ **What is the treatment for adult foodborne illness caused by *C. botulinum*? For infant botulism?**

For adults—Bivalent antitoxin A and B
For infants—Human-derived antitoxin

○ **If treating a botulism skinborne infection, what class of antibiotics should you avoid?**

Aminoglycosides, because they may potentiate the neurological symptoms.

○ **Is the motor paralysis induced by botulinum toxin reversible?**

It's an irreversible paralysis, and recovery is from axonal sprouting from old sarcolemmal area to a new locus.

○ **What is the sine-quo-non of botulism poisoning presentation?**

Bulbar palsy.

○ **What is the most common cause of sexually transmitted disease in the United States?**

Chlamydia trachomatis infections.

○ **Can *Chlamydia* bacteria grow on independently?**

No, they are obligate intracellular pathogens.

○ **What are the two most common forms of transmission of *Chlamydia*?**

Close contact either sexually or via the birth canal.

○ **A 23-year-old male patient is complaining of dysuria with a discharge that is clear and thin in appearance. What is the most likely pathogen that presents with this finding?**

Chlamydia urethritis infection.

○ **What is the drug of choice for the treatment of sexually transmitted *Chlamydia*?**

Azithromycin.

○ **What is the treatment of neonatal conjunctivitis caused by *C. trachomatis*?**

Erythromycin.

○   **Describe lesions associated with chlamydia:**

Painless, shallow ulcerations, papular or nodular lesions, and herpetiform vesicles that wax and wane.

○   **Describe the lesions associated with lymphogranuloma venereum (LV):**

LV caused by *Chlamydia* presents as painless skin lesions with lymphadenopathy. Lesions may be papular, nodular, or herpetiform vesicles. Sinus formation, involving the vagina and rectum, are common in women.

○   **On a recent medical mission trip to East Africa, you are caring for several members of a village who have had painless diarrhea, which has the appearance of colorless "rice water" stools. There is no abdominal pain, but the villagers are dehydrated and have suspected electrolyte abnormalities. What would be the leading diagnosis?**

Vibrio cholera outbreak.

○   **What is the most common mode of contamination of patients infected with *V. cholera*?**

Contaminated water or food (uncooked or raw shellfish, dried fish, and vegetables held in ambient heat).

○   **What is the treatment for a patient with confirmed or suspected cholera?**

Aggressive oral hydration along with electrolyte replenishment. If severe infection, oral doxycycline (one-time dose) or tetracycline can be used.

○   **What are the signs and symptoms of *diphtheria*?**

Acute onset of exudative pharyngitis, high fever, and malaise. A pseudomembrane may form in the oropharynx with possible respiratory compromise. Powerful exotoxins directly affect the heart, kidneys, and nervous system. Diphtheria infection may lead to paralysis of the intrinsic and extrinsic eye muscles, which may be confused with bulbar palsy caused by *Clostridium botulinum*. Botulism does not cause fever.

○   **What confirmatory test is run for the diagnosis of *diphtheria*?**

Culture, usually from the nose, throat, or mucous membrane lesion.

○   **What are the three considerations for the treatment of *diphtheria*?**

1.   Antitoxin—Before cultures are back and have high suspicion
2.   Antibiotics—Erythromycin or Penicillin G
3.   Immunization

○   **Do individuals with close contact to a *diphtheria* patient need to be watched?**

Yes. You must observe them for up to a week for any signs of infection, culture the throat for diphtheria, and prophylaxis with erythromycin for a 10-day course, or IM Penicillin G.

○   **What percentage of patients with *gonococcal* genital infections have concomitant *Chlamydia trichomatous* infections?**

45%. This is why treatment for *gonorrhea* includes ceftriaxone and doxycycline to cover both infections.

○ **What is the most common type of *gonorrhea* infection that can be seen in newborns?**

Conjunctivitis.

○ ***N. gonorrhea* is confirmed by what type of laboratory test?**

Gram stain and culture. You will see gram-negative diplococci.

○ **A 10-year-old girl presents to your facility with a history and physical examination that is consistent with vaginitis producing thick, purulent yellow discharge. What is the likely pathogen for this, and is this the only thing that you need to be worried about for the patient?**

The vaginitis with discharge as described is consistent with *N. gonorrhea* infection. A 10-year-old girl who present with this should give you a high suspicion for sexual abuse, as she should not get this type of infection.

○ **What is the recommended initial treatment for cases of gonorrhea?**

Third-generation cephalosporins (specifically ceftriaxone) plus either doxycycline (100 mg bid for 7 days) or azithromycin (1 g PO × 1 dose) for presumptive coinfection with *Chlamydia*.

○ **What is the most common physical examination finding in an adult patient with disseminated gonorrhea?**

Septic arthritis.

○ **Describe the skin lesions found in a patient with disseminated gonococcemia:**

Umbilicated pustules with red halos.

○ **What is the course of treatment for disseminated *gonorrhea*?**

7-day course of ceftriaxone or cefotaxime. If suspicion for meningitis, 10–14 days of treatment is recommended.

○ **What is the most common cause of bacterial enterocolitis in the United States?**

Salmonella infection.

○ **How is *Salmonella* transmitted?**

It is transmitted by humans and usually comes from contaminated water or food.

○ **Name the three types of infections that occur as a result of *Salmonella*:**

Enterocolitis, typhoid, and septicemia.

○ **What are the features of typhoid fever?**

Remember BIRDS FLEW:

Bradycardia	**F**ever
Insidious onset	**L**eukopenia
Rose spots	**E**pidemic
Dicrotic pulse	**W**idal reaction
Splenomegaly	

○ **Name the signs and symptoms for salmonella enterocolitis:**

Fever, diarrhea, and abdominal pain.

○ **What test do you order to confirm a diagnosis of *Salmonella*?**

Stool cultures most common. You can also obtain blood and urine cultures if examination is consistent.

○ **Which has a longer incubation period, staphylococci or salmonellae?**

Salmonellae; it is generally ingested in small doses and then multiplies in the GI tract. Symptoms occur 6–48 hours after ingestion. *Staphylococcus aureus* has an incubation period of just 3 hours.

○ **What is the first-line treatment for salmonella enterocolitis?**

Fluid and electrolyte replenishment.

○ **What is the pharmacological treatment for persistent salmonellosis?**

Ampicillin, TMP-SMX, chloramphenicol.

○ **Antibiotics should be avoided with what infectious diarrhea?**

Salmonella. Clear exceptions are severe cases of diarrhea in immunocompromised patients and in children younger than 6 months old.

○ **Which part of the GI tract does *Shigella* sp. infect more often?**

The colon.

○ **In a patient who presents with diarrhea, high fever, headache, lethargy, confusion, a normal lumbar puncture, 45% band forms on the differential of his white blood count, and a blood culture that is positive for *Escherichia coli*, what is the most likely cause of the diarrhea?**

Shigella. Blood cultures in shigella diarrhea are virtually never positive for shigella. When they are positive, they are more likely to be positive for *Escherichia coli*. Perhaps this is due to the fact that while Shigella is locally quite invasive at the mucosal level, it is very poorly invasive at the systemic level. Resident *E. coli* in the gut, however, take advantage of the disrupted mucosa and invade the blood stream.

○ **What is the microscopic makeup of *Shigella* sp.?**

It is an aerobic, gram-negative bacillus.

○ **What is the primary transmission route of *Shigella*?**

Fecal–oral.

○ **Does a stool sample culture give you a diagnosis for *Shigella*?**

No. It will show fecal leukocytes, which is consistent with a colitis picture.

○ **Do you treat *Shigella* with antibiotics?**

In general, no, if the disease is self-limiting to less than 72 hours. Should the infection be prolonged, if there is significant diarrhea, dysentery, or an immunocompromised patient, and then antibiotics are used to shorten the duration of the illness and reduce the amount of fecal leukocytes in the stool.

○ **What is the treatment for *Shigella sp.*?**

TMP-SMX or ciprofloxacin (if resistant).

○ **What causes tetanus?**

Clostridium tetani. This organism is a gram-positive rod; it is vegetative and a spore former. It produces tetanospasmin, an endotoxin, which induces the disinhibition of the motor and autonomic nervous systems and thus the exhibition of tetanus clinical symptoms.

○ **What is the incubation period of tetanus?**

Hours to months. The shorter the incubation period, the more severe the disease. The average age of incubation is 14 days.

○ **What is the most common presentation of tetanus?**

"Generalized tetanus" with pain and stiffness in the trunk and jaw muscles. Trismus develops and results in risus sardonicus ("The Devil's Smile").

○ **Outline the treatment for tetanus:**

Respiratory: Administer succinylcholine for immediate intubation if required.

Immunotherapy: Human tetanus immune globulin will neutralize circulating tetanospasmin and the toxin in the wound. However, it will not neutralize toxin fixed in the nervous system. Dose TIG 3000–5000 units. Prescribe tetanus toxoid, 0.6 mL IM, at 1 week and 6 weeks and 6 months.

Antibiotics: *Clostridium tetani* is sensitive to cephalosporins, tetracycline, erythromycin, and penicillin, but penicillin G is the drug of choice.

Muscle relaxants: Administer diazepam or dantrolene to help with the tetanic spasms.

Neuromuscular block: Prescribe pancuronium bromide, 2 mg plus sedation.

Autonomic dysfunction: Prescribe labetalol, 0.25–1.0 mg/min IV; or magnesium sulfate, 70 mg/kg IV load; then 1–4 g/hour continuous infusion is used to treat autonomic dysfunction. Administer MS, 5–30 mg IV infusion every 2–8 hours; and clonidine, .1.3 mg every 8 hour per NG.

Note: Fatal cardiovascular complications have occurred in patients treated with β-adrenergic blocking agents alone. Adrenergic blocking agents used to treat autonomic dysfunction may precipitate myocardial depression.

○ **Distinguish the key differences between strychnine and tetanus poisoning:**

Tetanus poisoning produces constant muscle tension, whereas strychnine produces tetany and convulsions with episodes of relaxation between muscle contractions.

○ **What are the signs and symptoms of tularemia?**

Indurated skin ulcers at the site of inoculation, regional lymphadenopathy, fever, shaking chills, cough, hemoptysis, SOB, rales or pleural rub, hepatosplenomegaly, and a maculopapular rash.

○ **What is the treatment for tularemia?**

Streptomycin. Mortality rate is 5% to 30% without antibiotic treatment.

○ **What is the most common symptom of tularemia?**

Skin sores at the site of inoculation and lymphadenopathy (75%). Other symptoms include pneumonia, lesions in the GI system, infection of the eyes, fever, and headache.

○ **How is tularemia most commonly transmitted?**

Via ticks and rabbits. Tularemia is caused by *F. tularensis*.

○ **What is the most common cause of cellulitis?**

Streptococcus pyogenes. Staphylococcus aureus can also cause cellulitis though it is generally less severe and more often associated with an open wound.

○ **What is the most common cause of cutaneous abscesses?**

Staphylococcus aureus.

○ **What percentage of dog and cat bites become infected?**

About 10% of dog bites and 50% of cat bites become infected. *Pasteurella multocida* are the causative agents for 30% of dog bites and 50% of cat bites.

○ **A 6-year-old child presents with headache, fever, malaise, and tender regional lymphadenopathy about a week after a cat bite. A tender papule develops at the site. What is the diagnosis?**

Cat-scratch disease. This condition usually develops 3 days to 6 weeks following a cat bite or scratch. The papule typically blisters and heals with eschar formation. A transient macular or vesicular rash may also develop.

○ **What is thought to be the mode of inoculation in cat-scratch disease?**

Rubbing the eye after contact with a cat.

○ **What is the probable cause of an animal bite infection arising that develops in less than 24 hours? More than 48 hours?**

Less than 24 hours: *Pasteurella multocida* or streptococci. More than 48 hours: *Staphylococcus aureus.*

○ **What is the most common cause of gas gangrene?**

Clostridium perfringens.

○ **What are the neurological features of brucellosis?**

Mainly a chronic meningitis and the vascular complications thereof. However, cranial neuropathies, demyelination and mycotic aneurysms have all been described.

○ **How is brucellosis spread?**

By ingestion of contaminated milk and milk products. It may also be spread by contact with an infected animal (usually cattle). *Brucella melitensis* is the culprit.

○ **A 31-year-old man stepped on a nail at his job. The nail pierced through his sneaker and into his foot. His tetanus status is up to date. What is your main concern?**

Infection with *Pseudomonas* that can lead to osteomyelitis. Pseudomonal infection is most commonly associated with hot, moist environments, such as sneakers and moisture in socks.

○ **What is the most common causative bacterium associated with right-sided endocarditis in IV drug abusers?**

Staphylococcus aureus. Left-sided endocarditis in IV drug abusers is usually due to *E. coli, Streptococcus, Klebsiella, Pseudomonas,* or *Candida.*

○ **What are the major Jones criteria used to diagnose rheumatic fever?**

Carditis, chorea (Sydenham), erythema marginatum, migratory polyarthritis, and subcutaneous nodules. The diagnosis requires either 2 major or 1 major and 2 minor with evidence of previous streptococcal infection.

○ **After finishing the prescribed dosage of penicillin for pharyngitis, your patient's repeat culture still grows *Streptococcus.* What should you do?**

Nothing. Most people are asymptomatic carriers and in most cases it is inconsequential.

○ **What is the cause of chancroid?**

Hemophilus ducreyi. Patients with this condition present with one or more painful necrotic lesions. Suppurating inguinal lymphadenopathy may also be present.

○ **What is the most common infectious disease complication of both measles and influenza?**

Pneumococcal pneumonia.

○ **Do household pets transmit *Yersinia*?**

Yes.

○ **On Tuesday, you are driving home from work in rural California and pass three dead squirrels. On Wednesday, taking a different route, you pass two more dead squirrels. The following morning you see a 26-year-old male patient with enlarged tender lymphadenitis and a 105°F fever. What illness might you suspect?**

Cases of human plague (*Yersinia pestis*) are sometimes heralded by squirrel die-offs. A squirrelly die-off occurs when the organism is introduced into a highly susceptible mammalian population, causing a high mortality rate among infected animals. This is referred to as epizootic plague.

○ **One day after a previously healthy adult has been admitted to the hospital after an accidental overdose of oral iron, she appears to become septic. What is the most likely organism causing her sepsis?**

Yersinia enterocolitica. The growth of *Y. enterocolitica* appears to be enhanced after exposure to excess iron. This combined with intestinal damage to the mucosa by the iron may play a role in pathogenesis.

○   **What is the treatment for *Yersinia* sp.?**

TMP-SMX, tetracycline, and third-generation cephalosporin.

○   **What is Weil disease?**

Weil syndrome is the less common variety of leptospirosis, with icterus, marked hepatic and renal involvement along with a bleeding diathesis being the main features, and hence the name leptospirosis-ictero-hemorrhagica.

○   **What is the most common neurological feature of leptospirosis?**

Aseptic meningitis (present in over 50%).

○   **What clinical feature of leptospirosis sets it apart from other infections of the nervous system and hints at the diagnosis?**

Hemorrhagic complications. These are not uncommon, and intraparenchymal and subarachnoid hemorrhages have been reported.

○   **Which organisms produce focal nervous system pathology via an exotoxin?**

Clostridium diphtheria, Clostridium botulinum, Clostridium tetani, Staphylococcus aureus plus wood and dog ticks (*Dermacentor* A and B).

○   **How should you treat a patient who has been bitten by a wild raccoon?**

Wound care, tetanus prophylaxis, RIG, 20 IU/kg (1/2 at bite site and 1/2 IM), and HDCV, 1 cc IM.

○   **Do animal bites from birds, reptiles, or rodents (hamster, squirrel, mouse, rat, gerbil, guinea pig, rabbit) require the rabies vaccine?**

No, these types of animal bites do not carry rabies.

○   **Describe the skin lesions associated with a *Pseudomonas aeruginosa* infection.**

Pale, erythematous lesions 1 cm in size with an ulcerated necrotic center.

○   **Why is needle aspiration preferred over incision and drainage for a fluctuant, acute cervical lymphadenitis?**

Development of a fistula tract is possible if the patient has atypical mycobacterium or cat-scratch fever instead of bacterial lymphadenitis.

○   **What is the cause of granuloma inguinale?**

The bacterium *Donovania granulomatis*, recently renamed *Calymmatobacterium granulomatis*.

○   **What triad is associated with Reiter syndrome?**

Nongonococcal urethritis, polyarthritis, and conjunctivitis. Conjunctivitis is the least common and occurs in only 30% of the patients. Acute attacks respond well to NSAIDs.

○ **What is the treatment for persistent *E. coli*?**

Trimethoprim with sulfamethoxazole (TMP-SMX).

○ **What is the treatment for *Giardia lamblia*?**

Quinacrine or metronidazole or furazolidone.

○ **What are the common features of *Vibrio parahaemolyticus*?**

This condition is caused by organisms associated with oysters, clams, and crabs. Symptoms include cramps, vomiting, dysentery, and explosive diarrhea. Severe infections are treated with tetracycline and chloramphenicol.

○ **What are the antibiotics of choice in a wound resulting from a skin diving incident?**

Ciprofloxacin or TMP-SMX.

○ **What is the most common gram-negative aerobe found in cutaneous abscesses?**

Proteus mirabilis.

○ **Describe the Gram stain appearance of *Staphylococcus aureus*:**

Gram-positive cocci in grapelike clusters.

○ **Which type of diarrhea-causing disease may be transmitted by pets?**

Yersinia.

○ **Does *H. influenzae* typically cause abscesses?**

No.

○ **What is the common pathogen in a cat bite?**

Pasteurella multocida.

○ **What percentage of untreated group A β-hemolytic streptococcal infections will progress to rheumatic fever?**

3%. Increased incidence of the disease is noted in lower socioeconomic areas.

○ **What is used to control outbreaks of meningococcal meningitis?**

Rifampin and ceftriaxone are used as chemoprophylaxis for contacts.

● ● ● MYCOBACTERIAL DISEASE ● ● ●

○ **Why does therapy for tuberculosis (TB) take several months, when other infections usually clear in a matter of days?**

Because the mycobacterium divide very slowly and have a long dormant phase, during which time they are not responsive to medications.

○ **What is the typical timeframe for symptoms to appear for patients with TB?**

1–6 months.

○ **What are some of the classic symptoms of TB?**

Fevers, chills, cough, night sweats, weight loss, or poor weight gain.

○ **What are some radiographic findings on chest X-ray in a patient with TB?**

Can be normal. Abnormalities can be increased markings of the hilar, mediastinal, and carinal nodes, atelectasis or infiltrate of a segment of a lobe; pleural effusions, cavitary lesions and miliary disease.

○ **What type of bacteria is TB?**

It is an acid-fast bacillus.

○ **Name the two types of lesions found in TB:**

1. Exudative lesions—Usually seen at the site of the lung that produces inflammatory reaction of the local tissue.
2. Granulomatous lesions—These are giant cells that have tubercle bacilli around the cells. Over time, these cells will heal but will leave fibrotic or calcified tissue behind.

○ **What percentages of TB infections are symptomatic?**

Only 10%.

○ **What is the main treatment drug for TB?**

Rifampin.

○ **What is the most common side effect of rifampin?**

Orange discoloration of urine and tears.

○ **What is the triple drug treatment for pulmonary TB, and for how long on each drug?**

Isoniazaid, 6 months

Rifampin, 6 months

Pyrazinamide, 2 months

For HIV+ patients, ethambutol is added with this regimen for 9–12 months duration.

○ **If the result of a patient's PPD is read as 3 mm of induration and then 15 mm of induration following the placement of the second PPD 2 weeks later, which study should be considered the more reliable?**

The second study with an induration of 15 mm. With time, the body's memory of the tuberculosis infection may wane. The placement of a PPD may stimulate that memory. This is what is referred to as the "booster phenomenon." The boosted result is considered to be the reliable result.

○ **List the four groups of atypical mycobacterium, the common bacteria in each group, where it is found, the physical effects, and what drug it used to treat:**

Group with Name	Name of Bacteria	Environment	Physical Effects	Drug of Choice
Group I	*M. kansasii*	Unknown	Resembles TB infections	Anti-TB drugs
Photochromogens	*M. marinum*	Swimming pools and aquariums	Ulcerating skin lesions at abrasions	Tetracycline, minocycline
Group II Scotochromogens	*M. scrofulaceum*	Environmental water sources	Cervical adenitis	Surgical excision of affected lymph node
Group III Nonchromogens	*M. avium* M. intracellulare	Water and soil Water and soil	Pulmonary infection similar to TB	Clarithromycin Plus one or more: ethambutol, rifabutin, or ciprofloxacin
Group IV	*M. fortuitum*	Soil and water	Skin and soft tissue punctures	Amikacin
Rapidly growing bacteria	M. chelonei	Soil and water	Immuno-compromised patients and patients with prosthetics and indwelling catheters	Plus doxycycline

○ **What regions of the United States have more cases of coccidiomycosis?**

Typically the Southwest states (Arizona, New Mexico, Southern California) and some in the Ohio valley. It is sometimes referred to as Valley fever or the San Joaquin fever

○ **How is the diagnosis of coccidiomycosis made?**

By culture or staining of sputum, bronchoalveolar lavage or tissue, and by a positive serology.

○ **What is the treatment for a pulmonary infection due to *coccidiomycosis*?**

Amphotericin B is used for serious infections. Minor infections do not require medications.

○ **What is the cause of granuloma inguinale?**

Calymmatobacterium granulomatis. Onset occurs with small papular, nodular, or vesicular lesions that develop slowly into ulcerative or granulomatous lesions. Lesions are painless and are located on mucous membranes of the genital, inguinal, and anal areas.

○ **A patient from the Philippines has a hypopigmented patch that is lacking in sensation. What is the most likely cause of his problem?**

Leprosy (*Mycobacterium leprae*).

○ **What is the mode of transmission for leprosy?**

It is human-to-human contact mostly but in prolonged contact with the patient.

○ **What are the two forms of leprosy?**

Tuberculin and lepromatous.

○ **What is the treatment for leprosy?**

Dapsone alone causes resistance. However, a combination of dapsone and rifampin is recommended.

• • • PARASITIC DISEASE • • •

○ **List three common protozoa that can cause diarrhea:**

1. *Entamoeba histolytica*—Found worldwide. Although half of the infected patients are asymptomatic, the usual symptoms consist of N/V/D/F, anorexia, abdominal pain, and leukocytosis. Determine the presence of this organism by ordering stool tests and performing an ELISA for extraintestinal infections. Treatment is with metronidazole or tinidazole followed by chloroquine phosphate.
2. *Giardia lamblia*—Found worldwide. This organism is one of the most common intestinal parasites in the United States. Symptoms include explosive watery diarrhea, flatus, abdominal distention, fatigue, and fever. The diagnosis is confirmed via a stool examination. Treatment is with metronidazole.
3. *Cryptosporidium parvum*—Found worldwide. Symptoms are profuse watery diarrhea, cramps, N/V/F, and weight loss. Treatment is supportive care. Medications may be needed for immunocompromised patients.

○ **What is the most common intestinal parasite in the United States?**

Giardia. Cysts are obtained from contaminated water or by hand-to-mouth transmission. Symptoms include explosive foul smelling diarrhea, abdominal distention, fever, fatigue, and weight loss. Cysts reside in the duodenum and upper jejunum.

○ **What are the characteristic features of cerebral amebiasis, and what is the pathogenic organism?**

Cerebral amebiasis is usually a secondary infection, and patients often have intestinal or hepatic amebiasis. The causative organism is *Entamoeba histolytica*. The clinical features are that of intracerebral abscesses causing focal neurological signs. Frontal lobes and basal nuclei are common sites of abscess formation.

○ **What is the treatment for amebiasis with neurological involvement?**

E. histolytica is treated with metronidazole, emetine, and chloroquine. *Naegleria* species is treated with amphotericin and rifampicin.

○ **Besides the intestinal and cerebral manifestations related to *Entamoeba histolytica*, what is another potential complication related to the parasite?**

It can also develop liver abscess. The signs and symptoms of these patients will have right upper quadrant pain, fevers, and weight loss with a tender, enlarged liver.

○ **Which parasite is found in 25%–50% of women, causes a watery, foul-smelling vaginal discharge, and microscopically appears as a pear-shaped organism with four flagellates anteriorly?**

Trichomonas vaginalis.

○ **What is the antibiotic of choice for this type of infection?**

Metronidazole.

○ **Where is the hookworm *Necator americanus* infection acquired?**

In areas where human fertilizer is used and people don't wear shoes. Patients present with chronic anemia, cough, low-grade fever, diarrhea, abdominal pain, weakness, weight loss, eosinophilia, and guaiac positive stools. A diagnosis is confirmed if ova are present in the stool. Treatment includes mebendazole or pyrantel pamoate.

○ **What are the signs and symptoms of *Trichuris trichiura*?**

This hookworm lives in the cecum. Complaints include anorexia, abdominal pain especially RUQ, insomnia, fever, diarrhea, flatulence, weight loss, pruritus, eosinophilia, and microcytic hypochromic anemia. Examining for ova in the stool makes a diagnosis. Mebendazole is the treatment of choice.

○ **A patient attended a walrus, bear, and pork roast. He now has N/V/D/F, urticaria, myalgia, splinter hemorrhages, muscle spasm, headache, and a stiff neck. What physical finding will clinch the diagnosis?**

Periorbital edema is pathognomonic for infection with *Trichinella spiralis*. Patients may have acute myocarditis, nonsuppurative meningitis, and catarrhal enteritis bronchopneumonia. Laboratory studies may reveal leukocytosis, eosinophilia, ECG changes, and elevated CPK. Diagnosis is confirmed with a latex agglutination, skin test, complement fixation, or bentonite flocculation test. A stool examination is not helpful after the initial GI phase for confirming the diagnosis.

○ **How are tapeworms transmitted into humans?**

They are usually acquired by ingesting undercooked fish, which has the larvae present. The larvae then proliferate. In the cases of cystircecosis and hydatid disease, the eggs are ingested.

○ **Which is the most common tapeworm in the United States?**

Hymenolepis nana (dwarf tapeworm). Infections are spread via fecal/oral spread and occur in institutionalized patients, typically children.

○ **Which intestinal parasites are known to cause anemia as their major manifestation?**

Hookworms. Three species of hookworms affect humans. These include *Ancylostoma duodenale, Necator americanus,* and *Ancylostoma ceylanicum.*

○ **Hookworm is associated with what sort of anemia?**

Iron deficiency anemia.

○ **Fish tapeworm (*Diphyllobothrium latum*) is associated with what type of anemia?**

Pernicious anemia.

○ **Roundworm is associated with what GI problem?**

Small bowel obstruction.

○ **In general, what kinds of education can you provide to patients to prevent infections that arise from hookworms?**

Beef and pork products must be cooked thoroughly as well as hands washed properly. Prevention from farmers to prevent ingestion of human waste by cows and pigs is also paramount.

○ **Name the four types of malaria; and which one is the most prevalent?**

1. *Plasmodium falciparum* (most prevalent)
2. *P. vivax*
3. *P. ovale*
4. *P. malariae*

○ **What is the most deadly form of malaria?**

Plasmodium falciparum.

○ **What is the vector for malaria?**

The female anopheline mosquito.

○ **What laboratory findings are expected for a patient with malaria?**

Normochromic normocytic anemia, a normal or depressed leukocyte count, thrombocytopenia, an elevated sedimentation rate, abnormal kidney and LFTs, hyponatremia, hypoglycemia, and a false-positive VDRL.

○ **How is malaria diagnosed?**

Visualization of parasites on Giemsa-stained blood smears. In early infection, especially with *P. falciparum,* parasitized erythrocytes may be sequestered and undetectable.

○ **How is *P. falciparum* diagnosed on blood smear?**

1. Small ring forms with double chromatin knobs within the erythrocyte
2. Multiple rings infected within red blood cells
3. Rare trophozoites and schizonts on smear
4. Pathognomonic crescent-shaped gametocytes
5. Parasitemia exceeding 4%

○ **What is the drug of choice for treating *P. vivax*, ovale, and malariae?**

Chloroquine.

○ **How is uncomplicated chloroquine-resistant *P. falciparum* treated?**

Quinine plus pyrimethamine-sulfadoxine plus doxycycline or mefloquine.

○ **What are the adverse effects of chloroquine?**

N/V/D/F, pruritus, headache, dizziness, rash, and hypotension.

○ **Which hemoglobin provides the greatest innate resistance to falciparum malaria?**

Erythrocytes of patients who are heterozygous for sickle cell hemoglobin (sickle cell trait) are resistant to malaria.

○ **What species of *Plasmodium* is resistant to chloroquine?**

Falciparum.

○ **A 5-year-old boy presents with his mother complaining of anal itching that has been present for the last 3 days. On examination, the child has small whitish worms that were obtained by the "Scotch tape" method. What diagnosis does this child have?**

Pinworms.

○ **What is the most common helminth in the United States?**

Enterobius.

○ **What is the most common physical complaint in individuals with an *Enterobius* infection?**

Perianal pruritus.

○ **What is the treatment for pinworms?**

Mebendazole as well as proper teaching about hand hygiene to the patient.

○ **Name the most common form of transmission for toxoplasmosis:**

Ingestion of the cysts via uncooked meat or feline feces.

○ **Is there a risk for transmission of toxoplasmosis from a pregnant woman to the fetus?**

Yes, but only if the mother gets infected during the pregnancy.

○ **Which types of pregnant women are at increased risk for developing toxoplasmosis?**

Women who are cat owners. They must be educated to refrain from cleaning out the cat litter as well as told to avoid eating uncooked meats.

○ **What pathological findings are seen in the brain biopsy of toxoplasma encephalitis?**

Presence of tachyzoites around the necrotic lesion.

○ **What are some important radiological differences between intracranial toxoplasmosis and lymphoma?**

  1. Intracranial toxoplasmosis is usually multiple, whereas lymphomas are usually solitary, at least in the beginning.
  2. Enhancement—Both may enhance with gadolinium on the MRI scan; however, toxoplasma lesions are usually round and discrete in comparison to the lymphoma.
  3. Thallium 201 SPECT scan—Lymphomas usually show increased activity in the thallium scans compared to toxoplasmosis, which has poor uptake.
  4. Location—Toxoplasmosis is usually in the deeper structures such as basal ganglia, or the gray white junction, whereas the lymphomas usually present themselves in the periventricular areas. However, biopsy is still necessary to make the diagnosis since imaging studies may overlap.

○ **What is the current recommended treatment for intracranial toxoplasmosis in HIV disease?**

This is usually a combination therapy with sulfadiazine, pyrimethamine, and folinic acid.

○ **How is Chagas disease transmitted?**

By the blood-sucking Reduviid "kissing" bug, blood transfusion, or breast feeding. A nodule or chagoma develops at the site. Symptoms include fever, headache, conjunctivitis, anorexia, and myocarditis. CHF and ventricular aneurysms can occur. The myenteric plexus is involved and may result in megacolon. Laboratory findings include anemia, leukocytosis, elevated sedimentation rate, and ECG changes, such as PR interval, heart block, T wave changes, and arrhythmias.

○ **What causes swimmer itch (Schistosome dermatitis)?**

An invading cercariae.

○ **What is the vector of trypanosomiasis?**

Tsetse fly.

○ **What is the infectious agent of elephantiasis?**

Nematode microfilaria.

○ **What vector transmits Chagas disease (*Trypanosoma cruzi*)?**

Reduviid (assassin or kissing bug).

○ **Cysticercosis is associated with:**

New onset seizure.

○ **Onchocerciasis (from *Onchocerca volvulus*) is associated with what visual deficit?**

Blindness. This is referred to as river blindness.

○ **Chagas disease is associated with:**

Acute myocarditis. *Trypanosoma cruzi* invades the myocardium resulting in myocarditis. Conduction defects may occur. The vector for this parasite is the insect reduviid.

○ **What is the most frequently transmitted tick-borne disease?**

Lyme disease. The causative agent is a spirochete (*Borrelia burgdorferi*), the vectors are *Ixodes dammini, I. pacificus, Amblyomma americanum,* and *Dermacentor variabilis.*

○ **What areas of the United States report the highest incidence of Lyme disease?**

New England, the middle Atlantic, and upper Midwestern states.

○ **What are the signs and symptoms of Lyme disease?**

Stage I: In the first month after the tick bite, patients can present with fever, fatigue, malaise, myalgia, headache, and a circular macule or papule lesion with a central clearing at the site of the tick bite that gradually enlarges (erythema chronicum migrans).

Stage II: (Weeks to months later) This stage involves neurological abnormalities such as meningoencephalitis, cranial neuropathies, peripheral neuropathies, myocarditis, and conjunctivitis to blindness.

Stage III: (Months to years) Migratory oligoarthritis of the large joints, neurological symptoms such as subtle encephalopathy (mood, memory, and sleep disturbances) polyneuropathy, cognitive dysfunction, and incapacitating fatigue.

○ **How is Lyme disease diagnosed?**

Immunofluorescent and immunoabsorbent assays identify the antibodies to the spirochete. Treatment includes doxycycline or tetracycline, amoxicillin, IV penicillin (V in pregnant patients), or erythromycin.

○ **What is the vector and causative organism of Lyme disease?**

The vector is *Ixodes dammini,* and the organism is *Borrelia burgdorferi.* It is the most frequently transmitted tick-borne disease.

○ **Which two diseases are transmitted by the deer tick, *Ixodes dammini*?**

Lyme disease and babesiosis.

○ **At which stage of Lyme disease does neurological involvement occur?**

The second and third stages. Second-stage cranial neuropathies, meningitis and radiculoneuritis. Third-stage encephalitis, and a variety of CNS manifestations including stroke like syndromes, extrapyramidal, and cerebellar involvement.

○ **Describe the skin lesion seen in Lyme disease:**

A large distinct circular skin lesion called erythema chronicum migrans. It is an annular erythematous lesion with central clearing.

○ **When does ECM show up in Lyme disease?**

Stage I, which is 3–32 days after the bite.

○ **How do patients present with babesia infection?**

Intermittent fever, splenomegaly, jaundice, and hemolysis. The disease may be fatal in patients without spleens. Treatment is with clindamycin and quinine.

○ **Which type of paralysis does tick paralysis cause?**

Ascending paralysis. The venom that causes the paralysis is probably a neurotoxin. A conduction block is induced at the peripheral motor nerve branches and thereby prevents the release of acetylcholine at the neuromuscular junction; 43 species of ticks have been implicated as causative agents.

○ **What tick-borne disease is also harbored in wild rabbits?**

Tularemia.

○ **A patient presents with sudden onset of fever, lethargy, a retro-orbital headache, myalgias, anorexia, nausea, and vomiting. She is extremely photophobic. The patient has been on a camping trip in Wyoming. What tick-borne disease might cause these symptoms?**

Colorado tick fever. This is caused by a virus of the genus *Orbivirus* and the family Reoviridae. The vector is the tick *D. andersoni*. The disease is self-limited; treatment is supportive.

○ *Dermacentor andersoni* **(wood tick) is a pesky arthropod associated with four tick-borne illnesses! Name these illnesses and the cause of each:**

1. Rocky Mountain spotted fever (RMSF)—caused by *Rickettsia rickettsii*; *Dermacentor andersoni* is a vector.
2. Tick paralysis—caused by a neurotoxin. The symptoms, consisting of ascending paralysis with decrease or loss of DTRs, are similar to those associated with Guillain-Barré syndrome.
3. Q fever—caused by *Coxiella burnetii* (a Rickettsiae).
4. Colorado tick fever—caused by an arbovirus.

○ **Which condition resembles Guillain-Barre syndrome, the appropriate treatment of which results in miraculous complete improvements often within a day?**

Tick paralysis, which results in an ascending paralysis within a few days of attack by the tick *Dermacentor* (hard tick). This releases a toxin in its saliva, which is responsible for the neuromuscular blockade. Removal of the tick results in resolution of the weakness that begins within hours.

○ **What is the common name for** *Dermacentor andersoni***?**

Wood tick.

○ **What causes Q fever?**

Coxiella burnetii, also known as *Rickettsia burnetii*. It is found in the *Dermacentor andersoni* tick.

○ **Describe a patient with tick paralysis:**

Bulbar paralysis, ascending flaccid paralysis, paresthesias of hands and feet, symmetric loss of deep tendon reflexes, and respiratory paralysis.

○ **What kind of tick transmits Rocky Mountain spotted fever (RMSF)?**

The female andersoni tick which transmits *Rickettsia rickettsii*.

○ **Where do the majority of Rocky Mountain spotted fever cases come from?**

North Carolina, South Carolina, Tennessee, Oklahoma, and Arkansas comprise 56% of all cases.

○ **What is the most common symptom in RMSF?**

Headache. This occurs in 90% of patients.

○ **A patient presents a 40°C fever and a erythematous, macular, and blanching rash which becomes deep red, dusky, papular, and petechial. The patient is vomiting and has a headache, myalgias, and cough. Where did the rash begin?**

Rocky Mountain spotted fever (RMSF) rash typically begins on the flexor surfaces of the ankles and wrists and spreads centripetally and centrifugally.

○ **Which test confirms RMSF?**

Immunofluorescent antibody staining of a skin biopsy or serologic fluorescent antibody titer. The Weil-Felix reaction and complement fixation tests are no longer recommended.

○ **Which antibiotics are prescribed for the treatment of RMSF?**

Tetracycline or chloramphenicol. Antibiotic therapy should not be withheld pending serologic confirmation.

○ **What antibiotic is used to treat Rocky Mountain spotted fever in a patient allergic to tetracycline?**

Chloramphenicol.

○ **A 24-year-old male patient presents with a painless ulcer to the glans penis. What is the likely diagnosis?**

Primary chancre from syphilis. These generally erupt within 2–10 weeks from exposure.

○ **What is the most common lesion that is seen in secondary syphilis?**

Condyloma lata. These are mainly found on the genital region.

○ **What are some signs and symptoms of secondary syphilis?**

Patchy alopecia, fevers, chills, myalgias, weight loss, headache, and malaise.

○ **A patient is infected with *Treponema pallidum*. What is the treatment?**

The type of treatment depends upon the stage of the infection. Primary and secondary syphilis are treated with benzathine penicillin G (2.4 million units IM × 1 dose) or doxycycline (100 mg bid PO for 14 day). Tertiary syphilis is treated with benzathine penicillin G, 2.4 million units IM × 3 doses 3 weeks apart.

○ **Is the vasculitis that is seen in syphilis, a large or a small vessel disease?**

Both. Large vessel (Heubner arteritis) is caused by adventitial lymphocytic proliferation of large vessels, and is commonly seen in the late meningovascular syphilis. The small vessel (Nissl-Alzheimer) vasculitis is the dominant vasculitic pattern in the paretic neurosyphilis.

○ **What is the recommended treatment for neurosyphilis?**

Intravenous penicillin G. Follow-up CSF examinations are mandatory.

○ **What complication may arise from aggressive treatment of neurosyphilis with penicillin?**

Jarisch-Herxheimer reaction. It is due to a release of endotoxin when large numbers of spirochete are lysed during the penicillin treatment, and consists of mild fever, malaise, headache, arthralgia, and may produce a temporary worsening of the neurological status.

○ **What are five infectious diseases that give false-positive treponemal tests (FTA, MHA-TP, TPI) for syphilis?**

Yaws, pinta, leptospirosis, rat-bite fever (*Spirillum minus*), and Lyme disease.

○ **What are five diseases that give false-positive non-treponema (VDRL, RPR) tests for syphilis?**

Infectious mononucleosis, connective tissue diseases, tuberculosis, endocarditis, and intravenous drug abuse.

○ **A woman comes to your office frantic because her husband has just received a positive VDRL result. They have been happily married for 35 years and she can't believe he has been unfaithful. Is it at all possible that he has been loyal to his wife?**

Yes. False-positive tests can occur if the patient has had a viral or mycoplasma infection in the near past, if the patient is an IV drug user, or if the patient has SLE. The presence or absence of syphilis can be confirmed with the fluorescent treponemal antibody absorption test (FTA-ABS).

● ● ● VIRAL DISEASE ● ● ●

○ **What is the most common cause of congenital anomalies in the United States?**

Cytomegalovirus (CMV).

○ **Name the forms of transmission of CMV in the different stages of life—fetus/infant, adolescent, and adult:**

Fetus/infant—across placenta, during birth from canal, or through breast milk
Adolescent—saliva
Adult—sexual contact; both semen and cervical discharge, blood transfusions, and organ transplants

○ **Name the forms of anomalies in infants with CMV, and what percentage of infants with CMV present with these problems?**

Seizures, deafness, jaundice, microcephaly, and purpura. About 20% of the infants with CMV will have one of these conditions.

○ **How is the diagnosis of CMV made?**

By the use of immunofluorescent antibody tests known as "shell vials." An alternative test is the PCR assay.

○ **Name two CMV-related illnesses that can affect AIDS patients:**

CMV colitis and retinitis. In other immunocompromised patients it can cause pneumonitis and hepatitis.

○ **What is the treatment for CMV infections?**

Ganciclovir is the first-line treatment. Valganciclovir can be used as an alternate drug and also in retinitis cases.

○ **What causes infectious mononucleosis?**

Epstein-Barr virus (EBV).

○ **Are there any other illnesses that EBV can cause?**

Yes, Burkitt lymphoma, nasopharyngeal cancer, B-cell lymphomas, and hairy leukoplakia seen more commonly in AIDS patients.

○ **How is EBV transmitted?**

Through the saliva.

○ **What percentage of Americans have the antibody to fight against EBV?**

90%.

○ **What patients are at risk to get the virus?**

Immunocompromised, first few years in life as a child, and lower socioeconomic classes.

○ **Name the hallmark characteristics seen in patients with EBV (infectious mononucleosis):**

Fever, sore throat, malaise, cervical lymphadenopathy, and anorexia.

○ **A 17-year-old adolescent boy who has recently been diagnosed with infectious mononucleosis. He is in high school and plays for the football team. What are some considerations that need to be addressed for all patients with mono, and what do you need to tell your patient?**

All patients who have infectious mono need to have a careful examination of the spleen, which can enlarge, and in some cases of mono rupture. In rare cases, hepatomegaly can occur. The patient has to be held from playing any contact sport until the virus has subsided and he has been reevaluated to resume contact sports.

○ **What is the average length of illness in infectious mononucleosis?**

56–60 days.

○ **How is the diagnosis of EBV made?**

Two methods: one by hematologic and measuring the numbers of abnormal lymphocytes on smear and second by immunologic. There is an heterophil antibody test and a EBV-specific antibody test.

○ **What is the treatment for EBV?**

Mainly supportive care, hydration, pain medications for sore throat, acetaminophen for fever, and prevention of injury of splenic injury.

○ **What causes erythema infectiosum?**

It is parvovirus B19 and is referred to as "fifth disease" or "slapped cheek syndrome."

○ **Is there a test that can determine erythema infectiosum?**

Yes, the detection of IgM antibodies could be run; however, it is mainly a diagnosis on examination.

○ **Is there a specific treatment for fifth disease?**

No, it is only supportive care of any symptoms.

○ **What is the most common site of a herpes simplex I infection?**

The lower lip. These lesions are painful and can frequently recur since the virus remains in the sensory ganglia. Recurrences are generally triggered by stress, sun, and illness.

○ **What is the main transmission of HSV-1 and HSV-2?**

HSV-1: Saliva
HSV-2: Sexual contact

○ **Where does HSV lie dormant within the body?**

It is held latent in the sensory ganglion cells.

○ **What STD pathogens cause painful ulcers?**

Type II genital herpes and chancroid.

STD	Ulcer	Node
Genital herpes	Painful	Painful
Chancroid	Painful	Painful
Syphilis	Painless	Less painful
Lymphogranuloma venereum	Painless	Moderately painful

○ **Name the different forms of HSV-1 and HSV-2:**

HSV-1	HSV-2
Gingivostomatitis	Genital herpes
Herpes labialis	Neonatal herpes
Keratoconjunctivitis	Aseptic meningitis
Encephalitis	
Herpetic whitlow	
Herpes gladiatorum (from wrestling contact)	
Esophagitis and pneumonia (in immunocompromised patients)	

○ **A 27-year-old woman who is 36 weeks pregnant and has a past history of HSV-2 but has been symptom free for the last several months. What considerations do you have to make in this patient's case?**

She may need a caesarean section if by term she has either active lesions present of positive viral cultures.

○ **What is the treatment for patients with HSV?**

Acyclovir.

○ **Is there any advantage for long-term suppressive therapy for a patient with HSV?**

Yes, long-term therapy can be helpful in reducing the number and severity of outbreaks. Valacyclovir and famciclovir are drugs of choice.

○ **Describe the pathophysiologic features of HIV:**

HIV attacks the T4 helper cells. The genetic material of HIV consists of single-stranded RNA. HIV has been found in semen, vaginal secretions, blood and blood products, saliva, urine, cerebrospinal fluid, tears, alveolar fluid, synovial fluid, breast milk, transplanted tissue, and amniotic fluid. There has been no documentation of infection from casual contact.

○ **How quickly do patients infected with HIV become symptomatic?**

5%–10% develop symptoms within 3 years of seroconversion. Predictive characteristics include a low CD4 count and a hematocrit less than 40. The mean incubation time is about 8.23 years for adults and 1.97 years for children younger than 5 years.

○ **A 22-year-old man, who has no significant medical history and is taking no medication, has a creamy white coat on his tongue. The substance easily rubs off, revealing an erythematous base. What should you be most concerned about?**

HIV. In a patient who has no obvious reason for having an overgrowth of oral candida, HIV should be suspected. Other causes for oral thrush overgrowth include cancer, systemic illness, neutropenia, diabetes, adrenal insufficiency, nutritional deficiencies, or an immunocompromised state.

○ **An HIV-positive patient presents with a history of weight loss, diarrhea, fever, anorexia, and malaise. She is also dyspneic. Laboratory studies reveal abnormal LFTs and anemia. What is the most likely diagnosis?**

Mycobacterium avium intracellulare. Laboratory confirmation is made by an acid-fast stain of body fluids or by a blood culture.

○ **What are the signs and symptoms of CNS cryptococcal infection in an AIDS patient?**

Headache, depression, lightheadedness, seizures, and cranial nerve palsies. A diagnosis is confirmed by an India ink prep, a fungal culture, or by a testing for the presence of cryptococcal antigens in the CSF.

○ **What is the most common eye finding in AIDS patients?**

Cotton wool spots. It has been proposed that the cotton wool spots are associated with PCP. These finding may be hard to differentiate from the fluffy, white, often perivascular retinal lesions that are associated with CMV.

○ **What is the most common cause of retinitis in AIDS patients?**

Cytomegalovirus. Findings include photophobia, redness, scotoma, pain, or a change in visual acuity. On examination, fluffy white retinal lesions may be evident.

○ **What is the most common opportunistic infection in AIDS patients?**

Pneumocystis carinii (PCP). Symptoms may include a nonproductive cough and dyspnea. A chest X-ray may reveal diffuse interstitial infiltrates, or it may be negative. Although Gallium scanning is more sensitive, false positives occur. Initial treatment includes TMP-SMX. Pentamidine is an alternative.

○ **What is HAART?**

HAART is an acronym for **H**ighly **A**ctive **A**nti**r**etroviral **T**herapy. This is a combination of antiretroviral medications that can nearly completely suppress HIV viral replication. Medications used are nucleoside reverse transcriptase inhibitors and protease inhibitors.

○ **What is PEP and when can it be used?**

PEP is an acronym for **P**ost **E**xposure **P**rophylaxis. It is a combination of HIV medications used to try to prevent HIV infection in individuals who have been exposed to the HIV virus. It should be used as soon as possible but definitely within 72 hours.

○ **What is the most common gastrointestinal complaint in AIDS patients?**

Diarrhea. Many of the medications used to treat HIV have GI side effects. Hepatomegaly and hepatitis are also typical. Conversely, jaundice is an uncommon finding. Cryptosporidium and Isospora are the common causes of prolonged watery diarrhea.

○ **What is the current recommended treatment for intracranial toxoplasmosis in HIV disease?**

This is usually a combination therapy with sulfadiazine, pyrimethamine, and folinic acid.

○ **What is the nature of CNS lymphoma in AIDS?**

They are almost all tumors of B cell origin. They may be large cell immunoblastic, or small noncleaved cell lymphoma.

○ **Which virus is considered responsible for AIDS associated CNS lymphoma?**

Epstein-Barr virus (EBV).

○ **What is the meaning of the term reverse transcriptase in the description of HIV?**

Under normal circumstances, the transcription of a protein in a human cell occurs in a forward direction going from DNA to RNA. In reverse transcriptase, the transcription proceeds from RNA to DNA. HIV is a reverse transcriptase or a "retrovirus" that needs to be incorporated into the human genome by the reverse transcription before replicating.

○ **What life-threatening infection is most commonly associated with AIDS patients?**

Pneumocystis carinii pneumonia (PCP).

○ **What often causes a change in visual acuity in AIDS patients?**

Cytomegalovirus.

○ **Which type of malignancy is most commonly associated with AIDS?**

Kaposi sarcoma, followed by non-Hodgkin lymphoma.

○ **How many years does a patient usually live after being diagnosed with HIV?**

It depends. Life expectancy in a 20-year-old on therapy is about 29 additional years. However, patients who start therapy and are diagnosed with a CD4 count lower than 100 cells/mm^3 have an average of 12 extra years, those with a count of 200 cells/mm^3 or higher have an average of 30 extra years, and those with a history of injectable drug use have comparatively lower extra years (12 years).

○ **Describe the AIDS dementia complex, which is also known as HIV-I encephalopathy:**

A progressive disease caused directly by HIV-I. It is present in one-third of AIDS patients and is characterized by recent memory impairment, concentration deficit, elevated DTRs, seizures, and frontal release signs.

○ **What is the most common cause of focal encephalitis in AIDS patients?**

Toxoplasma gondii.

○ **What is the risk of transmission of HIV from an HIV-infected person following a needle stick exposure?**

0.3%–0.5% on average. (Although this varies depending on needle gauge and depth and site of insertion.)

○ **What are the most common adverse effects of AZT in an AIDS patient?**

Granulocytopenia and anemia.

○ **What signs indicate an HIV-positive patient is at increased risk for opportunistic infections like PCP?**

An absolute CD4 count of less than 200 and a CD4 lymphocytic percentage of less than 20.

○ **What immunizations are recommended for patients with HIV?**

IPV and Td every 10 years
Influenza vaccine yearly
Pneumococcal vaccine once
Hepatitis B vaccine for at risk patients
Hib and MMR are optional

○ **At what point should AZT treatment begin in an asymptomatic patient with HIV?**

When the CD4$^+$ count reaches 300 cells/mm^3

○ **What is the prophylactic regime of choice for PCP in patients with AIDS?**

Trimethoprim-sulfamethoxazole DS should be started when the CD4$^+$ count reaches 200 cells/mm^3.

○ **At what point should prophylaxis treatment against** *Mycobacterium avium intracellulare* **and toxoplasmosis be started in patients with AIDS?**

When the CD4$^+$ count reaches 100 cells/mm^3.

○ **Immunocompromised patients can safely be given which vaccines?**

Killed or inactivated vaccines:

Diphtheria

H. influenzae

Influenza

Pneumococcal

Enhanced inactivated polio

Hepatitis

Pertussis

Tetanus

It may be easier to remember the vaccines that should be avoided. The following are live, attenuated vaccines: Oral polio and MMR.

○ **Human papillomavirus (HPV) originates as tumors from what type of cell?**

Squamous cells.

○ **How is HPV transmitted?**

Skin-to-skin contact, usually sexual contact.

○ **What is the cause of condylomata acuminata?**

Papilloma virus.

○ **Which types of HPV cause carcinoma of the cervix and penis?**

Types 16 and 18.

○ **What medium is used to detect occult premalignant lesions caused by HPV?**

Acetic acid prep.

○ **What is the main treatment for HPV?**

Podophyllin. Genital warts can be either burned off or cryotherapy be used.

○ **What is the vaccine for the prevention of HPV, and what types of HPV does it protect against?**

The vaccine Gardisil is available and protects against HPV 6 and 11 (genital warts) and 16 and 18 (cervical cancer). The vaccine is administered to females between the ages of 9 and 26 years.

○ **What strain of influenza is more common in adults? In children?**

Adults: Influenza A

Children: Influenza B

○   **What strain of influenza is most virulent?**

Influenza A.

○   **Influenza epidemics and pandemics are generally associated with which strain of influenza?**

Influenza A.

○   **Amantadine is 70%–90% effective in preventing which strain of influenza?**

Influenza A. Amantadine should be prescribed as chemoprophylaxis in immunocompromised patients who are not vaccinated or as a supplement to vaccination. It can also be given to healthy unvaccinated people who want to avoid the flu. Over the last few years, the use of amantidine for treatment of influenza has fallen out of favor due to higher resistance (over 90%) to the drug.

○   **When should the influenza vaccine be given?**

In September or October, about 1 to 2 months before the influenza season begins. The vaccine, unlike amantadine, is protective against influenza A and B.

○   **What is a contraindication to the administration of the influenza vaccine?**

A history of anaphylactic hypersensitivity to eggs or their products.

○   **How is the influenza virus transmitted?**

By respiratory droplets.

○   **Name the signs and symptoms of a patient with influenza:**

Fevers, chills, malaise, nonproductive cough, myalgias, headache, and sore throat.

○   **What is a potential respiratory complication to influenza?**

Bacterial pneumonia.

○   **What is the most common pathogen for this type of pneumonia?**

Staphylococcus aureus.

○   **Name two drugs approved for the treatment of influenza:**

Oseltamivir (Tamiflu) and zanamivir (Relenza).

○   **What is the most common clinical finding on examination in a patient with mumps?**

Parotid gland swelling.

○   **What are some prodromal symptoms in patients with mumps?**

Fevers, malaise, and anorexia.

○   **What is a key examination that must be done in a male patient with mumps?**

You must examine the scrotum to look for acute orchitis.

○ **Besides orchitis in men, what is another potentially serious complication related to mumps?**

Meningitis.

○ **How is mumps transmitted?**

Respiratory droplets. It has a high peak incidence in the winter months.

○ **What is the treatment for mumps?**

There is no treatment. If orchitis occurs, immediate consultation with a urologist in indicated. If suspicion for meningitis, appropriate treatment for the infection is warranted.

○ **How can mumps be prevented?**

By giving the live attenuated mumps vaccine as scheduled. This is usually the MMR vaccine.

○ **Explain the pathophysiology of rabies:**

Infection occurs within the myocytes for the first 48–96 hours. It then spreads across the motor endplate and ascends and replicates along the peripheral nervous system, axoplasm, and into the dorsal root ganglia, spinal cord, and CNS. From the gray matter, the virus spreads by peripheral nerves to tissues and organ systems.

○ **What is the characteristic histologic finding associated with rabies?**

Eosinophilic intracellular lesions within the cerebral neurons called Negri bodies are the sites of CNS viral replication. Although these lesions occur in 75% of rabies cases and are pathognomonic for rabies, their absence does not eliminate the possibility of rabies.

○ **What are the signs and symptoms of rabies?**

Incubation period of 12–700 days with an average of 20–90 days. Initial signs and systems are fever, headache, malaise, anorexia, sore throat, nausea, cough, and pain or paresthesias at the bite site.

In the CNS stage, agitation, restlessness, altered mental status, painful bulbar and peripheral muscular spasms, bulbar or focal motor paresis, and opisthotonos are exhibited. As in the Landry-Guillain-Barré syndrome, 20% develop ascending, symmetric flaccid and areflexic paralysis. In addition, hypersensitivity to water and sensory stimuli to light, touch, and noise may occur.

The progressive stage includes lucid and confused intervals with hyperpyrexia, lacrimation, salivation, and mydriasis along with brainstem dysfunction, hyperreflexia, and extensor planter response.

Final stages include coma, convulsions, and apnea, followed by death between the fourth and seventh day for the untreated patient.

○ **What is the diagnostic procedure of choice in rabies?**

Fluorescent antibody testing (FAT).

○ **How is rabies treated?**

Wound care includes debridement and irrigation. The wound must not be sutured; it should remain open. This will decrease the rabies infection by 90%. RIG 20 IU/kg, half at wound site and half in the deltoid muscle, should be administered along with HDCV, 1 mL doses IM on days 0, 3, 7, 14, and 28, also in the deltoid muscle.

○ **Describe the intracorporeal dissipation of the rabies virus:**

The virus spreads centripetally up the peripheral nerve into the CNS. The incubation period for rabies is usually 30–60 days with a range of 10 days to 1 year. Transmission usually occurs via infected secretions, saliva, or infected tissue. Stages of the disease include upper respiratory tract infection symptomatology, followed by encephalitis. The brainstem is affected last.

○ **What animals are the most prevalent vectors of rabies in the world? In the United States?**

Worldwide, dog is the most common carrier of rabies. In the United States, the skunk has become primary carrier. In descending order, bats, raccoons, cows, dogs, foxes, and cats are also sources.

○ **What would you expect to find in the hippocampus of a patient with rabies?**

Negri bodies. Incubation for rabies is 30–60 days. Treatment includes cleaning of the wound, rabies immune globulin, and human diploid cell vaccine. Remember, half the rabies immune globulin goes around the wound; the other half goes IM.

○ **Since 1980, how many individuals in the United States have survived from rabies without postexposure prophylaxis?**

None, it is 100% fatal.

○ **What is the etiology of roseola infantum?**

It is a virus caused by the herpes virus 6 or 7.

○ **What are the hallmark features of the virus?**

High spiking fevers up to a week followed by a rose-pink maculopapular rash.

○ **What is some other physical examination characteristics associated with roseola?**

Pharyngeal and tonsillar injection without exudates, and lymphadenopathy.

○ **Is there a specific treatment for this virus?**

No. Supportive care and treatment of the fever with acetaminophen is appropriate.

○ **What are the two types of rubella?**

Rubella (German measles) and congenital rubella syndrome.

○ **How is the virus spread?**

Through respiratory droplets and through the placenta in congenital rubella syndrome.

○ **Name some potential congenital defects as a result of rubella:**

Patent ductus arteriosus, cataracts, deafness, and mental retardation.

○ **At what stage are these defects more likely to occur in pregnancy?**

In the first trimester.

○ **How would you test for congenital rubella syndrome in a pregnant woman?**

The presence of IgM antibody indicates a recent infection. Amniocentesis analysis can detect if the virus is in the fluid.

○ **What measure can be taken for preventing rubella?**

Vaccination of the rubella live attenuated virus.

○ **What is the characteristic of a rash caused by measles?**

It is a maculopapular rash.

○ **How is the virus transmitted?**

Respiratory droplets from coughing and sneezing.

○ **Which vitamin deficiency will cause a worsening of the measles virus?**

Vitamin A.

○ **What are some prodromal signs and symptoms that present with measles?**

A course of 10–14 days will start a presentation of fevers, conjunctivitis, coryza, and coughing. The hallmark of Koplik spots will reveal themselves on the buccal mucosal surface.

○ **What are Koplik spots?**

The are bright-red lesions with a white central dot on the buccal mucosa.

○ **Name some complications of measles:**

Encephalitis, pneumonia, and otitis media.

○ **Describe the signs and symptoms of varicella (chicken pox):**

Onset of varicella rash 1–2 days after prodromal symptoms of slight malaise, anorexia, and fever. The rash begins on the trunk and scalp, appearing as faint macules and later becoming vesicles. Remember, dew drops on a rose petal appearance.

○ **What is zoster?**

Zoster is the recurrent infection of the Herpes virus. This virus will break out commonly in a single dermatome and begin with pain to the dermatome, followed by a vesicular, red-bordered rash that will crust over a 14-day period. Postherpetic neuralgia is a potential long-term complication.

○ **What is the most reliable method for diagnosing varicella-zoster?**

In a majority of cases the diagnosis is made clinically.

○ **What is the treatment in immunocompetent children and in adults?**

In children, no treatment is necessary, only supportive care.

In adults, course of acyclovir for varicella to reduce the course of the virus. In zoster, famciclovir and valacyclovir can be used.

○ **Which patients are recommended to receive the varicella vaccine and the zoster vaccine?**

Varicella—children aged 1 to 12 years.

Zoster—adults older than 60 years.

○ **What is the typical clinical presentation of progressive multifocal leukoencephalopathy (PML)?**

PML commonly presents with focal neurological signs such as hemisensory or motor signs, and visual field deficits.

○ **Which virus is responsible for causing PML?**

JC virus, which is a papovavirus that infects oligodendrocytes.

○ **PML is seen in which other immune disorders?**

Cell-mediated immune deficiency. It is thus seen in HIV disease, chronic myeloid leukemia, Hodgkin disease, chemotherapy patients, and rarely sarcoidosis.

○ **What are the common radiological features of PML?**

Hypodensities in the subcortical white matter on the CT scan. T1 images on the brain MRI are hypointense and T2 images are hyperintense. They are nonenhancing and usually start in the parietooccipital region of the subcortical white matter.

○ **Which virus is considered responsible for tropical spastic paraparesis (TSP)?**

Human T cell lymphotrophic virus type 1.

○ **What are the modes of transmission of HTLV 1?**

Vertical: mother to child. Horizontal: through sexual contact and blood transfusion.

○ **To which group of viruses does the poliovirus belong?**

Poliovirus is an enterovirus that belongs to the picornavirus group.

○ **What are four other infectious causes of paraparesis?**

Syphilis, tuberculosis with Pott disease of the spine, leptospirosis, and VZV.

○ **What is epidemic pleurodynia (Bornholm disease)?**

An upper respiratory tract infection followed by pleuritic chest pain and tender muscles. Coxsackie viruses are a group of enteroviruses responsible for the epidemic myalgia (Bornholm disease) where pleurodynia is also a common feature. Specifically, the disease is thought to occur due to a Coxsackie group B virus.

○ **What is the cerebral spinal fluid (CSF) characteristic of polio?**

In the acute stages, it is associated with a lymphocytic pleocytosis, elevated protein, and normal glucose. There may be a neutrophilic response very early in the disease. Chronic residual polio has normal CSF.

○ **What is the cause of epidemic keratoconjunctivitis?**

Adenovirus.

○ **What is the most common cause of foodborne viral gastroenteritis?**

Norwalk virus commonly found in shellfish.

○ **What is the Jarisch-Herxheimer reaction?**

Headache, fever, myalgia, hypotension, and an increased severity of syphilis symptoms that occurs after taking benzathine penicillin G for the treatment of syphilis. The reaction may result in neurological, auditory, or visual changes.

○ **How should a patient with a black widow spider bite be treated?**

Consider antivenin, IV calcium gluconate, and IV opiates plus IV benzodiazepines.

○ **How should a jellyfish sting be treated?**

Rinse with saline. Apply 5% acetic acid (vinegar) locally to the wound for approximately 30 minutes. In addition, corticosteroid agents may be applied topically. No antibiotics are necessary. Tetanus prophylaxis.

Chironex fleckeri antivenin only for this coelenterate.

○ **What is the differential diagnosis of a ring lesion on CT scan?**

Toxoplasmosis, lymphoma, fungal infection, TB, CMV, Kaposi sarcoma, and hemorrhage.

○ **Name four enterotoxin-producing organisms that can cause food poisoning:**

1. *Clostridium*
2. *Staphylococcus aureus*
3. *Vibrio cholerae*
4. *E. coli*

○ **What is the most common presentation of cryptococcosis?**

Fungal meningitis with *Cryptococcus neoformans*.

○ **What prophylactic medication would you recommend to a patient traveling to Costa Rica?**

Mefloquine, 250 mg, once a week. Treatment should begin 1 week before travel and continue 6 weeks after returning. Mefloquine, not chloroquine, is now the drug of choice due to the resistance of chloroquine in some regions. Check with the CDC for specific information.

○   **What preventive measures would you recommend to a patient planning a trip to Mexico?**

Avoidance of water, ice, foods prepared in water, and raw or prepeeled fruits and vegetables. Prophylactic antibiotics are not routinely recommended. However, if they are a necessity, ciprofloxacin is the drug of choice. Otherwise, treatment with antibiotics should begin with the onset of symptoms, as should rehydration.

○   **A friend is headed to Benin on the west coast of Africa. What immunizations and prophylactic treatments must she receive before departing?**

Hepatitis A vaccine
Oral polio vaccine
Tetanus-diphtheria vaccine
Live oral typhoid vaccine
Measles vaccine
Yellow fever vaccine
Mefloquine prophylaxis for malaria

○   **At what concentration is ozone damaging to your health?**

10 ppm. Initial effects are tearing, pulmonary edema, and pain in the trachea.

○   **Which immunizations do healthy senior citizens need?**

Tetanus booster every 10 years, influenza vaccination every year, and a pneumococcal vaccination.

○   **Which vaccine should be administered to postsplenectomy patients?**

Pneumococcal vaccine.

○   **What five vaccines should be administered to adults?**

1. Hepatitis B vaccine: Give to high-risk patients (health care workers, homosexuals, and IV drug users)
2. Influenza vaccine: Give annually to elderly patients and patients with chronic illnesses
3. MR: Give to all patients without immunity (most often required by school institutions)
4. Pneumococcal vaccine: Give once to patients older than 65 years and patients with chronic illnesses
5. Tetanus/diphtheria: Give all adults a primary series and a booster every 10 years

○   **Other than immunocompromised patients, who should not receive live vaccines?**

Pregnant women. Oral polio vaccine should be avoided in anyone in close contact with an immunocompromised person because of the virus's ability to spread.

○   **A patient comes in for vaccinations and has a URI and a fever of 37.5°C. Can you administer vaccines to this patient?**

Yes. URI or gastrointestinal illness is not a contraindication to vaccination. Fever may be as high as 38°C and the vaccine still administered. Likewise, use of antibiotics or recent exposure to illness is not a reason to delay vaccination.

○   **When administering the Mantoux skin test to a person with HIV, what induration indicates a positive reaction?**

>5 mm. In individuals with risk factors for TB, induration must be >10 mm. For those with no risk factors, induration must be >15 mm to be positive.

● ● ● **REFERENCES** ● ● ●

Fauci AS, Braunwald E, Kasper DL, et al., eds. *Harrison's Principles of Internal Medicine*, 17th ed. New York: McGraw-Hill; 2008. http://www. accessmedicine.com

Hall JB, Schmidt G, Wood LD. *Principles of Critical Care.* 3rd ed. New York, NY: McGraw-Hill; 2005.

Levinson W. *Review of Medical Microbiology and Immunology.* 10th ed. New York, NY: McGraw-Hill; 2008.

McPhee SJ, Papadakis MA, eds. *Current Medical Diagnosis and Treatment 2009.* New York, NY: McGraw-Hill; 2009.

McPhee SJ, Ganong WF. *Pathophysiology of Disease—An Introduction to Clinical Medicine.* 5th ed. New York, NY: McGraw-Hill; 2006.

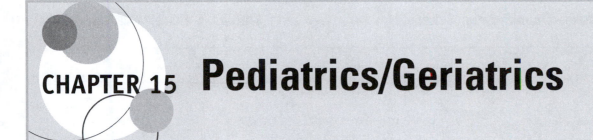

CHAPTER 15 Pediatrics/Geriatrics

Daniel Thibodeau, MHP, PA-C

● ● ● PEDIATRICS ● ● ●

○ **Describe some child development stages at the following ages: 1–2 months, 3–5 months, 6–8 months, 9–11 months, 1 year, and 18 months:**

1–2 months: Holds head erect, drops toys, follows objects, becomes alert with voices

3–5 months: Reaches for objects and brings to mouth, grasps cube (ulnar first then thumb), laughs, turns from back to side

6–8 months: Reaches with one hand, imitates "bye bye" babbles, inhibited by the word *no*

9–11 months: Stands alone, imitates peek-a-boo, uses thumb and index to pick up object, follows one step command like "come here"

1 year: Walks independently, says mama and dada, gives toys on request, says one to two words

18 months: Throws ball, sits self on chair, says 4–20 words, feeds self

○ **What are the three possible schedules from which to choose when deciding the set of polio vaccines a child needs?**

1. 2 doses of IPV followed by 2 doses of OPV

2. 4 doses of IPV

3. 4 doses of OPV

○ **A child is born to an HBsAg-negative mother. Which vaccine should the child receive?**

Recombivax (2.5) or Engerix-B (10). The second dose should be given at least 1 month after the first, and the third dose at least 2 months later (but not before the age of 6 months).

○ **An unvaccinated 13-year-old adolescent comes to your office. Should he receive a hepatitis vaccine if there are no known carriers in his family?**

Yes.

Recommended Immunization Schedule for Persons Aged 0 Through 6 Years—United States • 2009

For those who fall behind or start late, see the catch-up schedule

Vaccine ▼ Age ▶	Birth	1 month	2 months	4 months	6 months	12 months	15 months	18 months	19–23 months	2–3 years	4–6 years
Hepatitis B[1]	HepB	HepB		see footnote 1		HepB					
Rotavirus[2]			RV	RV	RV[2]						
Diphtheria, Tetanus, Pertussis[3]			DTaP	DTaP	DTaP	see footnote 3	DTaP				DTaP
Haemophilus influenzae type b[4]			Hib	Hib	Hib[4]	Hib					
Pneumococcal[5]			PCV	PCV	PCV	PCV				PPSV	
Inactivated Poliovirus			IPV	IPV		IPV					IPV
Influenza[6]						Influenza (Yearly)					
Measles, Mumps, Rubella[7]						MMR		see footnote 7			MMR
Varicella[8]						Varicella		see footnote 8			Varicella
Hepatitis A[9]						HepA (2 doses)				HepA Series	
Meningococcal[10]										MCV	

Range of recommended ages

Certain high-risk groups

This schedule indicates the recommended ages for routine administration of currently licensed vaccines, as of December 1, 2008, for children aged 0 through 6 years. Any dose not administered at the recommended age should be administered at a subsequent visit, when indicated and feasible. Licensed combination vaccines may be used whenever any component of the combination is indicated and other components are not contraindicated and if approved by the Food and Drug Administration for that dose of the series. Providers should consult the relevant Advisory Committee on Immunization Practices statement for detailed recommendations, including high-risk conditions: http://www.cdc.gov/vaccines/pubs/acip-list.htm. Clinically significant adverse events that follow immunization should be reported to the Vaccine Adverse Event Reporting System (VAERS). Guidance about how to obtain and complete a VAERS form is available at http://www.vaers.hhs.gov or by telephone, 800-822-7967.

1. Hepatitis B vaccine (HepB). *(Minimum age: birth)*
At birth:
- Administer monovalent HepB to all newborns before hospital discharge.
- If mother is hepatitis B surface antigen (HBsAg)-positive, administer HepB and 0.5 mL of hepatitis B immune globulin (HBIG) within 12 hours of birth.
- If mother's HBsAg status is unknown, administer HepB within 12 hours of birth. Determine mother's HBsAg status as soon as possible and, if HBsAg-positive, administer HBIG (no later than age 1 week).
After the birth dose:
- The HepB series should be completed with either monovalent HepB or a combination vaccine containing HepB. The second dose should be administered at age 1 or 2 months. The final dose should be administered no earlier than age 24 weeks.
- Infants born to HBsAg-positive mothers should be tested for HBsAg and antibody to HBsAg (anti-HBs) after completion of at least 3 doses of the HepB series, at age 9 through 18 months (generally at the next well-child visit).
4-month dose:
- Administration of 4 doses of HepB to infants is permissible when combination vaccines containing HepB are administered after the birth dose.

2. Rotavirus vaccine (RV). *(Minimum age: 6 weeks)*
- Administer the first dose at age 6 through 14 weeks (maximum age: 14 weeks 6 days). Vaccination should not be initiated for infants aged 15 weeks or older (i.e., 15 weeks 0 days or older).
- Administer the final dose in the series by age 8 months 0 days.
- If Rotarix® is administered at ages 2 and 4 months, a dose at 6 months is not indicated.

3. Diphtheria and tetanus toxoids and acellular pertussis vaccine (DTaP). *(Minimum age: 6 weeks)*
- The fourth dose may be administered as early as age 12 months, provided at least 6 months have elapsed since the third dose.
- Administer the final dose in the series at age 4 through 6 years.

4. Haemophilus influenzae type b conjugate vaccine (Hib). *(Minimum age: 6 weeks)*
- If PRP-OMP (PedvaxHIB® or Comvax® [HepB-Hib]) is administered at ages 2 and 4 months, a dose at age 6 months is not indicated.
- TriHiBit® (DTaP/Hib) should not be used for doses at ages 2, 4, or 6 months but can be used as the final dose in children aged 12 months or older.

5. Pneumococcal vaccine. *(Minimum age: 6 weeks for pneumococcal conjugate vaccine [PCV]; 2 years for pneumococcal polysaccharide vaccine [PPSV])*
- PCV is recommended for all children aged younger than 5 years. Administer 1 dose of PCV to all healthy children aged 24 through 59 months who are not completely vaccinated for their age.

- Administer PPSV to children aged 2 years or older with certain underlying medical conditions (see *MMWR* 2000;49[No. RR-9]), including a cochlear implant.

6. Influenza vaccine. *(Minimum age: 6 months for trivalent inactivated influenza vaccine [TIV]; 2 years for live, attenuated influenza vaccine [LAIV])*
- Administer annually to children aged 6 months through 18 years.
- For healthy nonpregnant persons (i.e., those who do not have underlying medical conditions that predispose them to influenza complications) aged 2 through 49 years, either LAIV or TIV may be used.
- Children receiving TIV should receive 0.25 mL if aged 6 through 35 months or 0.5 mL if aged 3 years or older.
- Administer 2 doses (separated by at least 4 weeks) to children aged younger than 9 years who are receiving influenza vaccine for the first time or who were vaccinated for the first time during the previous influenza season but only received 1 dose.

7. Measles, mumps, and rubella vaccine (MMR). *(Minimum age: 12 months)*
- Administer the second dose at age 4 through 6 years. However, the second dose may be administered before age 4, provided at least 28 days have elapsed since the first dose.

8. Varicella vaccine. *(Minimum age: 12 months)*
- Administer the second dose at age 4 through 6 years. However, the second dose may be administered before age 4, provided at least 3 months have elapsed since the first dose.
- For children aged 12 months through 12 years the minimum interval between doses is 3 months. However, if the second dose was administered at least 28 days after the first dose, it can be accepted as valid.

9. Hepatitis A vaccine (HepA). *(Minimum age: 12 months)*
- Administer to all children aged 1 year (i.e., aged 12 through 23 months). Administer 2 doses at least 6 months apart.
- Children not fully vaccinated by age 2 years can be vaccinated at subsequent visits.
- HepA also is recommended for children older than 1 year who live in areas where vaccination programs target older children or who are at increased risk of infection. See *MMWR* 2006;55(No. RR-7).

10. Meningococcal vaccine. *(Minimum age: 2 years for meningococcal conjugate vaccine [MCV] and for meningococcal polysaccharide vaccine [MPSV])*
- Administer MCV to children aged 2 through 10 years with terminal complement component deficiency, anatomic or functional asplenia, and certain other high-risk groups. See *MMWR* 2005;54(No. RR-7).
- Persons who received MPSV 3 or more years previously and who remain at increased risk for meningococcal disease should be revaccinated with MCV.

The Recommended Immunization Schedules for Persons Aged 0 Through 18 Years are approved by the Advisory Committee on Immunization Practices (www.cdc.gov/vaccines/recs/acip), the American Academy of Pediatrics (http://www.aap.org), and the American Academy of Family Physicians (http://www.aafp.org).
DEPARTMENT OF HEALTH AND HUMAN SERVICES • CENTERS FOR DISEASE CONTROL AND PREVENTION

CS103164

Recommended Immunization Schedule for Persons Aged 7 Through 18 Years—United States • 2009

For those who fall behind or start late, see the schedule below and the catch-up schedule

Vaccine ▼ Age ▶	7–10 years	11–12 years	13–18 years
Tetanus, Diphtheria, Pertussis[1]	*see footnote 1*	Tdap	Tdap
Human Papillomavirus[2]	*see footnote 2*	HPV (3 doses)	HPV Series
Meningococcal[3]	MCV	MCV	MCV
Influenza[4]	Influenza (Yearly)		
Pneumococcal[5]	PPSV		
Hepatitis A[6]	HepA Series		
Hepatitis B[7]	HepB Series		
Inactivated Poliovirus[8]	IPV Series		
Measles, Mumps, Rubella[9]	MMR Series		
Varicella[10]	Varicella Series		

Range of recommended ages

Catch-up immunization

Certain high-risk groups

This schedule indicates the recommended ages for routine administration of currently licensed vaccines, as of December 1, 2008, for children aged 7 through 18 years. Any dose not administered at the recommended age should be administered at a subsequent visit, when indicated and feasible. Licensed combination vaccines may be used whenever any component of the combination is indicated and other components are not contraindicated and if approved by the Food and Drug Administration for that dose of the series. Providers should consult the relevant Advisory Committee on Immunization Practices statement for detailed recommendations, including high-risk conditions: http://www.cdc.gov/vaccines/pubs/acip-list.htm. Clinically significant adverse events that follow immunization should be reported to the Vaccine Adverse Event Reporting System (VAERS). Guidance about how to obtain and complete a VAERS form is available at http://www.vaers.hhs.gov or by telephone, 800-822-7967.

1. Tetanus and diphtheria toxoids and acellular pertussis vaccine (Tdap). *(Minimum age: 10 years for BOOSTRIX® and 11 years for ADACEL®)*
- Administer at age 11 or 12 years for those who have completed the recommended childhood DTP/DTaP vaccination series and have not received a tetanus and diphtheria toxoid (Td) booster dose.
- Persons aged 13 through 18 years who have not received Tdap should receive a dose.
- A 5-year interval from the last Td dose is encouraged when Tdap is used as a booster dose; however, a shorter interval may be used if pertussis immunity is needed.

2. Human papillomavirus vaccine (HPV). *(Minimum age: 9 years)*
- Administer the first dose to females at age 11 or 12 years.
- Administer the second dose 2 months after the first dose and the third dose 6 months after the first dose (at least 24 weeks after the first dose).
- Administer the series to females at age 13 through 18 years if not previously vaccinated.

3. Meningococcal conjugate vaccine (MCV).
- Administer at age 11 or 12 years, or at age 13 through 18 years if not previously vaccinated.
- Administer to previously unvaccinated college freshmen living in a dormitory.
- MCV is recommended for children aged 2 through 10 years with terminal complement component deficiency, anatomic or functional asplenia, and certain other groups at high risk. See *MMWR* 2005;54(No. RR-7).
- Persons who received MPSV 5 or more years previously and remain at increased risk for meningococcal disease should be revaccinated with MCV.

4. Influenza vaccine.
- Administer annually to children aged 6 months through 18 years.
- For healthy nonpregnant persons (i.e., those who do not have underlying medical conditions that predispose them to influenza complications) aged 2 through 49 years, either LAIV or TIV may be used.
- Administer 2 doses (separated by at least 4 weeks) to children aged younger than 9 years who are receiving influenza vaccine for the first time or who were vaccinated for the first time during the previous influenza season but only received 1 dose.

5. Pneumococcal polysaccharide vaccine (PPSV).
- Administer to children with certain underlying medical conditions (see *MMWR* 1997;46[No. RR-8]), including a cochlear implant. A single revaccination should be administered to children with functional or anatomic asplenia or other immunocompromising condition after 5 years.

6. Hepatitis A vaccine (HepA).
- Administer 2 doses at least 6 months apart.
- HepA is recommended for children older than 1 year who live in areas where vaccination programs target older children or who are at increased risk of infection. See *MMWR* 2006;55(No. RR-7).

7. Hepatitis B vaccine (HepB).
- Administer the 3-dose series to those not previously vaccinated.
- A 2-dose series (separated by at least 4 months) of adult formulation Recombivax HB® is licensed for children aged 11 through 15 years.

8. Inactivated poliovirus vaccine (IPV).
- For children who received an all-IPV or all-oral poliovirus (OPV) series, a fourth dose is not necessary if the third dose was administered at age 4 years or older.
- If both OPV and IPV were administered as part of a series, a total of 4 doses should be administered, regardless of the child's current age.

9. Measles, mumps, and rubella vaccine (MMR).
- If not previously vaccinated, administer 2 doses or the second dose for those who have received only 1 dose, with at least 28 days between doses.

10. Varicella vaccine.
- For persons aged 7 through 18 years without evidence of immunity (see *MMWR* 2007;56[No. RR-4]), administer 2 doses if not previously vaccinated or the second dose if they have received only 1 dose.
- For persons aged 7 through 12 years, the minimum interval between doses is 3 months. However, if the second dose was administered at least 28 days after the first dose, it can be accepted as valid.
- For persons aged 13 years and older, the minimum interval between doses is 28 days.

The Recommended Immunization Schedules for Persons Aged 0 Through 18 Years are approved by the Advisory Committee on Immunization Practices (www.cdc.gov/vaccines/recs/acip), the American Academy of Pediatrics (http://www.aap.org), and the American Academy of Family Physicians (http://www.aafp.org).

DEPARTMENT OF HEALTH AND HUMAN SERVICES • CENTERS FOR DISEASE CONTROL AND PREVENTION

CS103164

○ **When is the MMR vaccine given?**

The first is given at 12–15 months of age and the second at 4–6 years. Children who have not yet received the second dose should not receive it after they are 11 or 12 years old.

○ **How common is vaccine-associated paralytic polio?**

1/2.4 million cases.

○ **Which polio vaccine can induce secondary transmission of vaccine virus?**

OPV.

○ **At what age do most children most commonly present with intestinal malrotation? Also, what are the common complications, signs, and symptoms?**

Malrotation usually occurs in children younger than 12 months. Volvulus is a common complication. Signs and symptoms include vomiting, blood-streaked stools, and abdominal pain.

○ **What are two unique clinical findings of tetralogy of Fallot?**

A boot-shaped heart on X-ray and exercise intolerance that is relieved by squatting. Treat shortness of breath by placing patient in the knee–chest position and administering morphine.

○ **What are the signs of left-sided heart failure in an infant?**

Increased respiratory rate, shortness of breath, and sweating during feeding.

○ **What is the most common cause of CHF in the second week of life?**

Coarctation of the aorta.

○ **What is the most common cause of pediatric bacteremia?**

Streptococcal pneumonia.

○ **What two viral illnesses are prodromes for Reye syndrome?**

Varicella (chicken pox) and influenzae B.

○ **What are the signs and symptoms of Reye syndrome?**

Irritability, combativeness, lethargy, right upper quadrant tenderness, history of influenzae B or recent chicken pox, papilledema, hypoglycemia, and seizures. Laboratory results reveal hypoglycemia, an ammonia level 20 times greater than normal, and a normal bilirubin level.

○ **Describe the five stages of Reye syndrome:**

Stage I: Vomiting, lethargy, and liver dysfunction

Stage II: Disorientation, combativeness, delirium, hyperventilation, increased deep tendon reflexes, liver dysfunction, hyperexcitable, tachypnea, fever, tachycardia, sweating, and pupillary dilatation

Stage III: Coma, decorticate rigidity, increased respiratory rate, and a mortality rate of 50%

Stage IV: Coma, decerebrate posturing, no ocular reflexes, loss of corneal reflexes, and liver damage

Stage V: Loss of deep tendon reflexes, seizures, flaccidity, respiratory arrest, and 95% mortality

○ **What are the first, second, and third drugs of choice for the treatment of seizures in children?**

Phenobarbital, phenytoin, and carbamazepine, respectively.

○ **What is the drug of choice for the treatment of a febrile seizure?**

Phenobarbital.

○ **Why is diazepam (Valium) avoided in neonatal seizures?**

It may cause hyperbilirubinemia by uncoupling the bilirubin–albumin complex.

○ **What is the most common cause of painless lower GI bleeding in an infant or child?**

Meckel diverticulum.

○ **A 16-month-old child presents with bilious vomiting, a distended abdomen, and blood in the stool. Diagnosis?**

Malrotation of the midgut.

○ **A child presents with periodic abdominal cramps, currant jelly stools, and a sausage-like tumor mass in the right lower quadrant. A contrast X-ray shows a coil spring sign. Diagnosis?**

Intussusception.

○ **A child presents with bluish discoloration of the gingiva. Probable diagnosis?**

Chronic lead poisoning. Expect the erythrocyte protoporphyrin level to be elevated with this condition.

○ **What is the current therapeutic regimen for treatment of meningitis in a neonate?**

Ampicillin and cefotaxime. A combination of these two antibiotics should be used in infants up to 2 months of age to cover coliform, group B streptococci, *Listeria,* and *Enterococcus.* In children aged 2 months to 6 years, cefotaxime alone is indicated.

○ **What is the most common cause of abdominal pain in children?**

Constipation.

○ **True/False: High fever in neonates with bacterial pneumonia usually follows a period of general fussiness and decreased feeding:**

True.

○ **Conjunctivitis is an associated finding in about what percentage of neonates with chlamydial pneumonia?**

About 50%.

○ **How many days after birth should newborns stop losing weight?**

About 6 days.

○ **True/False: A neonate stool color can be an important sign:**

False. Unless blood is evident, stool color is insignificant.

○ **What is the difference between vomiting and regurgitation?**

Very little once it's on you! Vomiting is caused by forceful diaphragmatic and abdominal muscle contraction. Regurgitation occurs without effort.

○ **Is regurgitation dangerous in an otherwise thriving neonate?**

No. However, it can be dangerous for newborns with failure to thrive or respiratory problems, and it may be associated with chronic aspiration.

○ **Projectile vomiting in the neonate is often associated with pyloric stenosis. When this is the case, such vomiting becomes a prominent sign at what age?**

2–3 weeks.

○ **Infectious diarrhea is usually viral. What are the two most common agents?**

Rotavirus and Norwalk agent.

○ **True/False: Bacterial and parasitic etiologies of diarrhea in the neonate are rare:**

True.

○ **What are some entities in the differential diagnosis of bloody diarrhea in the neonate?**

Necrotizing enterocolitis, bacterial enteritis, allergic reactions to milk, and iatrogenic causes secondary to antibiotics.

○ **What are some of the signs of sepsis to look for in babies with necrotizing enterocolitis?**

Poor feeding, lethargy, fever, jaundice, abdominal distention, and poor color.

○ **What should be considered in the case of a neonate who has never passed stool?**

Meconium ileus or plug, Hirschsprung disease, intestinal stenosis, or atresia.

○ **Anal stenosis, hypothyroidism, and Hirschsprung disease can all present with what clinical sign?**

Constipation, which was not present at birth but began before the infant was 1 month old.

○ **What is normal systolic blood pressure in a newborn?**

60 mm Hg.

○ **After the first month of life, what is the cause of meningitis and the number one cause of pneumonia in children?**

Meningitis: *H. influenzae.*

Pneumonia: *Streptococcus pneumoniae. H. influenzae* is the second most common cause.

○   **Discuss infantile spasms:**

Onset is by 3–9 months of age. It typically lasts seconds, and may occur in single episodes or bursts. The EEG is often abnormal. Almost 85% of these patients will be mentally handicapped.

○   **How much does the average teenager grow during adolescence?**

Teenagers generally increase their height by 15%–20% and double their weight.

○   **At what age do most people first have intercourse?**

Males: 16.1 years. Females: 16.9 years.

○   **By what age do most children stop wetting their beds?**

Age 4; 30% of 4 year olds and 10% of 6 year olds still wet their beds.

○   **What is the medical treatment for idiopathic enuresis?**

Desmopressin nose drops or imipramine. Most cases eventually resolve spontaneously.

○   **A 6-year-old boy consistently wets his pants. You tell his mother to reward the child with treats and praise during dry periods because this will help reinforce the desired behavior. What is this type of conditioning?**

Positive operant conditioning. The basic principles were defined by Pavlov:

Apert syndrome

Apnea (choanal stenosis)
Premature closure of cranial sutures (craniosynostosis)
Extremity (syndactyly, thumb anomalies)
Retarded
Tall forehead

Carpenter syndrome

Craniosynostosis
Acrocephaly
Retarded
Poly/syndactyly
Epicanthal folds
Narrow palate
Thorax (CHD)
Extremity anomaly
Renal/genital anomalies

Beckwith-Wiedemann syndrome

Weight >90% at birth

Insulin-like growth factor-2 involved

Ear creases or dysplasia

Defected umbilicus (omphalocele)

Enlarged liver

Macroglossia

Asymmetric extremities

Neonatal hypoglycemia

Neoplasm (Wilms tumor or hepatoblastoma)

Bloom syndrome

Breakage of chromosomes

Low birth weight

Overpigmented (café-au-lait spots)

Ocular/otic/odontic anomalies

Malignancy potential

Skin erythema of face

Cat-eye syndrome

Coloboma of iris

Anal atresia

TAPVR

Emotional retardation with mild MR

Yellow (jaundice) due to biliary atresia

Ear anomalies

Fetal alcohol syndrome

Microcephaly

Abnormal facies (short fissures, smooth philtrum)

Thorax (murmur, TOF, coarctation, ribs)

Extremity (joint laxity, palmar creases, clinodactyly)

Retarded growth

Neural-MR

ADHD

Learning disorder

Fetal rubella syndrome (German measles clinical features)

Mental retardation

Eyes (cataract)

Aortic coarctation or PDA

Skin rash (petechiae)

Liver (hepatitis)

Ears (deafness)

Small for gestational age

Fragile X syndrome

Fragile site

Retarded

Autistic/ADHD

Genital anomaly (macro-orchidism)

Increased mandible

Language problem

Ears (enlarged)

Fetal varicella syndrome (clinical features)

Hypoplastic limbs

Epidermal scars

Retarded (MR)

Prenatal growth deficiency (IUGR)

Eye (retinitis)

Seizure

Pyelonephritis (clinical features in newborn)

Poor feeding

Yellow (jaundice)

Emesis

Lethargy

Odorous urine

Trisomy 18

Extra chromosome 18

IQ low (MR)

Growth retardation (IUGR)

Hypertonia

Thorax (small chest/heart defects)

Eye/ear/extremities

Eating problem (always requires NGF)

Ninety percent die within first year

Turner syndrome

Thoracic aortic stenosis/coarctation

Underdeveloped gonads

Residual lymphedema

Neck webbing

Endocrine (GH and TSH deficiency)

Renal anomaly

Sexuality (delayed puberty)

● ● ● GERIATRICS ● ● ●

○ **Describe changes in vital signs in elderly patients.**

Blood pressure: Rise in systolic pressure due to arterial stiffening, and a widened pulse pressure. In some patients, orthostatic hypotension is seen.

Heart rate: Usually does not change elderly. Rhythms can change; most common is atrial arrhythmias (atrial fibrillation).

Respiratory rate: Usually remains unchanged.

Temperature: Patients more susceptible to hypothermia.

○ **What is the most common murmur heard in the elderly patient?**

Systolic aortic murmur.

○ **What percentage of elderly in the United States are older than 80 years?**

About 13%.

○ **Which gender and race has the highest life expectancy?**

White women.

○ **What are the two most prevalent diseases in the elderly older than age 60?**

Hypertension (60%–84%) and diabetes (18%–21%).

○ **What is the rate of cancer in patients older than age 65?**

There is a 10-fold increase.

○ **What are the 3 leading causes of death in the elderly?**

Heart disease (33%), cancer (22%), and cerebrovascular accident (8%).

○ **Name the 6 basic activities of daily living (ADLs).**

1. Dressing
2. Bathing
3. Feeding
4. Toileting
5. Transferring
6. Ambulating

○ **Name the 7 instrumental activities of daily living (IADLs).**

1. Money management
2. Medication administration
3. Using transportation
4. Using the telephone
5. Shopping
6. Housekeeping
7. Meal preparation

○ **At what age should all elderly start receiving an annual influenza vaccine?**

65 years of age.

○   **What percentage of the elderly are ambulatory?**

90%.

○   **What percentage of the elderly live in nursing homes?**

5%.

○   **What is the percentage of elderly older than 65 years who fall and older than 80 years who fall?**

About 30% of those older than 65 years fall, and it is 50% when older than 80 years.

○   **Which sex is more likely to have urinary incontinence in the elderly years?**

Women. However, as the age goes above 80 years, the percentage is equal.

○   **What is the most common form of incontinence in the elderly?**

Urge incontinence. It is more common in women and is due to detrusor hyperreflexia or decreased sensory capabilities.

○   **What drugs are used to treat stress incontinence?**

α-Adrenergic agonists and estrogen.

○   **Strokes, Parkinson disease, and Alzheimer disease are most commonly associated with which type of incontinence?**

Urge incontinence.

○   **What are some reversible conditions that you should consider that are related to urinary incontinence?**

Remember the mnemonic **DRIIIPP**:

Delirium
Restricted mobility—illness, injury, gait
Infection
Inflammation—atrophic vaginitis
Impaction
Polyuria
Pharmaceuticals (diuretics, anticholinergics, α-antagonists)

○   **What is the rate of mortality in an elderly patient with a pressure ulcer (bedsore)?**

The mortality increases fourfold.

○   **What percentage of women over the age of 80 has osteoporosis?**

70%.

○   **What percentage of prostate cancer deaths occur over the age of 65?**

92%.

○ **What may result from the administration of an aminoglycoside or cephalosporin to an elderly patient who is dehydrated?**

Acute renal failure secondary to tubulointerstitial injury. This may also occur if the above-mentioned drugs are given to an elderly patient on furosemide or with preexisting renal disease.

○ **What is the most common cause of hearing loss in the elderly?**

Presbycusis. Other causes include neoplasms, noise exposure, ototoxic drugs, and otosclerosis.

○ **Presbycusis is a hearing loss at which end of the audible range?**

The high end (4000–8000 Hz).

○ **Is the incidence of epidural and subdural hematomas higher or lower in elderly patients?**

Epidural hematomas are less common and subdural hematomas are more common.

○ **What geriatric population is at greatest risk for esophageal cancer?**

Elderly African Americans have a risk four times that of elderly Caucasian Americans. Other populations at risk include Chinese, Iranians, and South Africans.

○ **Who has a higher rupture rate in appendicitis, the very young or the very old?**

The very old. The rupture rate for geriatric patients is 65%–90% with an associated mortality of 15%. The pediatric population has a rupture rate of 15%–50% and an associated mortality rate of 3%.

○ **What is sundown syndrome?**

Hallucinations and delusions that occur at nighttime because of decreased sensory stimulation.

○ **What is the most common cause of large bowel obstruction in the elderly?**

Fecal impaction. Other causes are stenosing diverticula, neoplasms, and volvulus colon. Adhesions are rarely a cause of obstruction in the large bowel.

○ **The most common causes of dysphagia in the elderly population include:**

Hiatal hernia, reflux esophagitis, webs/rings, and cancer.

○ **An elderly patient with chronic COPD is most likely to contract what kind of pneumonia?**

H. influenzae pneumonia. Ampicillin is the drug of choice. This population is at risk and should be vaccinated.

○ **Giant cell arteritis is a chronic inflammation of the large blood vessels. What arteries are most commonly involved?**

The carotid and the cranial arteries. Blindness may result in 20% of afflicted patients. Treat with high dose corticosteroids. Those with a visual component must have an immediate ophthalmologic evaluation.

○ **What are the common neurologic signs and symptoms of giant cell arteritis?**

Amaurosis fugax, deafness, depression, and paralysis. Amaurosis fugax is the most dangerous because it can lead to permanent monocular or binocular blindness.

○ **What is the Trendelenburg test for varicose veins?**

Raise the leg above the heart, and then quickly lower it. If the leg veins become distended immediately after this test, there is valvular incompetency.

○ **What is the most common cause of cataract development?**

Old age. Cataracts occur congenitally, from medication or from trauma. Slit lamp examination may show absent red reflex and a gray clouding of the lens.

○ **What is the most common cause of blindness in the elderly?**

Senile macular degeneration. Such patients experience a gradual loss of central vision. The macula appears hemorrhagic or pigmented. This is due to atrophic degeneration of the retinal vessels that results in leaking vessels, fibrosis, and scarring of the retina.

○ **What is the most common nontraumatic cause of dementia?**

Alzheimer disease. At 65 years of age, 10% of the population has Alzheimer; by 85 years, 50% does. Multiinfarct dementia is the second most common cause of nontraumatic dementia.

○ **What is the first symptom of Alzheimer disease?**

Progressive memory loss. This is followed by disorientation, personality changes, language difficulty, and other symptoms of dementia.

○ **What is the prognosis for patients with Alzheimer disease?**

Alzheimer is an irreversible disease. Death occurs 5–10 years after presumptive diagnosis.

○ **Differentiate between dementia and delirium:**

Dementia: Irreversible, impaired functioning secondary to changes and deficits in memory, spatial concepts, personality, cognition, language, motor and sensory skills, judgment, or behavior. There is no change in consciousness.

Delirium: A reversible, organic mental syndrome reflecting deficits in attention, organized thinking, orientation, speech, memory, and perception. Patients are frequently confused, anxious, excited, and have hallucinations. A change in consciousness may be evident.

○ **How frequently should a patient at high risk for pressure ulcers be repositioned?**

Every 2 hours.

○ **What is the most common complication of a pressure ulcer?**

Sepsis.

○ **What is the most common presenting symptom in Parkinson disease:**

Tremor. The brain lesion is located in the substantia nigra.

○ **List, by order of initiation, drugs used for the treatment of Parkinson disease?**

Start with amantadine (Symmetrel) and trihexyphenidyl (Artane); if this fails, use a combination of levodopa and carbidopa. Pergolide and bromocriptine can be used to treat episodes of immobility.

○   **What is the drug of choice for treating depression in the elderly?**

Nortriptyline.

○   **A 65-year-old African American has hypertension and gout. What medications should be prescribed?**

Although diuretics are the most effective drugs for the treatment of hypertension in this race, the patient has gout, which will be exacerbated by the use of diuretics. ACE inhibitors or calcium channel blockers are better choices for this patient.

○   **What is the mortality rate for geriatric patients who have sustained a hip fracture?**

25% will die in the first year following the fracture.

○   **What is the most common cause of community-acquired pneumonia in the elderly?**

Streptococcus pneumoniae.

○   **How do you clinically differentiate between polymyalgia rheumatica and polymyositis?**

In polymyositis, there is proximal muscle pain, weakness, and tenderness, and elevated muscle enzymes. In contrast, polymyalgia rheumatica presents with an elevated sedimentation rate (also seen in giant cell arteritis, which is associated with polymyalgia rheumatica).

○   **What are the two pathologic findings used to confirm the diagnosis of Alzheimer disease?**

The quantity of neurofibrillary tangles and senile plaques. Other findings include neuronal loss and amyloid degeneration.

○   **What is the most common cause of UTIs in uncatheterized elderly patients?**

E. coli.

○   **What is the most common cause of relapsing UTIs in elderly patients?**

Chronic bacterial prostatitis, caused by *E. coli, Proteus, Klebsiella pneumoniae,* and enterococci.

○   **In the elderly, what is a common side effect of verapamil?**

Constipation.

○   **What is the most common pathophysiologic cause of delirium?**

Acetylcholine deficiency.

○   **Parkinson-like side effects are common with which class of drugs?**

Neuroleptics. Parkinson-like side effects can develop with perphenazine, chlorpromazine, reserpine, haloperidol, metoclopramide, and the illicit meperidine analog MPTP.

○   **In the elderly, what is the most common cause of death resulting from community-acquired infections? Institutional? Nosocomial?**

In the community and institutions, it is bacterial pneumonia; in hospitals, it is UTIs.

○ **What is the most common cause of drug-induced hallucinations in the geriatric population?**

Propranolol.

○ **Why is it unsafe to place a geriatric patient on digoxin and Lasix?**

Hypokalemia and digoxin toxicity may result. If this is the best choice for management, careful monitoring of both electrolytes and digoxin levels will be needed.

○ **What percentage of patients with primary Alzheimer disease will present with secondary depression?**

30%–35%.

○ **What is the most common cause of abdominal pain in the elderly?**

Constipation.

○ **What is the most common risk factor for Alzheimer disease?**

A family history of dementia.

○ **An elderly female presents with high blood pressure and a history of CHF. What is the antihypertensive drug of choice?**

ACE inhibitors. They will reduce both preload and afterload.

○ **Patients with which type of apolipoprotein are more likely to acquire Alzheimer disease?**

Type 4, apolipoprotein E.

○ **An elderly man presents with high blood pressure and a history of NIDDM. What is the antihypertensive drug of choice?**

ACE inhibitors. They have renal protective properties.

○ **What is the major risk of tricyclic antidepressants in the elderly?**

Orthostatic hypotension because this can lead to falls.

○ **An elderly African American man presents with high blood pressure and a history of angina. What is the antihypertensive drug of choice?**

Calcium channel blockers.

○ **What are the most common sources of sepsis in the elderly?**

Respiratory > urinary > intra-abdominal.

○ **Describe the common findings of benign essential tremors:**

Tremulousness of speech and nodding of head. This is an action tremor that is usually familial and is often treated with atenolol, propranolol, diazepam, and alcohol.

○ **What laboratory values increase with age?**

BUN/Cr, sedimentation rate, thyroxine (T4), and calcium (in women).

○ **What laboratory values decrease with age?**

Leukocyte count and creatinine phosphokinase.

○ **What is the incidence of morbidity and mortality in patients older than 60 years who present with syncope?**

1 in 5 will suffer significant morbidity or mortality within 6 months.

○ **What percentage of septic elderly patients do not present with a fever?**

25%.

○ **What drugs are most commonly associated with ADRS in the elderly?**

Analgesics, cardiovascular, and psychotropic drugs.

○ **What are the common adverse drug interactions of cimetidine in the elderly?**

Cimetidine inhibits the metabolism of phenytoin, Coumadin, and theophylline.

○ **What are the common adverse drug interactions of Coumadin?**

Metabolism is inhibited by allopurinol, trimethoprim-sulfamethoxazole, metronidazole, and quinolones.

○ **What is the most common cause of <u>acute</u> abdominal pain in the elderly?**

Acute cholecystitis. Approximately 50% of patients older than 65 years have gallstones.

○ **Describe the clinical features of appendicitis in the elderly:**

Anorexia and vomiting are less common, and migration of the pain to the RLQ is absent in up to 60% of elderly patients. The elderly account for 50% of the deaths as a result of appendicitis. Half of elderly patients with appendicitis have normal white counts upon presentation.

● ● ● REFERENCES ● ● ●

Crawford MH. *Current Medical Diagnosis and Treatment—Cardiology.* 3rd ed. New York, NY: McGraw-Hill; 2009.

Fauci AS, Braunwald E, Kasper DL, et al., eds. *Harrison's Principles of Internal Medicine,* 17th ed. New York: McGraw-Hill; 2008. http://www.accessmedicine.com

Hay WW Jr, Levin M, Sondheimer JM, Deterding R. *Current Medical Diagnosis and Treatment—Pediatrics.* 13th ed. New York, NY: McGraw-Hill; 2009.

McPhee SJ, Papadakis MA, eds. *Current Medical Diagnosis and Treatment 2009.* New York, NY: McGraw-Hill; 2009.

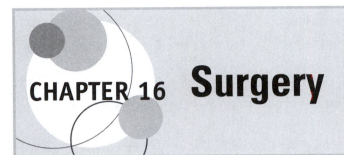

CHAPTER 16 Surgery

Jeffrey G. Yates, MPA, PA-C

○ **How many days should sutures remain in the following areas: face, scalp, trunk, hands, back, and extremities?**

Face: 3–5 days

Scalp: 5–7 days

Trunk: 7–10 days

Hands, back, and extremities: 10 days and 14 days if over a joint

○ **What is the onset of effect, duration, and maximum dose of the two most commonly used local anesthetics (LAs)?**

Lidocaine: 2–5 minute onset of effects with a 1–2 hour duration. The maximum dose of 4.5 and 7 mg/kg if epinephrine is added.

Bupivacaine: 3–7 minute onset of effects with a duration of 90 minutes to 6 hours. The maximum dose is 2 and 3 mg/kg if epinephrine is added.

○ **What are the lines of Langerhans?**

Lines of tension in the skin that incisions should follow when possible for the best cosmetic results. In the forehead, these lines run horizontally, while in the lower face they run vertically.

○ **Why is epinephrine added to local anesthesia?**

To increase the duration of the anesthesia and provide hemostasis. Epinephrine causes vasoconstriction and therefore decreases bleeding and slows the systemic absorption of lidocaine.

○ **Which is more painful to the patient, plain lidocaine or lidocaine with epinephrine?**

Lidocaine with epinephrine, because it has a very low pH. To avoid this pain, buffer the solution with sodium bicarbonate by adding 1 mL of sodium bicarbonate to 9 mL of lidocaine +/− epinephrine. The injection should be administered very slowly and subdermally.

○ **In what areas should you avoid the infiltrative administration of lidocaine with epinephrine?**

Lidocaine with epinephrine should not be used on fingers, toes, ears, nose, or the penis because the limited vascularity in these regions might be compromised.

○ **Where is a local anesthetic injected for an ulnar nerve block?**

On the anterior wrist, in the proximal volar skin crease, between the ulnar artery and the flexor carpi ulnaris.

○ **Where is a local anesthetic injected for a median nerve block?**

On the anterior wrist in the proximal volar skin crease, between the tendon of the palmaris longus and the flexor carpi radialis.

○ **What are the primary advantages of performing a digital nerve block?**

Less anesthetic agent is required, better anesthetic effects are obtained, and the tissues do not become distorted.

○ **What nerve block is used to anesthetize of the sole of the foot?**

Tibial nerve block. Tibial nerve block does not provide anesthesia to the lateral aspect of the heel and foot.

○ **What is the preferred route for anesthesia for deep lacerations of the anterior tongue?**

Lingual nerve block.

○ **How should hair be removed prior to wound repair?**

Clip the hair around the wound. A razor preparation can increase the infection rate.

○ **What three elements are common to a surgical infection?**

An infectious agent, a susceptible host, and a closed, poorly perfused space.

○ **Define the term closure by primary intention:**

Primary intention occurs when tissue is cleanly incised and reapproximated and repair occurs without complication. Primary healing is simpler and requires less time and material than secondary healing.

○ **What is meant when a wound is closed by secondary intention?**

Secondary intention occurs in open wounds through formation of granulation tissue and eventual coverage of the defect by spontaneous migration of epithelial cells. Most infected wounds and burns heal in this manner.

○ **What is delayed primary closure?**

When a wound is allowed to heal open under a carefully maintained, occlusive dressing for about 5 days and is then closed as if primarily. Such wounds are less likely to become infected than if closed immediately because their oxygen needs are better met.

○ **What components create the perfect host for a surgical wound infection?**

Areas with or surrounded by poorly vascularized tissue and that have a natural space. The common denominators are poor perfusion, local hypoxia, hypercapnia, and acidosis. Some natural spaces with narrow outlets, such as those of the appendix, gallbladder, ureters, and intestines, are especially prone to becoming obstructed and then infected. The peritoneal and pleural cavities are potential spaces, and their surfaces slide over one another, thereby dispersing contaminating bacteria.

○ **How long can a "clean" wound closure be delayed before proliferation of infection-causing bacteria develops?**

6 hours, though the high vascularity of the face and scalp can allow for longer delays in these areas.

○ **What factors increase the likelihood of wound infection?**

Dirty, contaminated wounds or wounds with retained foreign bodies. Stellate or crushing wounds, wounds longer than 5 cm, wounds older than 6 hours, and wounds in infection prone anatomic sites are at increased risk.

○ **A patient presents to your office after stepping on a nail that went right through the shoe and punctured the plantar aspect of the foot. What gram-negative organism would be most commonly involved in this type of injury?**

Pseudomonas aeruginosa.

○ **Which has greater resistance to infection, sutures or staples?**

There are no significant differences in the healing of wounds closed by suture or staples; however, staples do not provide a conduit for infective organisms thereby making them more resistant to infections.

○ **Which factors determine the ultimate appearance of a scar?**

The wounds alignment, either parallel or perpendicular, to the skins tension lines. Static and dynamic tension on surrounding skin. Static tension refers to the width of the wound at rest. Dynamic tension is determined by determining the width of the wound during range of motion of the involved body part.

○ **Can tetanus develop after surgical procedures?**

Yes. Although most cases of tetanus in the United States develop after minor trauma, there have also been reports of tetanus following general surgical procedures, especially those involving the abdomen and pelvis.

○ **What are the indications and contraindications to tetanus prophylaxis?**

Consideration for prophylaxis should be made on every patient presenting with a wound, however slight. Patients with clean, minor, wounds should be considered for prophylaxis if their previous dose was taken more than 10 years ago. Prophylaxis should be considered for all other wounds if their previous dose was taken more than 5 years ago. The only contraindication to tetanus prophylaxis is a history of severe systemic reaction after a previous dose.

○ **How long should a repaired laceration need be kept out of the sun?**

Patients should be instructed to keep the repaired area out of the sun during the time of healing, about 2–3 months, and also to cover the area with sunblock for the following 6–12 months. Sun exposure may case hyperpigmentation to the wound area.

○ **What organisms are most common in wound infections?**

Staphylococcus, primarily *S. aureus.*

○   **What is the most likely cause of a postoperative fever which occurs (1) the day after the operation (POD 1), (2) 3 days postoperative (POD 3), (3) 5 days postoperative (POD 5), (4) 7 days postoperative (POD 7), and (5) 2–3 weeks postoperative?**

　1. **W**IND: Atelectasis

　2. **W**ATER: Urinary tract infection (UTI)

　3. **W**ALK: Deep vein thrombosis (DVT)

　4. **W**OUND: Postoperative infection

　5. **W**ONDER DRUGS: Hypersensitivity reaction most common caused by antibiotics

Mnemonic: Wind, Water, Walk, Wound, and Wonder drugs

○   **What gas is used to create a pneumoperitoneum during a laparoscopy? Why is this gas used? What are the associated risks?**

Carbon dioxide (CO_2). CO_2 is noncombustible and has a high rate of diffusion, which results in a low risk of gas embolism. The use of CO_2 can also result in tachycardia, increased central venous pressure, hypertension, decreased cardiac output, and occasionally, transient arrhythmias due to its rapid rate of absorption into the systemic circulation, which increases PCO_2 and decreases pH. Alternative, and significantly less popular, gases include helium and argon.

○   **A 32-year-old female patient is under general anesthesia for a cholecystectomy. Part way into the operation her body tenses up, she develops tachycardia and a fever of 101.8°F. What anesthetic-related complication is she experiencing and what is the recommended treatment?**

This patient is suffering from malignant hyperthermia, a muscular response to general anesthetics that causes the release of calcium. A patient's susceptibility to malignant hyperthermia may be established with the caffeine-halothane contracture test. Dantrolene may be used prophylactically or in the acute treatment of patient's experiencing this complication. Its effects will inhibit the release of calcium while aiding in the prevention of acute renal failure.

○   **What is the maintenance IV fluid rate for a child weighing 30 kg?**

The 100/50/20 rule would apply in this patient:

100 mL/kg/day for the first 10 kg + 50 mL/kg/day for the next 10 kg + 20 mL/kg/day for the next 10 kg. This child should receive 1700 mL/day at an IV flow rate of 71mL/h.

○   **What is the appropriate bolus for a dehydrated child weighing 15 kg?**

The recommended IVFB for a child is calculated at 20 mL/kg.

20 mL × 15 kg = 300 mL

○   **What is the composition of sodium in normal saline and lactated ringers IV solutions?**

Normal saline (0.9% sodium chloride) 154 mEq/L
Lactated ringers 130 mEq/L

○   **What solutes determine serum osmolality?**

Sodium, chloride, bicarbonate, proteins, and glucose. To a much lesser extent magnesium, calcium, and potassium are also present.

○ **What are the laboratory criteria for intubating patients and placing them on mechanical ventilation?**

Room air $Pao_2 < 60$ mm Hg or $Paco_2 > 45$ mm Hg

Basing your decision to intubate on laboratory criteria alone is a critical error. The clinical indications of a respiratory rate > 36 breaths/min, labored respiratory efforts, the use of accessory muscles, and tachycardia are much more significant. The patient's clinical status provides the primary indication for intubation.

○ **What negative pressure must be generated by an intubated patient for weaning to be successful?**

At least 20–30 cm of H_2O. Other important factors include Pao_2, arterial saturation, pH, spontaneous respiratory rate, minute volume, tidal volume, and PEEP.

○ **What is the Whipple procedure?**

Pancreaticoduodenectomy. The procedure involves resection of the distal stomach, pylorus, duodenum, proximal pancreas, and the gallbladder, plus a truncal vagotomy. The jejunum is then anastomosed to the stomach, biliary, and pancreatic ducts. This procedure is used for treating pancreatic, duodenal, ampulla of Vater, and common bile duct cancers.

○ **What are the Billroth I and II procedures?**

Billroth I anastomosis is a gastroduodenostomy, and Billroth II is a gastrojejunostomy.

○ **What is the Roux-en-Y operative procedure?**

An end-to-side anastomosis between the distal segment of small bowel and the stomach or esophagus. This forms a Y shape. This procedure is used in gastric bypass surgery for obesity and to treat reflux of bile and pancreatic secretions into the stomach secondary to ductal tumors, injury, obstruction, or infection.

○ **Match the type of transplant to the most appropriate definition:**

1. **Autograft**
2. **Heterotrophic**
3. **Isograft**
4. **Orthotopic**
5. **Allograft**
6. **Xenograft**

a. **Donor and recipient are genetically the same**
b. **Donor and recipient are the same person**
c. **Donor and recipient are of the same species**
d. **Donor and recipient belong to different species**
e. **Transplantation to a normal anatomical position**
f. **Transplantation to a different anatomical position**

Answers: (1) b, (2) f, (3) a, (4) e, (5) c, and (6) d.

○ **What fungal infection is most common in transplant patients?**

Candida albicans.

○ **Differentiate between visceral and parietal pain:**

Visceral pain: Diffuse and poorly localized pain caused by the stretching of a hollow viscus. It is frequently associated with autonomic nervous system responses.

Parietal pain: Sharp and localized pain due to irritation or inflammation of a parietal surface and associated with guarding, rebound, and a rigid abdomen.

○ **What is the most common cause of bleeding in postoperative patients?**

Failure to achieve operative local hemostasis.

○ **A fire victim suffers from partial and full thickness burns over the complete surface of both legs, his entire back, and his entire right arm. What percentage of his body is burned?**

Follow the "rule of 9s".

Anterior/posterior legs = 18% × 2 36%

Entire back = 18%

Entire right arm = 9%

TBSA 63%

○ **A patient who has been burned over the entire top of his body (arms and torso, front and back) develops severe difficulty breathing and appears to be going into respiratory arrest. What should be done?**

An emergent escharotomy. The patient is most likely suffering ventilatory restriction due to the circumferential eschar about his chest resulting in constriction of the chest cavity. Anesthesia is rarely required when performing an escharotomies and frequently are performed at the bedside because of their emergent nature.

○ **What is the caloric requirement of a 100-kg firefighter who was burned over 20% of his body?**

3300 kcal. (25 kcal/kg of body weight + 40 kcal/1% burned surface.)

○ **What is the 24-hour fluid resuscitation requirement for the above patient?**

4 L in the first 8 hours (500 mL/h) and 4 L in the next 16 hours (250 mL/h). The Parkland formula gives the requirement as 4 mL per kg body weight X% burned (4 mL X of 100 kg X 20-8L). Give half the volume in the first 8 hours and the other half in the next 16 hours.

○ **What does an increase in pulmonary arterial wedge pressure indicate?**

Fluid overload. Normal pulmonary wedge pressure is 4–12 mm Hg. Higher levels can indicate left ventricular failure, constrictive pericarditis, or mitral regurgitation with stenosis.

○ **What are the two most commonly injured genitourinary organs?**

Kidneys and bladder.

○ **What should be checked prior to inserting a chest tube in an intubated patient with respiratory distress and decreased breath sounds on one side?**

Position of the ET tube.

○ **A patient presents with fever and shoulder pain 4 days following a splenectomy. What is the most probable postoperative complication?**

Subphrenic abscess. This condition can cause fever as well as irritation to the diaphragm and to the branch of the phrenic nerve that innervates it.

○ **What organisms are most commonly responsible for overwhelming postsplenectomy sepsis?**

Encapsulated organisms: pneumococcal (50%), meningococcal (12%), *E. coli* (11%), *H. influenza* (8%), staphylococcal (8%), and streptococcal (7%).

○ **What is a sentinel loop?**

A distended or dilated loop of bowel detected by X-ray that lies near a localized inflammatory process.

○ **What is a delphian node?**

A palpable node on the trachea, which is just above the thyroid isthmus. This is indicative of thyroid disease (malignancy or thyroiditis).

○ **Which types of nodules are more likely to be malignant on a thyroid scan, hot or cold?**

Cold. These cells most commonly do not produce thyroid hormones and do not absorb iodine. This procedure should not be considered confirmatory and fine-needle aspiration (biopsy) is strongly suggested to obtain a diagnosis.

○ **What test should be performed to distinguish a benign cystic nodule from a malignant nodule?**

Fine-needle aspiration with biopsy and cytological evaluation.

○ **Name the function and spinal innervation level of the biceps, triceps, flexor digitorum, interossei, quadriceps, extensor hallucis, biceps femoris, soleus and gastrocnemius, and rectal sphincter:**

Muscle	Action	Spinal level
Biceps	Forearm flexion	C5–C6
Triceps	Forearm extensors	C7
Flexor digitorum	Finger flexion	C8
Interossei	Finger adduction/abduction	T1
Quadriceps	Knee extension	L3–L4
Extensor hallucis	Great toe dorsiflexion	L5
Biceps femoris	Knee flexion	S1
Soleus & gastrocnemius	Foot plantar flexion	S1–S2
Rectal sphincter	Sphincter tone	S2–S4

○ **What dose of methylprednisolone should be used to treat acute spinal cord injury?**

30 mg/kg load over 15 minutes in the first hour, followed 45 minutes later by 5.4 mg/kg per hour over the next 23–47 hours.

○ **What is the sensory innervation to the nipple, umbilicus, and perianal region?**

Nipple: T4
Umbilicus: T10
Perianal: S2–S4

○ **What is the most common etiology of a solitary thyroid nodule?**

A nodular goiter (50%). Other possibilities to consider include cancer (20%), adenoma (20%), cyst (5%), or thyroiditis (5%).

○ **Which nerve must be located and then avoided when performing a thyroidectomy?**

The recurrent laryngeal nerves, which are located immediately posterior to the gland.

○ **What is the most common type of thyroid carcinoma?**

Papillary carcinoma accounts for about 75% of thyroid carcinomas and statistically present with an excellent prognosis.

○ **A 15-year-old female adolescent comes to your office complaining of a mass in the midline of her neck near the hyoid bone. It is tender and raises when she swallows or if she sticks her tongue out. What is your diagnosis?**

An infected thyroglossal duct cyst. This is a remnant from the embryological descent of the thyroid in the neck. Treatment includes antibiotics, drainage, then excision once the inflammation subsides if necessary.

○ **What is the most common benign salivary gland tumor?**

Pleomorphic adenomas make up about 85% of these tumors.

○ **What is the most common type of malignant parotid gland tumor?**

Mucoepidermoid carcinoma is the most common malignant tumor of the parotid gland, accounting for 30% of parotid malignancies

○ **What type of contrast medium should be used to evaluate the esophagus if a perforation is suspected?**

Gastrografin (diatrizoate meglumine). This is an iodinated, water-soluble media that is not harmful in the presence of a mucosal tear.

○ **What are the most significant risk factors for esophageal cancer?**

Age 65 or older, being male, smoking, heavy drinking of alcohol, diets low in the intake of fruits and vegetables, obesity, and acid reflux disease

○ **Cancer occurs more frequently in which third of the esophagus?**

Adenocarcinoma of the distal esophagus is the most common form of esophageal cancer in the United States.

○ **Which other forms of cancer cell types may occur in esophagus?**

Squamous cell carcinoma most frequently occurs in the proximal region of the esophagus and is less common in the United States but is the most common worldwide

○ **Which types of cancer metastasize to bone?**

Prostate, thyroid, breast, lung, and kidney. (Remember the mnemonic: "P.T. Barnum Loves Kids.")

○ **What is Hamman sign?**

This is associated with a tracheobronchial injury resulting in a pneumomediastinum or pneumopericardium. The sound is heard best over the left lateral position and has been described as a series of precordial crackles that correlate with the cardiac contraction and not respiration.

○ **What is the most common site of rupture in Boerhaave syndrome?**

The left posterolateral wall of the lower third of the esophagus, 2–3 cm proximal to the gastroesophageal junction.

○ **What is the most common acute surgical condition of the abdomen?**

Acute appendicitis.

○ **What is the most common cause of appendicitis?**

Fecaliths. Fecaliths are found in 40% of uncomplicated appendicitis cases, 65% of cases involving gangrenous appendices that have not ruptured, and 90% of cases involving ruptured appendices

○ **How does retrocecal appendicitis most commonly present?**

Dysuria, hematuria, and urinary frequency (due to the proximity of the appendix to the right ureter). Poorly localized abdominal pain, anorexia, nausea, vomiting, diarrhea, mild fever, and peritonitis are also common signs.

○ **Differentiate between McBurney point, Rovsing sign, the obturator sign, and the psoas sign:**

McBurney point: Point of maximal tenderness in a patient with appendicitis. The location is two-thirds the way between the umbilicus and the iliac crest on the right side of the abdomen.
Rovsing sign: Palpation of LLQ causes pain in the RLQ.
Obturator sign: Internal rotation of a flexed hip causes pain.
Psoas sign: These signs are all indicative of an inflamed appendix. Extension of the right thigh causes pain.

○ **What kind of wound closure should be used in a patient with a perforated appendix?**

Delayed primary closure with direct drainage of the infection. Wound infection occurs in 20% of patients with perforated appendices.

○ **A 27-year-old man who smokes heavily complains of tingling in his fingers. On examination he has cyanotic digits with ulcers forming. What is the diagnosis?**

Thromboangiitis obliterans or Buerger disease. This is a disease that affects young smokers (males 20–40 years of age). Inflammatory changes (vasculitis) in the small- to medium-sized vessels cause constriction or occlusions.

○ **Where is the most common site of intracranial aneurysms?**

The circle of Willis (most common in the anterior communicating artery.

○ **What are the clinical signs of CSF leakage?**

A headache that improves when supine and worsens when sitting up, otorrhea, and rhinorrhea.

○ **What is the most common type of brain tumor in adults?**

Glioblastoma multiforme (40%). This is additionally the most aggressive (malignant) type of primary brain tumor in adults.

○ **What is the most common primary central nervous system tumor that arises in childhood.**

Medulloblastoma.

○ **What are the most common microorganisms found in brain abscesses?**

Direct extension—Sinus, odontogenic, and otogenic sources: *Streptococcus* species (aerobic and anaerobic), *Bacteroides, Enterobacteriaceae*, and *Pseudomonas*.

Hematogenous spread (Pathogens depend on predisposing source)

Endocarditis—*Streptococcus viridans* and *Staphylococcus aureus*

Pulmonary infections—*Streptococcus, Fusobacterium, Corynebacterium,* and *Peptococcus* species

Cardiac defects with right-to-left shunt—*Streptococcus* species

Intra-abdominal infections—*Klebsiella* species, *E. coli,* other Enterobacteriaceae, *Streptococcus* species, and anaerobes

Urinary tract infections—Enterobacteriaceae and *Pseudomonas* species

Wound infection—*S. aureus*

Penetrating head trauma

S. aureus is most commonly isolated.

Enterobacteriaceae, other gram-negative bacilli, *S. epidermidis, Clostridium* species, anaerobes, and *Pseudomonas* species may also be found.

Opportunistic infection (organ transplant, HIV, and immunodeficiencies). Common organisms include *Toxoplasma gondii* and *Nocardia, Aspergillus,* and *Candida* species.

○ **How many minutes of cerebral anoxia will result in irreversible brain injury?**

Greater than 4–6 minutes.

○ **Match the following terms with their definitions:**

1. Neurapraxia   a. Damage to the axon, no damage to the sheath
2. Axonotmesis   b. Temporary loss of function, no damage to axon
3. Neurotmesis   c. Damage to axon and sheath

Answers: (1) b, (2) a, and (3) c.

○ **You detect hard mass in the upper outer quadrant of the right breast of a 45-year-old woman. What are the next steps?**

Mammogram followed by a biopsy. The options for biopsy are as follows:

Fine-needle aspiration with cytology—Easily performed, inexpensive, false negative rate ∼10%

Large-needle (core) biopsy—Cost-effective, office-based procedure with false negative rates secondary to sampling errors

Open biopsy—Reliable means of diagnosis when previous attempts are nondiagnostic; performed with local anesthetic through an open incision

○ **What is the most common histologic type of breast cancer?**

Infiltrating ductal carcinoma (80%–90%) with subtypes: medullary, colloid, papillary, and tubular.

○ **A 30-year-old woman comes to you worried that she has breast cancer in both breasts. She is concerned because she experiences soreness in the upper outer quadrants of her breasts and what she describes as "lumpy" feeling upon self-examination with a mild swelling that seems to come and go. Further questioning reveals that her pain begins 1 week before she menstruates then disappears when her menses is over. What do you tell her?**

She most likely has fibrocystic breast changes but these are frequently clinically indistinguishable from carcinoma. First, provide her reassurance and let her know that fibrocystic changes are not a premalignant syndrome. Secondly, schedule her for a mammogram with plans to perform fine-needle aspiration of suspicious lesions.

○ **Which is the most common type of noncystic breast tumor?**

Fibroadenomas. These are most common in women younger than 25 years and presents as round, rubbery, mobile, nontender masses of 1–5 cm in diameter.

○ **What does a high cathepsin D level indicate in a woman with breast cancer?**

These levels serve as an independent prognostic indicator and have been shown to be related to an increased risk of metastasis.

○ **What is the most aggressive form of lung cancer and most likely to be involved in metastasis?**

Small-cell lung cancer comprises about 15%–20% of lung cancers and is the most aggressive form of the disease. It frequently metastasizes to the liver, bone, and brain.

○ **What is Westermark sign?**

Decreased vascular markings on chest X-ray, indicative of pulmonary embolism.

○ **What do muffled heart tones, hypotension, and distended neck veins indicate?**

This is Beck triad and is classic for pericardial tamponade.

○ **What is the most common kidney tumor in a child's first year of life?**

Wilms tumor (nephroblastoma).

○ **What is the average age for pediatric patients to develop Wilms tumor?**

Peak occurrence is at 3 years and it is rare after 8 years of age. Children with a localized tumor have a 90% cure rate when treated with surgery and chemotherapy; or with surgery, radiation, and chemotherapy combined.

○ **One to two percent of patients with Wilms tumor will develop secondary malignancies. Which types are most common?**

Hepatocellular carcinoma, leukemia, lymphoma, and soft tissue sarcoma.

○ **What are Grey-Turner and Cullen signs?**

Cullen sign: Periumbilical ecchymosis indicative of intraperitoneal hemorrhage, first recognized in patients experiencing a ruptured ectopic hemorrhage.

Grey Turner sign: Flank ecchymosis that develops in 24–48 hours, and is indicative retroperitoneal or intraabdominal hemorrhage. This is most commonly associated with severe acute pancreatitis, abdominal aortic aneurysm, abdominal trauma, and ruptured ectopic pregnancies.

○ **Serum amylase is frequently elevated in acute pancreatitis. What other conditions can cause a similar rise in amylase?**

Bowel infarction, cholecystitis, mumps, perforated ulcer, and renal failure. Lipase is more specific to pancreatic etiologies.

○ **What are the most common causes of pancreatitis?**

Alcoholism (40%) and gallstone disease (40%). Additional causes pancreatitis are due to hypercalcemia, hyperlipidemia, iatrogenic pancreatitis, and protein deficiency.

○ **Name some abdominal X-ray findings associated with acute pancreatitis:**

Approximately two-thirds of patients will have an abnormal abdominal radiograph. The most common finding is the presence of a sentinel loop (either of the jejunum, transverse colon, or duodenum). Additionally a colon cutoff sign, an abrupt cessation of gas in the mid or left transverse colon due colonic spasm secondary to inflammation of the adjacent pancreas.

○ **What are Ranson criteria?**

A means of estimating the severity and prognosis for patients with acute pancreatitis.

Criteria at initial presentation:

Age > 55 years
LDH > 350 IU/L
WBC > 16,000/mm^3
AST > 250 UI/L
Serum glucose > 200 mg/dL

Criteria developing during first 24 hours:

Hematocrit falling > 10%
Increase in BUN > 8 mg/dL
Serum Ca$^+$ < 8 mg/dL
Arterial PO$_2$ < 60 mm Hg
Base deficit > 4 mEq/L
Fluid sequestration > 6 L

Morbidity and mortality:

0 to 2 criteria = 2% mortality
3 to 4 criteria = 15% mortality
5 to 6 criteria = 40% mortality
7 to 8 criteria = 100% mortality

○ **What is the most common cause of pancreatic pseudocysts in children and adults?**

Children: The etiology for pancreatitis in children is widely varied with abdominal trauma being the most common case at 23% of the cases. Additionally, anomalies of the pancreaticobiliary system (15%), multisystem disease (14%), drugs and toxins (12%), viral infections (10%), hereditary disorders (2%), and metabolic disorders (2%) are also involved in this etiology.

Adults: Acute pancreatitis secondary to alcoholism or gallstone disease are the most common etiologies.

Pseudocysts are generally filled with fluid and pancreatic enzymes that arise from the pancreas and should be suspected in patients who fail to improve within 1 week of appropriate treatment.

○ **What is the treatment for pancreatic pseudocysts?**

In the absence of symptoms and radiographic evidence of enlargement expectant management for the first 6–12 weeks is recommended. The spontaneous resolution is expected in 40% of these cases. For pseudocysts greater than 5 cm or those that persist greater than 12 weeks treatment with percutaneous catheter drainage or surgical drainage into the stomach or intestine is recommended.

○ **A 44-year-old gentleman presents with a deep, dull pain in the center of his abdomen that radiates to his back and will not go away. He states he has not "felt like himself" for a few weeks and that he has been kind of depressed. He also notes that he has lost a lot of weight, about 30 pounds in 3 weeks. On physical examination you notice that he has mild jaundice, a palpable hepatomegaly, and an abdominal mass in the epigastrium. What is your diagnosis?**

This presentation is classic for carcinoma of the head of the pancreas. The ability to palpate a mass suggests surgical incurability secondary to advanced disease progression.

○ **Where is the most common anatomic and histologic location of pancreatic cancer?**

Head of the pancreas (66%–75%). Pancreatic cancer is generally adenocarcinoma and located in the ducts.

○ **What gender and age group most commonly presents with pancreatic cancer?**

Middle-aged men, 35–55 years of age.

○ **What is the overall 5-year survival rate for pancreatic carcinoma?**

10%: However only 60% of these patients have had a complete tumor resection. Patients with metastatic pancreatic cancer who have symptoms of weight loss or pain, the chance of surviving 1 year is less than 20% for those undergoing chemotherapy and less than 5% for those who choose not to receive chemotherapy.

○ **What is Courvoisier law?**

This states that in the presence of (obstructive) jaundice if the gallbladder is palpable, then the jaundice is unlikely to be due to gallstones.

○ **What is the most common endocrine tumor of the pancreas?**

An insulinoma, only 10% are malignant. The classic diagnostic criteria is "Whipple triad":

1. Hypoglycemic symptoms produced by fasting
2. Blood glucose < 50 mg/dL during symptomatic episodes
3. Relief of symptoms with administration of IV glucose

○ **Where do Glucagonomas arise?**

A glucagonoma is a rare neuroendocrine tumor with nearly exclusive pancreatic localization. Malignant glucagonomas are islet cell pancreatic tumors that originate from the alpha-2 cells of the pancreas.

○ **Which type of operation is associated with a higher incidence of common bile duct injury, laparoscopic cholecystectomy or conventional cholecystectomy?**

Laparoscopic.

○ **What is the typical size of an adrenal carcinoma when diagnosed?**

The mean diameter is 12 cm with an average range of 3–30 cm.

○ **What compounds are produced by a Pheochromocytomas?**

Catecholamines. This group of chemicals trigger an increase in blood pressure, perspiration, heart palpitations, anxiety, and weight loss.

○ **If vanillylmandelic acid, normetanephrine, and metanephrine are detected in the urine, what is the likely cause?**

Pheochromocytoma.

○ **Where are the majority of pheochromocytomas located?**

90% are found in the adrenal medulla.

○ **What is the pheochromocytoma rule of 10s?**

10% are malignant; 10% are multiple or bilateral; 10% are extra-adrenal; 10% occur in children; 10% recur after surgical removal; 10% are familial.

○ **What is the most common benign liver tumor?**

Hemangioma is the most common benign tumor affecting the liver and are composed of masses of blood vessels that are atypical or irregular in arrangement and size

○ **All types of hepatomas are associated with underlying liver disease except:**

Fibrolamellar hepatocellular carcinoma, or fibrolamellar carcinoma, is an uncommon malignant neoplasm of the liver.

○ **Hepatic cancer most commonly metastasizes to where?**

The lungs (bronchiogenic carcinoma).

○ **What is the 5-year survival rate for patients with liver cancer who present with a single tumor less than 5 cm in diameter and undergo transplant surgery?**

70%.

○   **Where will colorectal cancer most commonly metastasize?**

The liver and the lungs.

○   **Alpha-fetoprotein (AFP) will be elevated in which types of tumors?**

Primary hepatic neoplasms and testicular tumors.

○   **What is the most common cause of portal hypertension?**

Cirrhosis (85%) secondary to heavy alcohol use. The second most common cause is extrahepatic portal venous thrombosis or occlusion.

○   **What are the most commonly isolated organisms in pyogenic hepatic abscesses?**

E. coli, Klebsiella pneumoniae, Proteus vulgaris, and *Enterobacter aerogenes* most commonly as a result of ascending cholangitis secondary to biliary obstruction.

○   **What clinical sign can assist in the diagnosis of cholecystitis?**

Murphy sign: pain on inspiration with palpation of the RUQ. As the patient breaths in, the gallbladder is lowered in the abdomen and comes in contact with the peritoneum just below the examiner's hand. This will aggravate an inflamed gallbladder, causing the patient to discontinue breathing deeply.

○   **What is the difference between cholelithiasis, cholangitis, cholecystitis, and choledocholithiasis?**

Cholelithiasis: Gallstones in the gallbladder.
Cholangitis: Inflammation of the common bile duct often secondary to bacterial infection or choledocholithiasis.
Cholecystitis: Inflammation of the gallbladder most commonly as a result of gallstones.
Choledocholithiasis: Gallstones that have migrated from the gallbladder to the common bile duct.

○   **What percentage of people with gallstones will eventually require surgery?**

About 30%.

○   **Which ethnic group has the largest proportion of people with symptomatic gallstones?**

Native Americans and Mexican American populations.

○   **What percentage of patients with cholangitis are also bacteremic?**

25%–40% of patients may present with or develop fever, chills, or rigors.

○   **What is the diagnostic test of choice for a patient suspected of having gallstones?**

Ultrasound is the diagnostic procedure of choice and is very sensitive at seeing abnormalities in the biliary system, including stones or signs of inflammation or infection.

○   **What is the most common etiology of cholecystitis?**

Obstruction of the cystic duct secondary to cholelithiasis.

○ **What is Charcot triad?**

1. Fever
2. Jaundice
3. Abdominal pain

*Hallmark of acute cholangitis.

○ **What is Reynolds pentad?**

Charcot triad plus hypotension and mental status changes.

*Hallmark of acute ascending cholangitis.

○ **What are the majority of gallstones composed of?**

Cholesterol stones are more common in the United States, making up about 80% of all gallstones. They form when there is too much cholesterol in the bile. The remaining are pigmented stones that form when there is excess bilirubin in the bile.

○ **What are the majority of kidney stones made of?**

Calcium oxalate (60%). The remainder consists of uric acid, struvite, cystine, and calcium phosphate.

○ **What percentage of patients with cancer of the gallbladder will also have cholelithiasis?**

75%–90% of patients diagnosed with gallbladder cancer will have cholelithiasis.

○ **What is the diagnostic test of choice for acute cholecystitis?**

Biliary scintigraphy (hydroxy iminodiacetic acid (HIDA) scan) is the gold standard. The HIDA scan uses a gamma-ray–emitting isotope that is selectively extracted by the liver into bile. The labeled bile can then be used to determine if there is cystic duct obstruction or extrahepatic bile duct obstruction, which is based whether the bile fills the gall bladder or enters the intestine. Clinically the diagnosis is most commonly made using clinical impressions, CBC, and RUQ ultrasound.

○ **How effective is oral dissolution therapy with bile acids for patients with symptomatic gallstones?**

Oral therapy with bile acids can be administered in monotherapy or in combination therapy with bile acids having different mechanisms of action. Monotherapy has shown results of complete dissolution in 19%–37% of patients while combination therapy provided complete dissolution in 63% of patients. The expected dissolution rate is approximately a 1-mm decrease in stone diameter per month of treatment and is assessed by ultrasound every 3–6 months. Common side effects with this treatment are diarrhea, increased serum cholesterol levels, and possible hepatotoxicity.

○ **What are the contraindications to extracorporeal shockwave lithotripsy (ESWL) lithotripsy?**

Absolute contraindications include

acute urinary tract infection or urosepsis

uncorrected bleeding disorders or coagulopathies

pregnancy

uncorrected obstruction distal to the stone

○ **What is the most common major complication associated with laparoscopic cholecystectomy?**

Bile duct injury.

○ **Is it possible for gallstones to form in patients' S/P cholecystectomy?**

Yes. Stones may form as a result of bile backing up in the duct and a narrowing of the duct after surgery.

○ **Where is the most common site for fibromuscular dysplasia?**

The renal arteries. Fibromuscular dysplasia is a rare arterial disease that presents in 4/1000 people and is more common in women than men.

○ **Where is the most common site of a hernia?**

Inguinal (groin) hernia: Making up 75% of all abdominal wall hernias and occurring up to 25 times more often in men than women, these hernias are divided into two different types, direct and indirect.

○ **Do infants and children most commonly present with direct or indirect inguinal hernias?**

Indirect inguinal hernia: An indirect hernia follows the pathway that the testicles made during fetal development, descending from the abdomen into the scrotum. If this pathway does not close it may remain a possible site for a hernia to develop in later life. Sometimes the hernia sac may protrude into the scrotum. An indirect inguinal hernia may occur at any age.

○ **Differentiate between reducible, incarcerated, strangulated, Richter, and complete hernias:**

Reducible: An uncomplicated hernia which returns, either spontaneously or after manipulation, to its original site.

Incarcerated: Contents of the hernia sac cannot be returned to the abdomen by manipulation.

Strangulated: An incarcerated hernia so tightly constricted as to compromise the blood supply of the hernial sac, leading to gangrene of the sac and its contents.

Richter: An incarcerated or strangulated hernia in which only part of the circumference of the bowel wall is involved.

Complete: A hernia in which the sac and its contents have passed through the hernial orifice.

○ **What are the boundaries of Hesselbach triangle?**

Medial to the inferior epigastric artery, superior to the inguinal ligament, and lateral to the rectus sheath. Hesselbach triangle is the site through which direct hernias pass.

○ **What weakened tissue does a direct hernia pass through?**

The transversalis fascia that makes up the floor of Hesselbach triangle.

○ **Indirect inguinal hernias occur secondary to what defect?**

A failure of embryonic closure of the internal inguinal ring after the testicle has passed through it. This forms a temporary connection called the process vaginalis, which the resulting hernia can then pass through.

○ **Which type of hernia is most common in females?**

Males are 25 times more likely to develop a hernia but in females the direct inguinal hernia is the most common. While femoral hernias are more common in females than in males, they are still less common than direct hernias.

○   **Of all hernias involving the abdominal wall, which is most likely to strangulate?**

Usually occurring in women, femoral hernias are particularly at risk of becoming irreducible and strangulated.

○   **What type of hiatal hernia is most common, sliding or paraesophageal?**

A sliding hiatal hernia where the stomach and the section of the esophagus that joins the stomach slide up into the chest through the hiatus.

○   **Where is the most common site of duodenal ulcers?**

The first portion of the duodenum (duodenal bulb) accounts for 95% of duodenal ulcers.

○   **What is the most common site for benign gastric ulcers?**

The most common site is the lesser curvature of the stomach; however, they can occur anywhere. Malignant ulcers usually have irregular heaped-up margins that protrude into the lumen of the stomach.

○   **What are the signs and symptoms of intestinal obstruction in the newborn?**

Signs and symptoms of newborn proximal bowel obstruction can be subtle and nonspecific; however, the most common presentation in distal obstruction involves abdominal distention, delayed passage of meconium, and absence of transitional stools (meconium mixed with normal stool content).

○   **What amount of residual volume suctioned from the stomach of a newborn is diagnostic of obstruction?**

> 25–40 mL.

○   **A newborn's vomit will be stained with bile if the obstruction is distal to what anatomical structure?**

The ampulla of Vater.

○   **What is the differential diagnosis for neonatal intestinal obstruction?**

Disorders of the small intestine:

Duodenal atresia

Jejunoileal atresia

Malrotation and volvulus

Meconium ileus

Disorders of the large intestine:

Meconium plug syndrome

Anorectal malformation

Hirschsprung disease

Small left colon syndrome

Other causes:

Narcotics

Electrolyte abnormalities; hypermagnesemia, hypokalemia, hypercalcemia

Hypothyroidism

Sepsis

Congestive heart failure

○ **Where is the most prevalent location for atresia of the bowel?**

The duodenum (40%) is twice as common as in the jejunum (20%) and ileum (20%). In nearly half of all cases multiple congenital anomalies are present (Down Syndrome, being the most common).

○ **What is the "double bubble" sign?**

The appearance of a distended stomach and duodenum on the X-ray of a patient with duodenal obstruction. This is classically seen in duodenal atresia of the newborn.

○ **What is the most common cause of bowel obstruction in children?**

Intussusception is the most common cause of intestinal obstruction in infants and children aged 3 months to 6 years.

○ **What are the most common causes of small bowel obstruction in adults?**

The most common causes of mechanical obstruction are adhesions, hernias, and tumors.

○ **Volvulus of the colon most frequently involves which segment?**

The sigmoid colon is the most common site for colonic volvulus (65%) occurring often in patients older than 60 years, with a history of chronic constipation.

○ **Where is the most common site of intestinal obstruction secondary to gallstones?**

Gallstone Ileus occurs in the terminal ileum in 55%–60% of patients. A clinical presentation involves Rigler triad of pneumobilia, small bowel obstruction, and impacted gallstones at the ileocecal valve.

○ **What is the differential diagnosis for a 65-year-old man who has abdominal pain and bloody diarrhea a few days after the repair of an abdominal aortic aneurysm?**

Ischemic colitis is the most likely condition. The most common etiology resulting in this condition is diminished bowel perfusion resulting from low cardiac output and is often seen in patients with cardiac disease or in patients with prolonged shock of any etiology.

○ **Is colovesicular fistula more common among men or women?**

Men (3:1) more than women because a woman's uterus lies between her colon and bladder. This is condition is occasionally seen in women S/P hysterectomy.

○ **What is Osler-Weber-Rendu syndrome?**

Also known as hereditary hemorrhagic telangiectasia (HHT) is an autosomal dominant disorder typically identified by the triad of telangiectasia, recurrent epistaxis, and a positive family history for the disorder. The major cause of morbidity and mortality due to this disorder lies in the presence of multiorgan arteriovenous malformations (AVMs) and the associated hemorrhage that may accompany them.

○ **How much blood must be lost in the GI tract to cause melena?**

Between 50 and 100 mL. Normal healthy patients lose 2.5 mL of blood per day in their stools.

○ **What are the most common causes of upper GI bleeding?**

Peptic ulcer disease (PUD), esophageal varices, gastritis, and Mallory-Weiss syndrome account for 90% of all etiologies.

○ **What percentage of patients with upper GI bleeds will stop bleeding within hours of hospitalization?**

About 85% of UGIB will spontaneously stop bleeding within a few hours.

○ **What are the most common causes of rebleeding in patients with upper GI bleeds?**

PUD, esophageal varices, amenia, or shock. Most cases of rebleeding occur within 2 days from the time of the first episode.

○ **What percentage of patients with PUD bleed from their ulcers?**

About 20%, which result in 40% of the deaths related to this condition.

○ **Bleeding ulcers are more predominant in patients with which blood type?**

Type O. The reason is not known.

○ **Where are bleeding duodenal ulcers most commonly located?**

On the posterior surface of the duodenal bulb.

○ **How soon after an episode of duodenal bleeding has occurred can an ulcer patient be fed?**

12–24 hours after the bleeding has stopped in a patient that feels hungry.

○ **Which type of ulcer is more likely to rebleed?**

Gastric ulcers are three times more likely to rebleed compared to duodenal ulcers.

○ **What is the surgical treatment of choice for a bleeding peptic ulcer?**

Oversewing the ulcer combined with a bilateral truncal vagotomy and pyloroplasty. Other treatments are proximal gastric vagotomy and Billroth II gastrojejunostomy. The decision to perform surgery is based on the rate of bleed, not on the location of the bleed.

○ **What percentage of patients with large intestinal bleeding will spontaneously stop before transfusion requirements exceed two units?**

90%.

○ **If blood is recovered from the stomach after an NG tube is inserted, where is the most likely location of the bleed?**

A site above the ligament of Treitz (Upper GI Bleed).

○ **Where do the majority of Mallory-Weiss tears occur?**

In the stomach (gastric cardia), the esophagogastric junction, and the distal esophagus (5%).

○ **What is angiodysplasia and where is it most frequently found?**

It is an acquired condition of focal submucosal vascular ectasia that has a propensity to bleed spontaneously. Most frequently it is located in the cecum and proximal ascending colon. Lesions are generally singular; bleeding is intermittent and seldom massive.

○ **What is the major cause of death in patients with Hirschsprung disease?**

Nonbacterial/nonviral enterocolitis.

○ **Is Hirschsprung disease more common in men or women?**

Men (4:1 men-to-women-ratio).

○ **Are tumors located in the jejunum and ileum more likely malignant or benign?**

Benign. Tumors of the jejunum and ileum comprise only 1%–5% of all GI tumors. The majority (90%) are asymptomatic.

○ **What is the most common remnant of the omphalomesenteric (vitelline) duct?**

Meckel diverticulum.

○ **What is the Meckel diverticulum rule of 2s?**

2% of the population has it; it is 2 inches long; 2 feet from the ileocecal valve; occurs most commonly in children under 2; and is symptomatic in 2% of patients.

○ **What is the most likely cause of rectal bleeding in a patient with Meckel diverticulum?**

Peptic ulceration of the adjacent ileum caused by ectopic gastric mucosa.

○ **What is the most likely cause of cellulitis of the umbilicus in a pediatric patient with an acute abdomen?**

A perforated Meckel diverticulum.

○ **What is the difference in the prognosis between familial polyposis and Gardner disease?**

Although both are inheritable conditions of colonic polyps, Gardner disease rarely results in malignancy, while familial polyposis virtually always results in malignancy.

○ **Clinically, how is right-sided colon cancer differentiated from left-sided?**

Right-sided lesions present with occult blood in the feces, unexplained weakness or anemia, dyspepsia, palpable abdominal mass, and dull abdominal pain. **Left-sided lesions** present with gross rectal bleeding, obstructive symptoms, and noticeable changes in bowel habits with the common presentation of "Pencil thin" stools.

○ **Adenocarcinoma develops from adenomatous polyps. What percent of asymptomatic patients have adenomatous polyps when a routine colonoscopy is performed?**

25% with the prevalence increasing with age: At age 50: 30%, age 60: 40%; age 70: 50%; and age 80: 55%.

○ **The advancement to adenocarcinoma of the colon from adenoma is significantly related to the size of the adenoma. What is the risk of developing cancer if a 1.5 cm polyp is found upon colonoscopic examination?**

10%. The risk for developing adenocarcinoma is 1% if the polyp is less than 1 cm, 10% if it is 1 to 2 cm, and 45% if the polyp is greater than 2 cm.

○ **Is a villous, tubulovillous, or tubular adenoma more likely to become malignant?**

40% of villous adenomas will become malignant, compared to 22% of tubulovillous adenomas and 5% of tubular adenomas.

○ **Which are more likely to turn malignant, pedunculated or sessile lesions?**

Sessile lesions are more likely to become malignant.

○ **Where are the majority of colorectal cancers found?**

In the rectum (30%), ascending colon (25%), sigmoid colon (20%), descending colon (15%), and transverse colon (10%).

○ **What is the surgical treatment of choice for cecal cancer?**

Colonic resection from the vermiform appendix to the junction of the ascending and transverse colon.

○ **What is the treatment of choice for a plantar wart?**

Cryosurgery with liquid nitrogen. Additional options include electrodesiccation and curettage, surgical excision, and laser therapy.

○ **Where are soft tissue sarcomas most often found?**

About 60% occur in the arms, legs, hands, or feet.

○ **A 41-year-old patient complains of severe but short rectal spasms but has not noticed any bleeding. He is known to be stressed and overtaxed at work. What is your diagnosis?**

Proctalgia fugax. Proctalgia fugax is transient, severe rectal pain related to spasm of levator ani and coccygeal muscles that may last seconds or up to 20 minutes.

○ **A patient complains of severe pain when defecating. He is constipated, has blood-streaked stools, and a bloody discharge following bowel movements. What is the diagnosis?**

Anal fissure.

○ **Differentiate between mucosal rectal prolapse, complete rectal prolapse, and occult rectal prolapse:**

Mucosal rectal prolapse: Involves only a small portion of the rectum protruding through the anus and have the appearance of radial folds.

Complete rectal prolapse: Involves all the layers of the rectum protruding through the anus. Clinically, this condition appears as concentric folds.

Occult rectal prolapse: Does not involve protrusion through the anus but rather intussusception.

○ **Which are more painful, internal or external hemorrhoids?**

External. The nerves above the pectinate or dentate line are supplied by the autonomic nervous system and have no sensory fibers. The nerves below the pectinate line are supplied by the inferior rectal nerve and have sensory fibers.

○ **Differentiate between first-, second-, third-, and fourth-degree internal hemorrhoids:**

Classification is based upon the following history:

First degree: Presence of only bleeding

Second degree: Bleed and prolapse but reduce spontaneously

Third degree: Bleed, prolapse, and require manual reduction

Fourth degree: Bleed, cannot be reduced, and may strangulate

○ **What portion of the colon most common presents with diverticular disease?**

The sigmoid colon is involved in 95% of patients.

○ **What percentage of patients with diverticula are symptomatic?**

20% and most commonly diagnosed by barium enema radiography or endoscopic procedures.

○ **What percentage of 40 year olds will have diverticula?**

10% and 65% will have diverticular by the age of 80.

○ **What are the signs and symptoms of diverticulitis?**

Abdominal pain, generally in the left lower quadrant with significant tenderness to palpation, a low-grade temperature, change in bowel habits, nausea, and vomiting. If perforated, patients may have peritoneal signs and appear toxic.

○ **What is the treatment for diverticulitis?**

Specific details of the treatment depend upon the severity of the patient's condition. Generally patients are hospitalized, made NPO, NG tube placed to suction, IV fluids are initiated with broad-spectrum IV antibiotics.
   Surgical treatment should be considered for patients who do not improve with medical therapies or develop signs of peritonitis.

○ **Ulcerative colitis has two peaks of incidence. When do they occur?**

The most significant peak is in the second (15–30 years old) decade. A second lower peak occurs during the sixth to eigth decades of life.

○ **What are some extraintestinal manifestations of ulcerative colitis?**

Lesions of the skin and mucus membranes: Erythema nodosum, erythema multiforme, pyoderma gangrenosum, pustular dermatitis, and aphthous stomatitis.

Ocular: Uveitis.

Bone and joint lesions: Arthralgia, arthritis, and ankylosing spondylitis.

Hepatobiliary and pancreatic lesions: Fatty infiltration, pericholangitis, cirrhosis, sclerosis cholangitis, bile duct carcinoma, gallstones, and pancreatic insufficiency.

Hematologic: Anemia (Most commonly iron deficiency anemia).

○ **Kultschitzsky cells are the precursors to what tumor?**

Carcinoid tumors arise from *Kultschitzsky cells*, granular *cells* within the intestinal and bronchial.

○ **What is the most probable cause of colovesicular fistulas?**

Diverticulitis.

○ **A 47-year-old man complains of impotence as well as pain and coldness in both legs after exercise. What would you expect to find on examination?**

This patient probably has Leriche syndrome, which is a vascular disorder marked by gradual occlusion of the terminal aorta, bilateral iliac arteries, or both; intermittent claudication in the buttocks, thighs, or calves; absence of pulsation in femoral arteries; pallor and coldness of the legs; gangrene of the toes; and, in men, impotence. Symptoms are the result of chronic tissue hypoxia caused by inadequate arterial perfusion of the affected areas.

○ **What is the most commonly obstructed artery in the lower extremity?**

The superficial femoral, which is a branch of the common femoral.

○ **A 64-year-old man presents with jaundice, upper GI bleeding, anemia, a palpable nontender gallbladder, a palpable liver, and rapid weight loss. What is your initial diagnosis and what confirmatory test would you order?**

This is the clinical picture of a tumor of the ampulla of Vater and the results of an ERCP would demonstrate the tumor as an exophytic papillary lesion, an ulcerating tumor, or an infiltrating mass. You would also expect to identify dilation of the biliary and pancreatic ducts.

○ **Testicular torsion occurs most commonly in what age group?**

Teens with the left testicle most commonly involved.

○ **What is the maximum amount of time a testicle can remain torsed without being irreversibly damaged?**

4–6 hours.

○ **What is definitive treatment for testicular torsion?**

Medical: The "Open Book Maneuver."
Surgical: Emergent surgical scrotal exploration.

○ **What percentage of palpable prostate nodules are malignant?**

Nearly 50%. Surgical cure of patients who present with asymptomatic nodules and no metastasis is attempted with radical prostatectomy or radiation therapy.

○ **What are mycotic aneurysms?**

A mycotic aneurysms is a localized, irreversible arterial dilatation due to destruction of the vessel wall by infection. A mycotic aneurysm can develop either when a new aneurysm is produced by infection of the arterial wall or when a preexisting aneurysm becomes secondarily infected.

○ **Where is mesenteric ischemia more serious, in the small or the large bowel?**

The small bowel. Embolization in the superior mesenteric artery affects the entire small bowel with mortality from small bowel ischemia being nearly 60%. Embolization to the large bowel is not as serious due to collateral circulation and ischemia of the large bowel rarely result in a full thickness injury or perforation.

○ **Where do glomus tumors develop?**

Glomus jugulare tumors are rare, slow-growing, hypervascular tumors that arise within the jugular foramen of the temporal bone.

○ **What is an ABI, and why is it significant?**

The ankle-brachial index (ABI) is a quick screening test used to evaluate peripheral vascular disease or traumatic arterial injury. It consists of measuring the resting systolic BP in the brachial artery and comparing it to the resting systolic BP in the posterior tibial or dorsalis pedis arteries of the lower extremity. The ABI is calculated by dividing the LE systolic BP by the brachial artery BP. A normal ABI is 1 or greater while a value of less than 1 indicates occlusive disease or arterial injury.

○ **What technical factors can affect the accuracy of the ABI?**

Doppler probe pressure, rapid deflation of the BP cuff, and arterial wall calcifications.

○ **Cricothyroidotomy is not recommended in children under what age?**

Children younger than 10–12 years old pose a relative contraindication to this procedure.

○ **Is succinylcholine a depolarizing or a nondepolarizing neuromuscular blocking agent?**

Depolarizing. Succinylcholine is the only commonly used depolarizing agent. It binds to postsynaptic acetylcholine receptors, thereby causing depolarization. The material is enzymatically degraded by pseudocholinesterase (serum cholinesterase). Onset is within 1 minute; paralysis last 7–10 minutes. The recommended adult dose is 1–2 mg/kg.

○ **What is the rationale for pretreating a patient with a subpolarizing (defasciculating) dose of a nondepolarizing agent prior to treatment with succinylcholine?**

This primarily reduces the fasciculations secondary to succinylcholine-induced depolarization. Additionally it may also be helpful in decreasing intracranial and intraocular pressure is associated with the administration of succinylcholine.

○ **What dosage of midazolam (Versed) causes a loss of consciousness and amnesia during rapid sequence induction?**

0.1 mg/kg; 5 mg is effective for most people.

○ **Etomidate is the recommended agent to obtain sedation and induction while performing Rapid Sequence Intubation. What is the appropriate adult dose?**

0.2–0.3 mg/kg.

○ **What is the "defasciculating" or the "priming" dose of vecuronium?**

~ 0.01 mg/kg or commonly 1 mg or 1/10th of the total dose.

○ **What dose of vecuronium should be administered for paralysis (no "priming")?**

0.08–0.1 mg/kg providing a NMR effects for 15–30 minutes.

○ **What is the appropriate initial dose of pancuronium (Pavulon)?**

0.04–0.1 mg/kg, which commonly provides 45 minutes of NMR.

○ **What pain medications are not recommended for the treatment of pain arising from acute diverticulitis?**

Opioid pain medications should be avoided, if possible. Their use may increase intraluminal colonic pressure and precipitate constipation and decreased bowel motility.

○ **What are the most common causes of large bowel obstruction?**

Carcinoma, followed by volvulus, diverticulitis inflammatory disorders, and fecal impaction, all of which most commonly occur in the sigmoid.

○ **What is the most common cause of massive upper GI tract hemorrhage?**

Duodenal ulcers.

○ **What layers of the bowel wall and mesentery are affected by regional enteritis?**

All layers.

○ **Which hernia is the most common in women?**

Inguinal hernia. It is also the most common in men.

○ **What is the most common cause of paralytic ileus?**

Abdominal surgery. This is a routine complication following abdominal surgery.

○ **An elderly woman presents with pain in the knee and medial aspect of the thigh. What GI diagnosis should be considered?**

Obturator hernia. This presentation is most common in elderly women and is difficult to diagnose and is frequently missed, which makes these the most lethal of all abdominal hernias (mortality 13%–40%).

○ **Where is the most common site of volvulus?**

The sigmoid colon in nearly 65% of patients.

○ **Describe the location of an indirect inguinal hernia:**

Lateral to the epigastric vessels, protruding through the inguinal canal and commonly into the scrotum.

○ **Describe the location of a femoral hernia:**

Descends through the femoral canal and beneath the inguinal ligament.

○ **Describe the location of a spigelian hernia:**

This is an acquired ventral hernia through the linea semilunaris, the line where the sheaths of the lateral abdominal muscles fuse to form the lateral rectus.

○ **What is a pantaloon hernia?**

A hernia with both direct and indirect inguinal hernia components that occur on the same side.

○ **What is a sliding hernia?**

A hernia in which one wall of the hernia sac includes viscus.

○ **Describe a Richter hernia:**

A hernia involving only one sidewall of the bowel, which can more easily result in bowel strangulation.

○ **Which is the most common type of hernia in children?**

Indirect. Direct inguinal hernias are more common in the elderly.

○ **In the pediatric esophagus, where is a foreign body most commonly lodged?**

The most common site of esophageal impaction is at the thoracic inlet, defined as the area between the clavicles on chest radiograph, this is the site of anatomical change from the skeletal muscle to the smooth muscle of the esophagus. More specifically most foreign bodies (70%) lodge at the cricopharyngeus sling.

○ **Of the following, which is not a common cause of large bowel obstruction: diverticulitis, adhesions, sigmoid volvulus, or neoplasms?**

Adhesions. Adhesions are the most common cause of small bowel obstructions are uncommon in the colon.

○ **Describe the clinical presentation of a patient with sigmoid volvulus:**

Most common in geriatric patients presenting with colicky abdominal pain with a dull discomfort between spasms. Patients commonly have abdominal distention and occasionally vomiting. Characteristic abdominal X-ray findings are a significantly dilated cecum with a distended loop that assumes a "coffee bean" shape.

○ **Describe a typical patient with intussusception:**

It usually occurs in children ages 3 months to 6 years, although the majority are 7–8 months old. It is more common in boys (3:1). The typical presentation is a previously healthy infant boy aged 6–12 months with sudden onset of colicky abdominal pain 10–20 minutes apart with vomiting.

○ **What is the most common anatomical abnormality in the arterial blood supply to the liver?**

The right hepatic artery branches from the superior mesenteric instead of the common hepatic, which arises from the proper hepatic in 15%–20% of the population.

○ **What is Kehr sign?**

Pain in the shoulder made worse in Trendelenburg. Pain in the left shoulder is a classic presentation indicating splenic injury.

○ **What spinal level provides motor innervation to the diaphragm?**

C3, C4, C5. (Phrenic nerve.) Remember: "3, 4, and 5 keep the diaphragm alive!"

○ **Where are the most common sites of the hematologic spread of breast cancer?**

Bones, liver, and brain.

○ **What characteristics are associated with the best prognosis in breast cancer?**

The (TNM) staging of breast cancer is the most reliable indicator of prognosis.

T1 Tumor < 2 cm

N0 No Regional lymph node metastasis

M0 No distant metastasis

○ **What is the most commonly injured nerve during parotidectomies?**

Most serious complications result from damage to the facial nerve (either temporary or permanent paralysis). Injury to the greater auricular nerve results in hypesthesia of the ear.

○ **If medical management fails to relieve symptoms of gastroesophageal reflux after a 1-year trial period, what surgical methods might be attempted?**

Previously antireflux surgery as considered only for patients that did not respond to medical treatment. Currently the following indications are considered:

Young patients who require chronic therapy with proton pump inhibitors for control of symptoms.

Patient in whom regurgitation persists during therapy.

Patients with respiratory symptoms (cough).

Patients with vocal cord damage.

Patients with Barrett esophagus.

The goal of surgical therapy is to restore the competence of the lower esophageal sphincter and the surgical procedure of choice is a laparoscopic Nissen fundoplication.

○ **Other than laparotomy, what invasive examination will confirm suspected mesenteric ischemia?**

For many years, angiography has been considered to be the criterion standard for the diagnosis of acute arterial occlusion with reported sensitivities 74%–100% and specificity 100%. Currently the nonevasive multidetector row CT has emerged as a valuable tool for the evaluation of mesenteric ischemia.

○ **What is the most common cause of postsplenectomy (postsplenic) sepsis?**

Streptococcus pneumonia and *Haemophilus influenza* to a lesser extent. All postsplenectomy patients should receive the pneumococcal conjugate vaccine (Prevnar), Hib vaccine, and the meningococcal vaccine.

○ **What are the X-ray findings in ischemic bowel disease?**

"Thumb printing" (mucosal dilation) on plain film with dilation of the colon and thickening of the valvulae conniventes.

○ **Which local anesthetic, ester or amide, is responsible for most allergic reactions?**

Ester (Procaine). However, allergic reactions that occur are usually not in response to Procaine, but rather to para-aminobenzoic acid (PABA), which is a major metabolic product of all ester-type local anesthetics.

○ **What are the most common signs and symptoms of mild, moderate, and severe dehydration?**

Symptom/sign	Mild dehydration	Moderate dehydration	Severe dehydration
Level of consciousness	Alert	Lethargic	Obtunded
Capillary refill*	2 seconds	2–4 seconds	Greater than 4 seconds, cool limbs
Mucous membranes	Normal	Dry	Parched, cracked
Tears	Normal	Decreased	Absent
Heart rate	Slightly increased	Increased	Very increased
Respiratory rate/pattern*	Normal	Increased	Increased and hyperpnea
Blood pressure	Normal	Normal, but orthostasis	Decreased
Pulse	Normal	Thready	Faint or impalpable
Skin turgor*	Normal	Slow	Tenting
Fontanel	Normal	Depressed	Sunken
Eyes	Normal	Sunken	Very sunken
Urine output	Decreased	Oliguria	Oliguria/anuria

● ● ● **REFERENCES** ● ● ●

Britt L, Trunkey DD, Feliciano DV *Acute Care Surgery—Principles and Practice.* New York, NY: Springer-Verlag; 2007.

Doherty GM, Way L. *Current Surgical Diagnosis and Treatment.* 12th ed. New York, NY: McGraw-Hill; 2006.

Tintinalli MJ, Kelen MG, Stapczynski MJ, Ma MO, Cline MD. *Tintinalli's Emergency Medicine—A Comprehensive Study Guide.* 6th ed. New York, NY: McGraw-Hill; 2004.

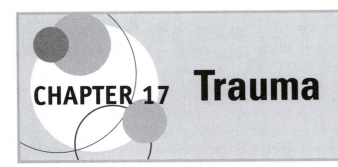

Jeffrey G. Yates, MPA, PA-C

○ **What percentage of cervical fractures are visualized on lateral, odontoid, and AP films of the neck?**

Cross-table lateral: 85%–90%

Odontoid: 10%

Anterior/Posterior: <5%

○ **Describe the three types of fractures involving the odontoid process:**

Type I odontoid fracture is an avulsion of the tip of the dens at the insertion site of the alar ligament. Although a type I fracture is mechanically stable, it often is seen in association with atlanto-occipital dislocation and must be ruled out because of this potentially life-threatening complication.

Type II fractures occur at the base of the dens and are the most common type of odontoid fracture. This type is associated with a high prevalence of nonunion due to the limited vascular supply and small area of cancellous bone.

Type III odontoid fracture occurs when the fracture line extends into the body of the axis.

○ **What are the two clinical decision-making criteria used to assess the need for radiographic imaging of the C-spine?**

1. To be clinically cleared using the Canadian C-Spine Rules (CCR), a patient must be alert (GCS 15), not intoxicated, and not have a distracting injury (e.g., long bone fracture, large laceration). The patient can be clinically cleared providing the following:
   ○ The patient is not high risk (age >65 years or dangerous mechanism or paresthesias in extremities).
   ○ A low-risk factor that allows safe assessment of range of motion exists. This includes simple rear end motor vehicle collision, seated position in the emergency department, ambulation at any time posttrauma, delayed onset of neck pain, and the absence of midline cervical spine tenderness.
   ○ The patient is able to actively rotate their neck 45° left and right.

2. The NEXUS criteria states that a patient with suspected C-spine injury can be cleared provided the following are met:
   ○ No posterior midline cervical spine tenderness is present.
   ○ No evidence of intoxication is present.
   ○ The patient has a normal level of alertness.
   ○ No focal neurologic deficit is present.
   ○ The patient does not have a painful distracting injury.

○ **On a lateral C-spine X-ray, how much soft tissue prevertebral swelling is normal from C2 through C4?**

Prevertebral space extends between the anterior border of the vertebra to the posterior wall of the pharynx in the upper vertebral level (C2-C4) or to the trachea in the lower vertebral level (C6).

- At the level of C2, prevertebral space should not exceed 7 mm.
- At the level of C3 and C4, it should not exceed 5 mm, or it should be less than half the width of the involved vertebrae.
- At the level of C6, prevertebral space is widened by the presence of the esophagus and cricopharyngeal muscle. At this level, the space should be no more than 22 mm in adults or 14 mm in children younger than 15 years.
  - Children younger than 24 months may exhibit a physiologic widening of the prevertebral space during expiration; therefore, obtain images in small children during inspiration to assess prevertebral space adequately.

If the prevertebral space is widened at any level, a hematoma secondary to a fracture is the most likely diagnosis.

○ **On a lateral C-spine X-ray, how much soft tissue predental soft tissue swelling is normal?**

The predental space, also known as the atlantodental interval, is the distance between the anterior aspect of the odontoid and the posterior aspect of the anterior arch of C1. This space should be no more than 3 mm in an adult and 5 mm in a child. Suspect transverse ligament disruption if these limits are exceeded.

○ **How much anterior subluxation is allowable on an adult lateral C-spine and still within the normal limits?**

3.5 mm.

○ **How much angulation is normal on an adult lateral C-spine, measured across a single interspace?**

Up to 11°.

○ **On a lateral C-spine, what does "fanning" of the spinous processes suggest?**

This is evident as an exaggerated widening of the space between two spinous process tips and suggests posterior ligamentous disruption.

○ **What are the three most unstable C-spine injuries?**

1. Rupture of the transverse ligament of the atlas.
2. Fracture of the dens (odontoid fracture).
3. Burst fracture with posterior ligamentous disruption (flexion teardrop fracture).

○ **Describe a Jefferson fracture:**

This fracture is caused by a compressive downward force that is transmitted evenly through the occipital condyles to the superior articular surfaces of the lateral masses of C1. The process displaces the masses laterally and causes fractures of the anterior and posterior arches, along with possible disruption of the transverse ligament.

Radiographically, the fracture is characterized by bilateral lateral displacement of the articular masses of C1. The odontoid view shows unilateral or bilateral displacement of the lateral masses of C1 with respect to the articular pillars of C2.

○ **Describe a hangman fracture:**

The name of this injury is derived from the typical fracture that occurs after hangings. Presently, it commonly is caused by motor vehicle collisions and entails bilateral fractures through the pedicles of C2 due to hyperextension.

Radiographically, a fracture line should be evident extending through the pedicles of C2 along with obvious disruption of the spinolaminar contour line

○ **What is a clay-shoveler fracture?**

Abrupt flexion of the neck, combined with a heavy upper body and lower neck muscular contraction, results in an oblique fracture of the base of the spinous process, which is avulsed by the intact supraspinous ligament. Fracture also occurs with direct blows to the spinous process or with trauma to the occiput that causes forced flexion of the neck

Radiographically, this injury is commonly observed in a lateral view, since the avulsed fragment is readily evident

○ **Describe the key features of spinal (neurogenic) shock:**

An acute onset of flaccidity and areflexia with the loss of anal sphincter tone and fecal incontinence. A priapism or loss of bulbocavernosus reflex may also occur. Hypotension with SBPs in the 80–100 mm Hg range is common with paradoxical bradycardia at 40–60 beat per minute. The classic skin findings are the presence of flushed, dry, and warm peripheral skin.

○ **A trauma patient presents with a decreasing level of consciousness and an enlarging right pupil. What is your diagnosis?**

Probable uncal herniation with oculomotor nerve compression.

○ **The corneal reflex tests what nerves?**

The ophthalmic branch (V1) of the trigeminal (fifth) nerve (afferent), and the facial (seventh) nerve (efferent).

○ **Name five clinical signs of basilar skull fracture:**

1. Periorbital ecchymosis (raccoon eyes)
2. Retroauricular ecchymosis (Battle sign)
3. Otorrhea or rhinorrhea
4. Hemotympanum or bloody ear discharge
5. First, second, seventh, and eighth CN deficits

○ **A trauma patient presents with anisocoria, neurological deterioration, and/or lateralizing motor findings. What should be the immediate treatment?**

1. Immediate intubation (maintain continued C-spine immobilization) with a controlled ventilatory rate. The use of routine hyperventilation should be avoided.
   ○ Consider pharmacologic paralysis and sedation

2. Obtain venous access and restore intravascular volume.

3. Monitor blood pressure (ICP), oxygen saturation, and neurologic status constantly while obtaining non–contrast-enhanced CT scan.
   ○ GOALS: MAP between 90 and 100 mm Hg, Oxygen saturation 100%, ICP < 20 mm Hg, $Paco_2$ = 33–37, Hct = 30–34, CVP = 8–14.

4. Control rising intracranial pressures (ICPs)
   ○ Elevate head of bed (HOB) 30°
   ○ Consider mannitol 25–50 g IV q4h
   ○ Consider phenytoin during the first 7 days only for patients with significant risk factors for posttraumatic seizures (cortical contusion, SDH, penetrating head wound).
   ○ Determine if the placement of a ventriculostomy catheter is warranted.

5. Determine the need for any acute neurosurgical procedures.

6. Repeat head CT in 24 hours.

○ **How is posterior column function tested? Why is it significant?**

Position and vibration sensation are carried in the posterior columns and are usually spared in anterior cord syndrome. Light touch sensation may also be spared. Pain and temperature sensation cross near the level of entry and are carried in the more posterior spinothalamic tract.

○ **Define increased intracranial pressure:**

Intracranial pressure (ICP) > 20 mm Hg.

○ **Where is the most common site of a basilar skull fracture?**

Through the floor of the anterior cranial fossa.

○ **What cardiovascular injury is commonly associated with a sternal fracture?**

Myocardial contusions (blunt myocardial injury).

○ **Which valve is most commonly injured during blunt trauma?**

Aortic valve.

○ **What plain film X-ray finding most accurately indicates traumatic rupture of the aorta?**

Widening of the mediastinum > 8 cm.

○ **What is the differential diagnosis of distended neck veins in a trauma patient?**

Tension pneumothorax and pericardial tamponade are the primary conditions with additional possibilities being pulmonary embolism right heart failure. It should be fully understood that JVD may not be present in a hypovolemic patient.

○ **What is the most sensitive indicator of compensated shock in children?**

Because cardiac output (CO) depends on both stroke volume (SV) and heart rate (HR), the body typically tries to maintain CO when SV decreases by increasing the HR. A patient in the early stages of shock is typically tachycardic.

○ **What initial fluid bolus should be administered to children in shock?**

20 mL/kg.

○ **A radial pulse on examination indicates a BP of at least what level?**

Approximately 80 mm Hg.

○ **A femoral pulse on examination indicates a BP of at least what level?**

70 mm Hg.

○ **A carotid pulse indicates a BP of at least what level?**

60 mm Hg.

○ **What is the most common complaint of patients with a traumatic aortic injury?**

For those patient that are still alive, they frequently complain of retrosternal or intrascapular pain. The most common signs and symptoms are those of acute exsanguinating hemorrhage and shock.

○ **When should amputation be considered in a lower extremity injury?**

Severe open fractures with popliteal artery and posterior tibial nerve injuries can be treated with current techniques; however, treatment is at a high cost and multiple surgeries are required. The result is often a leg that is painful, nonfunctional, and less efficient than a prosthesis.

○ **How long does it take to prepare fully cross-matched blood?**

30–60 minutes at a minimum.

○ **Should a chest tube be placed into an entrance or exit wound in the appropriate anatomical location rather than making a surgical incision in the chest?**

No. The tube might follow the bullet track into the diaphragm or lung.

○ **Why do simple through-and-through wounds of the extremities fare better regardless of the velocity of the bullet?**

The bullet's short path in the tissue results in (1) little or no deformation of slower bullets and (2) less time for higher velocity bullet to yaw, which results in less tissue damage.

○ **Is the heat from firing a bullet significant enough to sterilize a bullet and its wound?**

No, contaminants from the body surface and viscera can be carried along the bullet's path.

○ **Should intra-articular bullets be removed?**

In most cases they should be removed because of the potential for synovitis to develop, leading to severe damage of articular cartilage.

○ **What artery is usually involved in an epidural hematoma?**

The middle meningeal artery.

○ **Where are epidural hematomas located?**

Between the dura and inner table of the skull.

○ **Where are subdural hematomas located?**

Beneath the dura, over the brain, and in the arachnoid.

○ **What risk is associated with not treating a septal hematoma of the nose?**

Aseptic necrosis followed by absorption of the septal cartilage, resulting in septal perforation referred to as a "saddle-nose deformity."

○ **What are the most commonly injured organs as a result of blunt trauma?**

The spleen, liver, and retroperitoneum.

○ **A patient who was recently hit in the eye during a bar room brawl complains of diplopia when looking up. The injured eye does not appear able to look up. What is the diagnosis?**

Orbital blowout fracture with entrapment of inferior rectus or inferior oblique.

○ **What is the LD50 for falling in adults?**

25–30 feet.

○ **What clinical history and physical examination findings are most suggestive of a laryngeal fracture?**

Obtaining a mechanism of injury (MOI) of the patient sustaining a direct blow to the anterior or anterolateral neck is highly suggestive of a possible laryngeal injury. The physical examination findings of subcutaneous emphysema, the loss of the normal contour of the thyroid cartilage, and a palpable tracheal defect are most concerning for this condition.

○ **What formula should be used to calculate the fluid requirements for resuscitation of an adult burn victim during the first 24 hours of care?**

The Parkland formula: 2–4 mL × kg × % BSA involved. One half of this is given in the first 8 hours, and the second half is given over the next 16 hours.

○ **What is the adult dose of epinephrine for acute anaphylactic shock?**

0.3 mg of 1:10,000 IV or 0.3 mg of 1:1000 SQ.

○   **How should neurogenic shock be managed?**

The treatment of all patients with a suspected etiology of shock should start with the ABCs of **A**irway, **B**reathing, and **C**irculation. Additionally, appropriate fluid resuscitation should be instituted to restore the intravascular volume, blood pressure, and perfusion to vital organs. The use of vasopressors may prove beneficial, and typically vasopressors are required only for a brief 24–72 hours. Invasive hemodynamic monitoring may also be indicated but should be based upon the patient's age, associated injuries, and chronic medical conditions.

○   **What is the most common cause of airway obstruction in trauma?**

Unconscious patients: Tongue

Conscious patients: Dentures, avulsed teeth or other foreign bodies, oral secretions, and blood are the most common

○   **How much lactated Ringer solution should be infused while performing a diagnostic peritoneal lavage?**

Adults: 1 L of warmed normal saline

Children: 10 cc/kg of warmed normal saline

○   **What abdominal injuries are generally not recognized with the diagnostic peritoneal lavage (DPL) procedure?**

Diaphragmatic and retroperitoneal injuries.

○   **What two organs that do not typically bleed enough to produce a positive DPL when injured?**

The bladder and the small bowel.

○   **What criteria is used to indicate a positive diagnostic peritoneal lavage (DPL)?**

10 mL of gross blood on initial aspiration

>100,000 RBCs

>500 WBCs

Bacteria

Bile

Food particles

○   **Identify the zones of the neck and the appropriate method of evaluation for penetrating injuries to each zone:**

ZONE I: Extends from the clavicles to the cricoid cartilage

ZONE II: Extends from the cricoid cartilage to the angle of the mandible

ZONE III: Extends from the angle of the mandible to the base of the skull

For zone II injuries in patients who present with hemodynamic instability or with "hard signs" (rapidly expanding hematoma), immediate surgical exploration is strongly indicated. Stable patients may be evaluated in the same manner as stable zone I or III injured patients.

For stable patients presenting with injuries in zone I or III, an initial nonoperative evaluation is indicated, most frequently with the use of angiography. Other considerations are the use of computed tomographic (CT) or magnetic resonance (MR) angiography. There is also an emerging role for the use of bedside duplex ultrasound depending upon the experience of the clinician. Any unstable patient with a zone I or III related injury should undergo immediate surgical exploration.

○ **What is the etiology for the cause of death in an untreated tension pneumothorax?**

Decreased cardiac output. As a result of the mediastinal shift, the superior and inferior vena cava is compressed creating an impaired venus return and decreased cardiac output.

○ **What is the best method to open an airway while maintaining C-spine precautions?**

The jaw thrust maneuver.

○ **What is the formula for determining the appropriate ET tube size for children older than 1 year?**

The internal diameter of the appropriate endotracheal tube for a child will roughly equal the size of that child's little finger.

Uncuffed ET tube size = (age in years/4) + 4

Cuffed ET tube size = (age in years/4) + 3

○ **What is the correct ET tube size for a 1-year-old child?**

4.0–4.5 mm.

○ **What is the correct ET tube size for a 6-month-old child?**

4.0 mm.

○ **What is the average distance from the mouth to 2 cm above the carina in men and in women?**

Men: 23 cm; women: 21 cm.

○ **When should blood products be supplemented with fresh frozen plasma for a trauma patient receiving multiple units of transfused blood?**

A significant amount of ongoing research is being conducted on this topic and the common conclusion is that the higher the fresh frozen plasma to packed red blood cell ratio (FFP:PRBC) the higher the patient survivability. The current recommendation is for a ratio of 1:3, for every three units of PRBC, a single unit of FFP should be infused.

For each 5 units of transfused blood, fresh frozen plasma should be given.

○ **What is the Cushing reflex?**

The Cushing reflex is a hypothalamic response to ischemia in the brain. It consists of an increase in sympathetic outflow to the heart as an attempt to increase arterial blood pressure and total peripheral resistance, accompanied by bradycardia. The primary features of this reflex are increased systolic blood pressure and bradycardia.

○ **A core temperature of less than 33°C (mild hypothermia) is commonly associated with what complications?**

Metabolic acidosis, tachypnea, tachycardia, mental status changes, impaired coagulation, and decreased urine output.

○ **What are the six most lethal conditions involved with blunt force thoracic trauma?**

1. Airway obstruction
2. Tension pneumothorax
3. Cardia tamponade
4. Open pneumothorax
5. Massive hemothorax
6. Flail chest

○ **What, potentially life-threatening, conditions are most difficult to diagnose in patients experiencing blunt chest trauma?**

- Traumatic rupture of the aorta
- Major tracheobronchial disruption
- Blunt cardia injury
- Diaphragmatic tear
- Esophageal perforation
- Pulmonary contusion

○ **What are the three components to the Glasgow coma scale, and how many points is each worth?**

1. Eye opening: 4 points
2. Verbal response: 5 points
3. Motor response: 6 points

○ **What responses are measured while determining the Glasgow coma scale in a patient and what are their numerical values?**

	1	2	3	4	5	6
Eyes	Does not open eyes	Opens eyes in response to painful stimuli	Opens eyes in response to voice	Opens eyes spontaneously	N/A	N/A
Verbal	Makes no sounds	Incomprehensible sounds	Utters inappropriate words	Confused, disorientated	Oriented, converses normally	N/A
Motor	Makes no movements	Extension to painful stimuli	Abnormal flexion to painful stimuli	Flexion/withdrawal to painful stimuli	Localizes painful stimuli	Obeys commands

○ **What results are normal in the oculocephalic reflex?**

Conjugate eye movement is opposite to the direction of head rotation.

○ **When testing a patient's oculovestibular reflex, which direction of nystagmus is anticipated in response to cold water irrigation: toward or away from the irrigated ear?**

Away from the irrigated ear. Recall that nystagmus is defined as the direction of the fast component of saccadic eye movement. (*Remember*: COWS = **C**old **O**pposite, **W**arm **S**ame.)

○ **What does tonic eye movement toward an irrigated ear in response to warm caloric testing in a comatose patient signify?**

Life.

○ **What common finding on a sinus X-ray suggests a basilar skull fracture?**

Blood in the sphenoid sinus with a transsphenoid fracture pattern.

○ **The best view of the zygomatic arch on a face X-ray is:**

Standard facial series are the norm and are obtained with varying angulation of the X-ray beam vector. The Caldwell projection allows for visualization of the orbital floor and zygomatic process above the dense petrous pyramids. A submental vertex view affords excellent detail of the zygomatic arches. However, computed tomography (CT) scans have replaced radiographs in the evaluation of midfacial trauma and are the current modality of choice.

○ **Describe central cord syndrome:**

Traumatically, most commonly caused by severe neck hyperextension and injury to the ligamentum flavum with the following patient presentation:

Arm > leg weakness

Distil > proximal arm weakness

Variable sensory deficits

Bladder dysfunction

Frequently presents with a gradual improvement with traumatic mechanism of injury

○ **Under what conditions does trench (immersion) foot develop?**

Trench foot occurs when the extremity is exposed for several days to wet or cold conditions at temperatures that are above freezing. The extremity develops superficial damage resembling partial thickness burns.

○ **Describe pernio (chilblain):**

Exposure of an extremity for a prolonged period of time to dry, cold but above freezing temperatures. Patients develop superficial, small, edematous, painful ulcerations over the chronically exposed areas, most commonly the feet. Sensitivity of the surrounding skin, erythema, and pruritus may also develop.

○ **Describe frostnip:**

The skin becomes numb and blanched and then cessation of discomfort occurs. A sudden loss of the "cold" sensation at the location of injury is a reliable sign of precipitant frostbite. Frostnip will proceed to frostbite if treatment is not initiated.

○ **How is frostnip treated?**

It is treated by warming the affected area(s) by using the hands, breathing on the skin, or by placing the exposed extremities under the armpit. The affected part should not be rubbed because this treatment does not thaw the tissues completely.

○ **What are the proper classifications of frostbite?**

Superficial (first-degree injury): Erythema, edema, waxy appearance, hard white plaques, and sensory deficit.

Partial full-thickness (second-degree injury): Erythema, edema, and formation of blisters filled with clear or milky fluid and which are high in thromboxane. (These blisters form within 24 hours of injury.)

Complete full-thickness (third-degree injury): Damage affecting muscles, tendons, and bone, with resultant tissue loss.

○ **What is the appropriate treatment for frostbite?**

Do not use dry heat! The exposed extremity should be rewarmed rapidly by immersing the affected area in 38–41°C circulating water for 20 minutes or until flushing is observed. Elevation of the extremity will minimize the possibility of developing edema. Refreezing thawed tissue greatly increases damage. Remember to provide tetanus prophylaxis.

○ **What are the signs/symptoms of anterior cord syndrome?**

The common etiology is related to an anterior spinal artery infarction or injury. Patients presents with paralysis with loss of pain and temperature sensation below the level of the lesion that spares touch, vibration, and proprioception because that blood supply received from the posterior spinal arteries.

○ **What are some common complications of frostbite?**

Wound infection primary with *Staphylococcus aureus*, beta-hemolytic streptococci, gram-negative rods, or anaerobes. Tetanus (frostbite is considered a high-risk wound), hyperglycemia, metabolic acidosis, and tissue loss. In rare cases, rhabdomyolysis and compartment syndrome.

○ **What is the half-life of carboxyhemoglobin?**

4–6 hours on room air but can be reduced to approximately 40 minutes with the administration of 100% oxygen.

○ **What is the best method for transporting an amputated extremity?**

Wrap the extremity in sterile gauze, place it in waterproof plastic bag, and then immerse in ice.

○ **What organ is most severely affected in a blast injury?**

The lungs.

○ **What organ is most commonly affected in a blast injury?**

The middle and inner ear.

○ **What is the most effective method for decontaminating the skin following radiation exposure?**

Wash with soap and water after removing all clothes.

○ **What is the best emergency treatment of an Ellis III dental fracture in an adult?**

Cover the exposed surface with a calcium hydroxide composition (e.g., Dycal) or a glass ionomer.

Provide immediate dental follow-up and analgesics as needed.

Initiate antibiotics with coverage of intraoral flora (e.g., penicillin, clindamycin).

○ **What are the classic findings of shaken baby syndrome?**
- Failure to thrive
- Lethargy
- Seizures
- Retinal hemorrhages
- CT may show subarachnoid hemorrhage or subdural hematoma from torn bridging veins

○ **How do you treat a patient with a severe, high concentration hydrofluoric acid burn?**

Ensure that the caregivers are adequately protected. Decontaminate the patient with copious amounts of clean water while removing all of their clothing. If calcium gluconate gel is available, apply liberally to the affected area. For digital burns, if calcium gluconate gel is not available, the fingers may be soaked in magnesium hydroxide (Mylanta). Treat inhalation injuries with oxygen and 2.5% calcium gluconate nebulizer.

○ **How should an ocular burn secondary to hydrofluoric acid be treated?**

Generously irrigate with sterile water or saline for at least 15 minutes. Local anesthetic may be required. If pain persists, irrigate with a 1% solution of calcium gluconate.

○ **What electrolyte is depleted in a victim of a hydrofluoric acid burn?**

Hypocalcemia.

○ **An unconscious 60-year-old patient presents to the emergency department with a head injury. An ECG shows significant ST segment elevation. What is your main concern?**

Although MI should be considered and is quite probable, do not forget the possibility of an intracerebral hemorrhage. This may also cause significant ST segment elevation.

○ **A near-drowning victim is comatose and intubated. A diagnosis of severe pulmonary edema is made. What specific pulmonary treatment should be provided in the emergency department?**

It is important to give these patients PEEP early to increase alveolar pressure and alveolar volume. The increased lung volume increases the surface area by reopening and stabilizing collapsed or unstable alveoli.

○ **What laboratory abnormalities may be found with heat stroke?**

ABG analysis may reveal respiratory alkalosis due to direct CNS stimulation and metabolic acidosis due to lactic acidosis, hypoglycemia, hypernatremia, hypokalemia, and hypophosphatemia. CK levels exceeding 100,000 IU/mL are common. Elevated white blood cell counts are common as well as serum uric acid levels, blood urea nitrogen, and serum creatinine in patients whose course is complicated by renal failure myoglobinuria and proteinuria are frequently found on urinalysis.

○ **What distinguishes heat stroke from heat exhaustion?**

Heatstroke is the most severe form of the heat-related illnesses and is defined as a body temperature higher than 41.1°C (106°F) associated with neurologic dysfunction. Heat exhaustion is a milder form of heat-related illness that develops after several hours or days of exposure to high temperatures and inadequate or unbalanced replacement of fluids.

○ **How should a patient with heat stroke be treated?**

Heatstroke is a medical emergency and the rapid reduction of the core body temperature is the cornerstone of treatment because the duration of hyperthermia is the primary determinant of outcome.

Appropriate considerations include removal of restrictive clothing and spraying water on the body, covering the patient with ice water–soaked sheets, or placing ice packs in the axillae and groin may reduce the patient's temperature significantly. Patients who are unable to protect their airway should be intubated. Patients who are awake and responsive should receive supplemental oxygen. Intravenous lines may be placed in anticipation of fluid resuscitation and for the infusion of dextrose and thiamine if indicated.

○ **What complications can result from heat stroke?**

Renal failure, rhabdomyolysis, DIC, and seizures. *Remember*: Antipyretics are not recommended to reduce the core body temperature.

○ **A young boy presents for evaluation after suffering a coral snake bite. He has no complaints and appears to be in no distress. What is appropriate management?**

The onset of symptoms may be delayed up to 10 to 12 hours but may then be rapidly progressive. Admit this patient to the intensive care unit and monitor for impending respiratory failure. Coral snake venom has significant neurotoxicity and neuromuscular dysfunction is common.

○ **Describe the appearance of a coral snake:**

This is a round snake with red, yellow, and black stripes and a black spot on the head, which can easily be mistaken for the nonvenomous milk snake. The mnemonic "Red on yellow, kill a fellow; red on black, venom lack,"

○ **Which type of rattlesnake bite leads to most deaths?**

The Western diamond back rattlesnake accounts for nearly all lethal snakebites in the United States. However, it accounts for only 3% of the snakebites seen. Treat with 10 to 20 vials of antivenin.

○ **What are the physical attributes of a pit viper?**

The deep pits on each side of the triangular shaped head between the eye and the nostril tend to be a commonly recognizable feature. Research indicates that the pits are very sensitive detectors of radiant heat, thereby enabling the snake to find warm-blooded prey in the dark. Additionally, a pair of elongated fangs that are folded back against the palate of their triangular shaped head are a key feature.

○ **What is the recommended dose for steroids for treating patients with acute spinal cord injuries?**

Give high dose methylprednisolone (Solu-Medrol) 30 mg/kg bolus over 15 minutes followed by 45 minutes normal saline drip. Over the subsequent 23 hours, the patient should receive an infusion of 5.4 mg/kg/h of methylprednisolone.

○   **A patient with a temperature of 29°C develops ventricular fibrillation. Is defibrillation likely to be successful?**

Defibrillation is not indicated for patients experiencing severe hypothermia until they have been appropriated warmed.

○   **A straight (Miller) blade is preferred for intubating children of less than what age?**

Approximately 4 years of age.

○   **What is the Parkland formula for treating a pediatric burn victim weighing less than 25 kg?**

Ringer lactate at 3–4 mL/% TBSA burned/kg. One half of this should be infused over the first 8 hours with the remaining infused over the next 16 hours.

○   **How much fluid is required for maintenance of pediatric patients?**

100 mL/kg/day for each kg up to 10 kg, 50 mL/kg/day for each kg from 10 to 20 kg, and 20 mL/kg/day for each kg thereafter.

○   **A trauma patient, from a high speed MVC, presents with a complaint of a severe burning pain in the upper extremities and associated neck pain. On physical examination, the patient has good strength in his upper extremities and a significant decrease in sensation at his fingertips. There are no obvious neurologic deficits in the lower extremities with normal rectal tone. Radiographically, the patient's C-spine series is negative. What condition do you suspect and what diagnostic test should you order?**

Central cord syndrome. This injury is common with a hyperextension injury of the spinal cord. Impairment in the upper extremities is usually greater than in the lower extremities and is especially prevalent in the muscles of the hand. Pain and temperature sensations, as well as the sensation of light touch and of position sense, may be impaired below the level of injury. Neck pain and urinary retention are common complaints. MRIs demonstrates direct evidence of spinal cord impingement from bone, a disc, or a hematoma and are the diagnostic modality of choice. CT scanning of the cervical spine shows spinal canal compromise and allows the indirect approximation of the degree of spinal cord impingement.

○   **What is the common patient presentation of a laryngeal fracture and how are they diagnosed?**

Common signs of laryngeal injury include stridor, subcutaneous emphysema, hemoptysis, hematoma, ecchymosis, laryngeal tenderness, vocal cord immobility, loss of anatomical landmarks, and bony crepitus. CT scanning is the imaging modality of choice to assess laryngeal anatomy. The Schaefer classification of laryngeal injuries is based on a combination of the CT and endoscopic findings, which dictate treatment modalities.

○   **When does dysbaric air embolism (DAE) typically occur?**

DAE develops within minutes of surfacing after SCUBA diving. Symptoms are sudden and dramatic; they include loss of consciousness, focal neurologic symptoms (such as monoplegia, convulsions, blindness, and confusion), and sensory disturbances. Sudden loss of consciousness or other acute neurologic deficits immediately after surfacing is because of DAE unless proven otherwise. Treatment includes high flow oxygen and rapid transport for hyperbaric oxygen treatment.

○ **A 2-year-old has jammed a pencil into her lateral soft palate. What complication might develop?**

Penetrating injury to the internal carotid artery (ICA) with resultant neurologic deficit is a well-documented complication in children. In addition to the potential of thrombotic injury, the development of a collection of air in the retropharyngeal space can result in mediastinitis.

○ **In a trauma patient, what is the physical examination finding of dimpling of the unilateral cheek associated with?**

Zygomatic arch fracture.

○ **A patient sustains blunt force trauma to his face and mouth and you observe that a tooth has been fractured. Upon closer examination you note that blood is originating from the tooth and there is no additional intraoral injury. What is the Ellis classification?**

Ellis III fractures involve enamel, dentin, and pulp; patients complain of pain with manipulation, air, and temperature. Pinkish or reddish markings around surrounding dentin or blood in the center of the tooth from the exposed pulp may present.

○ **What is the most common location involved in the malposition of an orotracheal endotracheal tube?**

The right mainstem bronchus is the common location for a tube placed in the trachea; however, the most common location for an improperly placed endotracheal tube is the esophagus.

○ **A diver descends to 33 feet. How many atmospheres of pressure is he experiencing?**

2 atmospheres. Sea level is considered 1 atm and atmospheric pressure doubles every 33 ft. 2 atm = 33 feet; 3 atm = 66 feet.

○ **What are the most common complaints in patients with carbon monoxide poisoning?**

A headache is most common, followed by dizziness, weakness, and nausea.

○ **A patient presents after experiencing trauma to the head. He has an elevated systolic blood pressure and bradycardia. What is this reflex?**

Cushing reflex.

○ **What is the name for a flexion mechanism fracture through the anterior aspect of a vertebral body that is associated with ligamentous damage and an anterior cord syndrome?**

A flexion teardrop fracture occurs when flexion of the spine, along with vertical axial compression, causes a fracture of the anteroinferior aspect of the vertebral body. This fragment is displaced anteriorly and resembles a teardrop. For this fragment to be produced, significant posterior ligamentous disruption must occur. Since the fragment displaces anteriorly, a significant degree of anterior ligamentous disruption exists. This injury involves disruption of all three columns, making this an extremely unstable fracture that frequently is associated with spinal cord injury.

○ **What nerves control the corneal reflex?**

The afferent limb is V1 (ophthalmic) of the trigeminal nerve; the efferent limb is the facial or 7th cranial nerve.

○ **A patient presents with a hypertension-type neck injury after receiving a blow to the forehead. She complains of weakness in her arms and no weakness in her lower extremities. What is the most likely diagnosis?**

Central cord syndrome.

○ **You are evaluating a patient with an obvious traumatic spinal cord injury. On physical examination, he has motor paralysis, loss of gross proprioception, loss of vibratory sensation on one side, and loss of pain and temperature sensation on the opposite side. What is the likely diagnosis?**

Brown-Séquard syndrome.

○ **A patient presents after sustaining a high-speed traumatic injury to the chest. A systolic murmur over the precordium is auscultated and the patient has a slightly hoarse voice, and her pulse is stronger in the upper extremities. What is the most likely diagnosis?**

Traumatic rupture of the aorta.

○ **What is the most common X-ray finding in traumatic rupture of the aorta?**

Widening of the superior mediastinum.

○ **A patient presents with a history of blunt chest trauma, a 5/6 systolic murmur that radiates to the axillae, and an infarct pattern on ECG. What is the likely diagnosis?**

Traumatic ventricular septal defect.

○ **A patient who has been involved in a motor vehicle accident has X-ray findings of retroperitoneal air with obliteration of the right psoas margin on a flat plate of the abdomen. What is a likely diagnosis?**

Duodenal injury. Patients that are hemodynamically normal should undergo an Upper Gastrointestinal (UGI) study with a water-soluble contrast (Gastrografin).

○ **About how many liters of blood can a patient lose in the retroperitoneal space after sustaining a pelvic fracture?**

4 L before venous tamponade occurs.

○ **What is the most common cause of superior vena cava obstruction?**

Bronchogenic carcinoma.

○ **What laboratory abnormalities are found in times of stress?**

Increased cortisol, glucose intolerance, cholesterol, and platelet adhesion plus impaired lipoprotein ratios

○ **A patient opens his eyes to voice, makes incomprehensible sounds, and withdraws from painful stimulus. What is his GCS?**

E 3, V 2, M 4 = **9.**

○ **What acronym is commonly used during the evaluation of a patient with suspected rhabdomyolysis?**

MUSCLE = Rhabdomyolysis (evaluation)

Myoglobinuria
Urinalysis
Serum potassium
Creatinine
Lysis sign on CBC (hemolysis)
Enzyme (CPK) increase

○ **A trauma patient has blood at the urinary meatus. What test should be ordered?**

Retrograde urethrogram; 10 mL of radiocontrast solution should be injected into the urinary meatus.

○ **In blunt trauma, what is the most common renal pedicle injury?**

Renal artery thrombosis.

○ **A trauma patient presents with a "rocking horse" type of ventilation. What is the diagnosis?**

Probable high spinal cord injury with intercostal muscle paralysis.

○ **What is the differential diagnosis for a trauma patient presenting with subcutaneous emphysema.**

Pneumothorax, tension pneumothorax, tracheal/bronchial injury, or pneumomediastinum.

○ **What rib fracture has the worst prognosis?**

The first rib. First and second rib fractures are associated with bronchial tears, vascular injury, and myocardial contusions.

○ **A patient presents to the emergency department after a motor vehicle accident with hematuria and fractures of the tenth and eleventh ribs. What internal organ might be damaged?**

The spleen is the most commonly injured organ in blunt trauma and be especially suspicious of splenic trauma if the tenth or eleventh ribs are fractured and the patient has hematuria.

○ **For a trauma victim, what test is most helpful for evaluating retroperitoneal organs?**

CT.

○ **Where should the incision be made to perform a DPL on a trauma patient with a suspected pelvic fracture?**

A supraumbilical incision should be made to avoid insertion of the DPL catheter into a contained pelvic hematoma. Performing a FAST examination may be more clinically appropriate especially if the patient does not have hemodynamically normal vital signs.

○ **What is an absolute contraindication to DPL?**

The only absolute contraindication is the obvious need for laparotomy. Relative contraindications are previous abdominal surgery, morbid obesity, and pregnancy.

○ **What findings represent a positive DPL in blunt trauma?**

RBC > 100,000 cells/mm^3, WBC > 500 cells/mm^3, bile, bacteria, or vegetable material.

○ **What type of intracranial hemorrhage is more common in the geriatric patient?**

Subdural hematomas are most common.

○ **The inability to pass a nasogastric tube in a trauma victim suggests damage to what organ?**

A rupture of the left hemidiaphragm secondary to a diaphragmatic hernia.

● ● ● **REFERENCES** ● ● ●

Britt L, Trunkey DD, Feliciano DV *Acute Care Surgery—Principles and Practice.* New York, NY: Springer-Verlag; 2007.

Doherty GM, Way L. *Current Surgical Diagnosis and Treatment.* 12th ed. New York, NY: McGraw-Hill; 2006.

Peitzman AB, Rhodes M, Schwab CW, Yealy DM, Fabian TC. *The Trauma Manual.* 2nd ed. Philadelphia, PA: Lippincott, Williams & Wilkins; 2002.

Tintinalli MJ, Kelen MG, Stapczynski MJ, Ma MO, Cline MD. *Tintinalli's Emergency Medicine—A Comprehensive Study Guide.* 6th ed. New York, NY: McGraw-Hill; 2004.

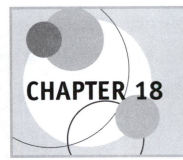

CHAPTER 18   Pharmacology/ Toxicology

Daniel Thibodeau, MHP, PA-C

● ● ● GENERAL PRINCIPLES ● ● ●

○ **What are the two mechanisms of drug metabolism and breakdown?**

Hepatic and renal.

○ **Which enzyme is mostly responsible for drug breakdown in the liver?**

Cytochrome P-450.

○ **What are the three methods of drug excretion from the kidneys?**

Glomerular filtration, proximal renal secretion, and distal tubule reabsorbtion.

● ● ● AUTONOMIC NERVOUS SYSTEM ● ● ●

○ **Which transmitter is released at all preganglionic and postganglionic receptors?**

Acetylcholine. This interaction of acetylcholine with pre- and postganglionic receptors gives the "flight or fight" responses.

○ **What are the two receptors of acetylcholine?**

Muscarinic and nicotinic.

○ **What effect does the sympathetic nervous system have on the cardiovascular system?**

Increases heart rate and contractility. Parasympathetic system would then reverse this and decrease heart rate.

○ **Which organs have both sympathetic and parasympathetic innervation?**

Heart, eyes, bronchial smooth muscle, and GI and GU smooth muscle.

○ **What are some of the main activities of β₁-, β₂-, and α-receptors?**

β₁-Heart regulation

β₂-Smooth muscle relaxation

α-Contraction and constriction, mostly vasoconstriction

○ **What effect does the activation of presynaptic α₂-receptors cause?**

It facilitates the release of norepinephrine.

○ **What are some common anticholinergics side effects?**

Dry eyes, dry mouth, blurred vision, constipation, and urinary retention.

○ **What are some uses of muscarinic antagonists?**

They can be used for problems with urinary frequency, urgency, as well as incontinence.

○ **Name the mechanism of action for neuromuscular blockers:**

They act as competitive blockers at the nicotinic receptors to cause muscle relaxation.

○ **What is the mechanism of action for succinylcholine?**

It is a depolarizing neuromuscular blocker.

○ **What is the one potentially fatal side effect of succinylcholine?**

It can cause malignant hyperthermia.

○ **What are the two substances that can activate both α- and β-receptors?**

Epinephrine and norepinephrine. However, norepinephrine has less of an effect on β₂-receptors, making it less effective on actions of bronchospasm like that of epinephrine.

○ **What is the main effect of dopamine?**

It causes renal and coronary vasodilation as well as activates the β₁-receptors of the heart at low doses.

○ **Name the two major actions that norepinephrine plays on the cardiovascular system:**

It causes an increase in total peripheral resistance and increases mean arterial pressure.

○ **α-agonists have what type of effect on the cardiovascular system?**

They act by reducing the sympathetic nerve activity, thus lowering blood pressure.

○ **What are the major side effects of α-agonists?**

As you could imagine, postural hypotension and reflex tachycardia.

○ **Why should you worry about giving a β-blocker to a diabetic patient?**

They can stimulate the sympathetic activity of glycogenolysis, gluconeogenesis, as well as lipolysis.

○ **What are some other side effects of β-blockers?**

Bronchoconstriction and decreased heart rate.

○ **What is the clinical presentation of anticholinergic poisoning?**

Mydriasis, tachycardia, hypoactive bowel sounds, urinary retention, dry axilla, hyperthermia, and mental status changes. *Remember*:

Dry as a bone

Red as a beet

Mad as a hatter

Hot as Hades

Blind as a bat

○ **Name a few substances that have anticholinergic properties:**

Antihistamines, cyclic antidepressants, phenothiazine, atropine, and, jimson weed.

○ **What ECG abnormality is most common in patients who suffer from anticholinergic toxicity?**

Sinus tachycardia. Other dangerous arrhythmias include conduction problems and V-Tach.

○ **What are the common anticholinergic compounds?**

Atropine, tricyclic antidepressants, antihistamines, phenothiazine, antiparkinsonian drugs, belladonna alkaloids, and some Solanaceae plants (i.e., deadly nightshade and jimson weed).

• • • CARDIOVASCULAR SYSTEM • • •

○ **What are the three groups of diuretics?**

Thiazide, loop, and potassium-sparing diuretics.

○ **How do the thiazide diuretics function?**

They limit the sodium and chloride reabsorption in the ascending loop. This in turn increases the urine production.

○ **What drug is the treatment of choice in hypertension?**

Thiazide diuretics.

○ **What is a main side effect of thiazide diuretics?**

Hypokalemia.

○ **How does the potassium sparing diuretics function?**

They act as an antagonist of aldosterone, which will lead to sodium retention.

○ **The use of ACE inhibitors functions to lower blood pressure by what mechanism?**

They convert angiotensin I to angiotensin II, which acts as an aldosterone antagonist, which in turn lowers pressure by retaining sodium.

○ **Unlike β-blockers, what advantage does ACE inhibitors have for the treatment of hypertension?**

They are ideal for diabetics because they do not affect gluconeogenesis.

○ **Name some major side effects of ACE inhibitors:**

Headache, dizziness, abdominal pain, confusion, renal failure, and erectile dysfunction.

○ **What is one of the most common side effects of ACE inhibitors?**

Cough.

○ **Do angiotensin II receptor antagonists cause cough?**

No.

○ **What is the main physiological effect by calcium channel blockers?**

They reduce cardiac afterload by blocking calcium entrance into cells.

○ **Name some of the most common side effects of calcium channel blockers:**

Headaches, dizziness, hypotension. Anything that you can imagine with the action of vasodilation can occur in calcium channel blockers.

○ **What action do nitrates have on blood vessels and the cardiac cycle?**

They vasodilate, which in turn causes a reduction in cardiac preload. At higher concentrations, nitrates will decrease afterload also.

○ **What drug is the treatment of choice for relieving coronary vasospasm?**

Nitroglycerine.

○ **What forms of nitrates can be given?**

Oral, intravenous, sublingual, and transdermal.

○ **Which nitrate when metabolized turns into cyanide?**

Sodium nitroprusside.

○ **What are the two main side effects of nitrates?**

Headache and hypotension. Another possible side effect is postural hypotension.

○ **What is the main goal in the treatment of coronary artery disease?**

Reduction of myocardial oxygen demand.

○ **What are the three pharmacologic principles in the treatment of heart failure?**

Decreasing the cardiac workload, controlling excess fluid, and enhancement of myocardial contractility.

○ **What are the main effects of ACE inhibitors with regard to heart failure?**

They reduce cardiac workload. This will slow the progression of heart failure, which in turn prolongs survival.

○ **What class of drugs is used as a mainstay in controlling the excess fluid accumulation in heart failure?**

Diuretics.

○ **How do the cardiac glycosides (digoxin and digitoxin) function to improve myocardial contractility?**

They inhibit the Na^+-K^+-ATPase pump, which improves contractility.

○ **A 77-year-old male patient with a history of heart failure has been taking both furosemide and digoxin for several months. Over the past 3 weeks, he has noticed having nausea, fatigue, drowsiness, and blurred vision. What could be the possible problem in this patient?**

Digoxin toxicity.

○ **What effect, if any, do diuretics play on the role of digoxin?**

If a patient on diuretics is not closely monitored for hypokalemia, lower serum potassium levels can have higher than normal therapeutic levels of digoxin, thus leading to possible toxicity.

○ **What are some of the common side effects resulting from digoxin toxicity?**

Arrhythmias, anorexia, nauseam diarrhea, drowsiness, fatigue, and visual disturbances (including a yellow visual appearance).

○ **What is the mechanism of dobutamine in the use of heart failure?**

It increases cardiac output and can be used in cardiac shock.

○ **Name three nonpharmacologic treatments for arrhythmias:**

Pacemakers, implantable defibrillators, and ablation therapy.

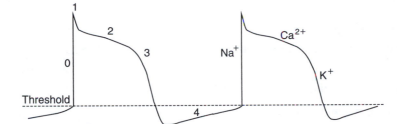

Figure 18-1 (Cardiac action potential. Note the first action potential shows the class of antiarrhythmics and where they have action. Note the second action potential and what electrolyte plays a major role in that part of the action potential. (Reproduced, with permission, from Stringer JL. *Basic Concepts in Pharmacology.* 3rd ed. New York, NY: McGraw-Hill; 2006: Fig 13-1.))

○ **What is the role of class I antiarrhythmic drugs?**

They are sodium channel blockers.

○ **Class IA drugs such as procainamide and quinidine are useful in what type of arrhythmias?**

Both atrial and ventricular arrhythmias.

○ **Lidocaine is an IB antiarrhythmic. What type of arrhythmias does this drug work best?**

Treatment of ventricular arrhythmias such as ventricular tachycardia, ventricular fibrillation, and ventricular ectopy.

○ **Are drugs like lidocaine effective in the treatment of supraventricular tachycardia?**

No, they have almost no effect on this type of arrhythmia.

○ **What is the mechanism by the class IC medications?**

They are used to suppress ventricular arrhythmias.

○ **What effects do β-blockers have on the sinoatrial (SA) and atrioventricular (AV) nodes?**

They slow the conduction at these sites, thus slowing the refractory period.

○ **β-blockers are useful in the treatment of which arrhythmias?**

They are useful in tachyarrhythmias as they can slow transmission.

○ **Amiodarone is a potassium channel blocker. Describe how this drug functions as an antiarrhythmic:**

It acts by slowing the repolarization of the action potential without impairing the resting potential prior to depolarization.

○ **Are calcium channel blockers more effective toward atrial or ventricular arrhythmias?**

Atrial. They slow the conduction at the AV node, which increases the refractory period.

○ **What drug is the treatment of choice for paroxysmal supraventricular tachycardia?**

Adenosine.

○ **Does adenosine have a long half-life?**

No, in fact, it is only seconds long, which is why it is favorable in converting SVT.

○ **What are three drugs that will increase heart rate?**

Atropine, epinephrine, and isoproterenol.

○ **What is the first-line pharmacologic treatment of hypercholesterolemia?**

HMG-CoA reductase inhibitors. These are referred to as the "statins."

○ **What is the effect of statins with respect to cholesterol?**

It lowers serum LDL and plasma cholesterol.

○ **What does niacin do for overall cholesterol levels?**

It lowers both overall cholesterol as well as triglycerides.

○ **What are the two side effects of niacin?**

Flushing of the skin and liver toxicity.

○ **If you have a patient who gets the typical flushing of the skin with the taking of niacin, what can you instruct the patient to do to help reduce this side effect?**

Usually, taking the medication with an 81 mg aspirin will help as well as instructing the patient to take the medication at night.

○ **Gemfibrozil, fenofibrate, and clofibrate, the so-called "fibrates," act to lower what to lipid values?**

They can lower triglycerides and HDL.

○ **Hemostasis consists of what three phases?**

Vascular (from tissue injury), platelet, and coagulation phases.

○ **What is the main synthesis component, which causes the formation of coagulation?**

Thromboxane A_2.

○ **What is the action of nonsteroidal anti-inflammatory drugs?**

They inhibit prostaglandins, which inhibit platelet aggregation and prolong bleeding time.

○ **How do drugs like ticlopidine and clopidogrel work as "blood thinners"?**

They inactivate the platelet adenosine diphosphate receptors, which in turn inhibit platelet aggregation.

○ **Which receptors are critical for the formation of platelet aggregation?**

Glycoprotein IIb/IIIa receptors. They prevent platelet aggregation by blocking fibrinogen and von Willebrand factors.

○ **What is the main side effect of all platelet inhibitors?**

They all can cause bleeding. That is also the main side effect of anticoagulants.

○ **Does heparin interact with the intrinsic or extrinsic coagulation pathway?**

Actually, both. It binds to antithrombin III and inactivates IIa, IXa, Xa, XIa, XIIa, XIII, and III.

○ **What anticoagulant has a longer half-life: heparin or low-molecular-weight heparin (LMWH)?**

Low-molecular-weight heparin.

○ **Which types of patients should avoid the use of LMWH?**

Those with renal impairment or those with bleeding abnormalities.

○ **What is the antidote to heparin?**

Protamine sulfate.

○ **What is the mechanism of action of warfarin?**

It is an antagonist of vitamin K.

○ **If administration of vitamin K is the antidote for warfarin overdose, how long does it take for the anticoagulant properties to take effect?**

At a minimum, 24 hours. Additional measures such as fresh frozen plasma and platelet transfusions can be given if emergency measures are required.

○ **What is the mechanism of action on thrombolytic agents?**

They act as plasminogen activators to lyse clots that have already formed. The plasminogen will convert to plasmin, which then causes the degradation of fibrin.

○ **What is the main side effect of thrombolytic agents?**

Bleeding, naturally.

○ **What can be a serious life-threatening side effect from streptokinase?**

An allergic-anaphylactic reaction. This is usually because streptokinase is created from a bacterial origin.

○ **Which drugs cause methemoglobinemia?**

Oxidant drugs, such as antimalarials, dapsone, nitrites/nitrates (nitroprusside), and local anesthetics (lidocaine). Methemoglobinemia occurs when the iron moiety of hemoglobin is oxidated from the ferrous to the ferric state.

○ **Which common enzyme deficiency predisposes to the development of methemoglobinemia in the presence of the above drugs?**

G6PD deficiency.

○ **What drugs can induce a chronic cough?**

ACE inhibitors cause chronic cough as a result of the accumulation of prostaglandins, kinins, or substances that excite the cough receptors. (Remember that ACE sitting next to you at the boards!!). β-Blockers evoke bronchoconstriction, and thus coughing, by blocking β-2 receptors. Never give β-blockers to asthmatic patients or other patients with an airway disease.

○ **What is the incidence of cough induced by captopril?**

1% to 2%.

○ **What is the incidence of enalapril-induced cough?**

24.7%.

○ **True/False: Generally, the cough related to ACE inhibitors resolves within a few days of withdrawal of the drug:**

False. The resolution of cough may be slow, taking several weeks.

○ **How does treatment for a cocaine-induced MI differ from a typical MI?**

Both are treated the same except that β-blockers are <u>not</u> used for a cocaine-induced MI secondary to potential unopposed α-adrenergic activity. The tachycardia of a cocaine-associated MI is first treated with benzodiazepine sedation.

○ **A patient has an arterial pH of 7.5 through alkalization, but her urine pH is still low. What electrolyte is probably responsible?**

Potassium. When reabsorbing sodium, the renal tubules will preferentially excrete hydrogen ions into the tubular lumen rather than potassium ions. Thus, potassium should be maintained at 4.0 mmol/L.

○ **What are the absolute indications for Digibind administration in digoxin poisoning?**

Ventricular arrhythmias, hemodynamically significant bradyarrhythmias that are unresponsive to standard therapy, and a potassium level greater than 5.0 mEq/L.

○ **A patient on Digoxin is bradycardic and hypotensive with significantly peaked T waves. What is the initial line of treatment?**

Administer 10 vials of Digibind intravenously while simultaneously treating the presumed hyperkalemia with insulin and glucose, sodium bicarbonate, and Kayexalate. After the Digibind is administered, hyperkalemic-induced arrhythmias may safely be treated with calcium chloride.

○ **What is the antidote for β-blocker poisoning?**

Glucagon. Glucagon receptors, located on myocardial cells, are G protein coupled receptors that activate adenylate cyclase, leading to increased levels of intracellular cAMP. Thus, glucagon administration causes the same intracellular effect as β-agonist.

○ **What are potential treatment modalities for a calcium channel blocker poisoning?**

Therapeutic interventions include IV calcium, isoproterenol, glucagon, transvenous pacer, atropine, and vasopressors, such as norepinephrine, epinephrine, or dopamine.

○ **What is the mechanism and treatment for clonidine-induced hypotension?**

Treatment: Includes IV fluid administration and dopamine.

Mechanism: Decreased cardiac output secondary to a decreased sympathetic outflow from the CNS.

○ **What typical eye response is related to clonidine poisoning?**

Pinpoint pupils.

○ **Clonidine is a centrally acting presynaptic α-2 adrenergic agonist that decreases the central sympathetic outflow. Although its primary use is to treat hypertension, clonidine has additional emergency value in blunting withdrawal symptoms from opiates and ethanol. A clonidine overdose closely resembles an overdose with which other class of drugs?**

Opiates.

○ **Toxicity from clonidine (Catapres) usually occurs within what time period?**

Within 4 hours.

○ **Which agent is a useful "antidote" for clonidine overdose?**

Naloxone (Narcan)

○ **True/False: A patient with acute digitalis OD presents with frequent multifocal PVCs, peaked T waves, and a K+ of 6.2 mEq/L. The correct treatment is to first administer $CaCl_2$, as this is the fastest-acting agent for reducing hyperkalemia:**

False! Although $CaCl_2$ is the fastest-acting agent for decreasing hyperkalemia, don't give any more Ca+ to a patient with digitalis-induced cardiac toxicity.

○ **β-Adrenergic antagonists have three main effects on the heart. Name these effects:**

1. Negative chronotropy
2. Negative inotropy
3. Decrease AV nodal conduction velocity (negative dromotropy)

○ **True/False: β-adrenergic antagonists can cause mental status changes and seizures:**

True.

○ **A cocaine addict presents with chest pain but his ECG is normal. What are the odds that he will have abnormal CPK and CPK-MB isoenzymes?**

6%–19%.

○ **What is the most common arrhythmia induced by chronic, heavy ethanol bingeing ?**

Atrial fibrillation.

○ **What is the antidote for nitrites?**

Methylene blue 1%, 0.2 mL/kg IV over 5 minutes. Severe methemoglobinemia requires an exchange transfusion.

○ **What are the effects of dopamine at various doses?**

1–10 mg/kg: Renal, mesenteric, coronary, and cerebral vasodilation
10–20 mg/kg: Both α- and β-adrenergic
20 mg/kg: Primarily α-adrenergic

○ **Methylene blue is used to treat:**

Methemoglobinemia.

○ **What are the signs and symptoms of isopropanol poisoning?**

Sweet breath odor (acetone), hypotension, hemorrhagic gastritis, and CNS depression from isopropanol and from its metabolite, acetone.

● ● ● **CENTRAL NERVOUS SYSTEM** ● ● ●

○ **What is the main pharmacologic goal in the treatment of Alzheimer disease?**

It is to maintain or elevate the level of acetylcholine by preventing the breakdown of acetylcholine.

○ **Define the following terms: Tolerance, cross-tolerance, and dependence:**

Tolerance is the state by which there is a reduced drug effect with repeated use of the medication. This will necessitate the requirement for more of a medication to produce the same desired result.

Cross-tolerance refers to a patient who is tolerant to one drug will also be tolerant to drugs that are in the same class.

Dependence is signs and symptoms of withdrawal when drug levels fall.

○ **Name the type of medication to use for the following specific seizures: generalized convulsive, partial (simple, complex, secondary), and generalized nonconvulsive:**

Seizure type	Medication of choice
Generalized convulsive	Valproate
	Carbamazepine
Partial (includes simple, complex, and secondarily generalized)	Carbamazepine
	Phenytoin
Generalized nonconvulsive	Ethosuximide
	Valproate

○ **How are all these antiepileptic medications metabolized?**

Hepatic.

○ **What are two major conditions that can be seen with the use of carbamazepine?**

Granulocyte suppression and apastic anemia.

○ **Name some common side effects of phenytoin:**

Hirsutism, coarse facial features, and gingival hyperplasia. With higher doses, it can cause ataxia and nystagmus.

○ **Are antipsychotic and neuroleptic drugs considered to be medications that can cure these diseases?**

No. They are not curative; they only allow the patient to function in a more normal state.

○ **What is the mechanism of neuroleptics?**

They are α-blockers, muscarinic, and histamine antagonists.

○ **What is a common side effect with most antipsychotic drugs?**

Extrapyramidal side effects (EPS).

○ **Name the more common EPSs and give some examples of each:**

Dystonia—spasms of the face, neck, tongue, and back

Parkinsonism—rigidity, shuffling gait, and tremor

Akathisia—motor restlessness

Tardive dyskinesia—lip smacking, jaw movements, darting of the tongue, and quick involuntary movements

○ **What is neuroleptic malignant syndrome?**

It is a rare syndrome that is potentially fatal as a result of the use of neuroleptic medications. It becomes more common as the doses of medications increase.

○ **What are some of the signs of neuroleptic malignant syndrome?**

These will present with severe forms of parkinsonism, catatonia, autonomic instability, and in some cases stupor.

○ **What is the mortality rate for a patient with neuroleptic malignant syndrome?**

About 10% to 20%.

○ **What are the three targets for the pharmacologic treatment of Parkinson disease?**

Dopamine replacement therapy, dopamine agonist therapy, and anticholinergic therapy.

○ **Which dopamine crosses the blood brain barrier (BBB)?**

Levodopa.

○ **Carbidopa does not cross the BBB. How does this drug function?**

It reduces the peripheral metabolism of l-dopa in the bloodstream, which in turn will increase the amount of dopamine going to the brain.

○ **Anticholinergics therapy reduces the effectiveness of uninhibited cholinergic neurons. Describe some of the side effects that these drugs commonly have:**

They are all the muscarinic side effects that you should be familiar with; dry mouth, confusion, constipation, and urinary retention.

○ **The two main anxiolytic and hypnotic drug classes are barbiturates and benzodiazepines. What are the main side effects of these two classes of drugs?**

Sedation and most induce sleep or hypnosis. At higher doses, they can induce medullary depression and death.

○ **What is the mechanism of action of barbiturates?**

They enhance the function of γ-aminobutyric acid (GABA) in the CNS.

○ **What are some potential side effects of barbiturates if not taken appropriately?**

Sedation, hypnosis, coma, suppression of respiration, and death.

○ **A 42-year-old male patient who has been on phenobarbital for the last several years arrives to the emergency department with nausea, vomiting, hypotension, and acute psychosis. By history, you have been told that he has not been taking his phenobarbital that he is normally prescribed. What is the probable diagnosis?**

Withdrawal symptoms secondary to barbiturate use. Other signs and symptoms include seizures and cardiovascular collapse, which can lead to death.

○ **What is the mechanism of action of benzodiazepines?**

They block a specific site associated with $GABA_A$ receptors which increases inhibition.

○ **A 23-year-old female patient presents to the emergency department with a suspected benzodiazepine overdose. She has shallow respirations, is hypoxic, and also has confusion, agitation, and restlessness. What is the antidote that could be given in this scenario?**

Flumazenil.

○ **Name one benzodiazepine does not produce dependence:**

Buspirone.

○ **What is the common mechanism of action of antidepressants and lithium?**

They all act by increasing the concentration of norepinephrine and serotonin.

○ **What are some indications for prescribing serotonin-selective reuptake inhibitors (SSRI)?**

Depression, eating disorders, panic disorders, obsessive–compulsive, and borderline personality disorders.

○ **What is the usual onset of improvement of symptoms after starting tricyclic antidepressants?**

It usually takes 2–3 weeks for patients to have a noticeable difference.

○ **How do heterocyclics work as antidepressants?**

They are potent muscarinic cholinergic antagonists, and have weak α_1 and H_1 antagonist properties.

○ **What is the mechanism of action of monoamine oxidase inhibitors?**

They increase levels of norepinephrine, serotonin, and dopamine by preventing the degradation of these products.

○ **What is the one major complication in taking an MAO inhibitor?**

They can cause a fatal hypertensive crisis.

○ **What are some foods that patients on MAO inhibitors should avoid?**

Cheeses, beer, and red wines. Any foods that have higher levels of tyramine or other active amines should be avoided.

○ **What are the three most common drugs that are used in the treatment of bipolar disease?**

Lithium, carbamazepine, and valproate.

○ **What is the major receptor for the mediation of pain?**

μ(mu)-Receptors. The other receptors that have less activity are kappa(κ) and delta(δ).

○ **What are the three main types of narcotics? Give some examples of each:**

1. Agonists—codeine, fentanyl, heroin, morphine, methadone, meperidine
2. Mixed agonist–antagonist—pentazocine, buprenorphine, nalbuphine
3. Antagonists—naloxone, naltrexone, and nalmefene

○ **Name some signs and symptoms from narcotic withdraw:**

Hyperactivity, nausea, vomiting, chills, fever, tearing, runny nose, tremor, abdominal pain, and cramps.

○ **What are the main effects of morphine?**

Analgesia, respiratory depression, spasm of the smooth muscle of the GI and GU tracts, and pinpoint pupils.

○ **What is the potency of fentanyl when compared to morphine?**

It is 80 times more potent but has a much shorter half-life.

○ **What is the indication for the use of methadone?**

It is used for narcotic withdraw and dependence. It acts by reducing the craving for narcotics.

○ **What is the drug of choice to reverse a narcotic overdose?**

Naloxone.

○ **What factors influence the elimination of inhaled anesthetics?**

The rate of ventilation, blood flow, and the solubility of the gas itself.

○ **What is the mechanism of action for local anesthetics?**

They block nerve conduction by the local application of the drug. They do this by blocking the sodium channel of the nerve membrane.

○ **Why should not the 600 mg/day of thioridazine (Mellaril) be exceeded?**

Exceeding this dosage causes retinitis pigmentosa. Thioridazine is a piperidine phenothiazine with low frequency extrapyramidal effects.

○ **Why is haloperidol one of the preferred neuroleptics?**

It can be used IM in emergencies, plus it has few side effects. It does, however, have a high frequency of extrapyramidal effects.

○ **What is the only neuroleptic with tardive dyskinesia as a side effect?**

Clozapine. Unfortunately, patients taking clozapine can develop agranulocytosis and are at a higher risk for seizures than patients on other neuroleptics. Other side effects include hypotension, anticholinergic symptoms, and oversedation.

○ **What happens when ethanol is combined with an anxiolytic (benzodiazepine)?**

Death can occur due to the combined respiratory depressive effects.

○ **Name another contraindication to benzodiazepine use:**

Known hypersensitivity, acute narrow angle glaucoma, and pregnancy, especially in the first trimester.

○ **What should be used to treat a hypertensive crisis caused by the combination of MAO inhibitors with a known toxin?**

An α- and β-adrenergic antagonist, such as labetalol. Also consider nifedipine or nitroglycerin. If unsuccessful, consider IV phentolamine or sodium nitroprusside.

○ **Name some drugs contraindicated in a patient on MAO inhibitors:**

Meperidine (Demerol) and dextromethorphan can cause toxic reactions, such as excitation and hyperpyrexia. The effects of indirect-acting adrenergic drugs are potentiated, including ephedrine, sympathomimetic amines in cold remedies, amphetamines, cocaine, and methylphenidate (Ritalin).

○ **Name the three common MAO inhibitors (chemical and brand name):**

1. Phenelzine (Nardil)
2. Isocarboxazid (Marplan)
3. Tranylcypromine (Parnate)

○ **Name eight drugs that decrease sexual desire:**

1. Antidepressants
2. Antihypertensives
3. Anticonvulsants
4. Neuroleptics
5. Cimetidine
6. Digitalis
7. Clofibrate
8. High doses or chronic ingestion of alcohol or street drugs

○ **What is the first cardiac finding in a cyclic antidepressant overdose?**

Sinus tachycardia.

○ **How long should a tricyclic antidepressant overdose patient, demonstrating tachycardia and conduction disturbances, be monitored?**

24 hours.

○ **What major tranquilizer displays the most hypotensive tendency?**

Thorazine.

○ **What is the most significant pathophysiologic mechanism of death from cyclic antidepressants?**

Myocardial depression, including hypotension and conduction blocks.

○ **What antibiotic may either increase or decrease lithium secretion?**

Tetracycline.

○ **How is lithium overdose treated?**

Lavage, saline diuresis, furosemide, and hemodialysis. Alkalinization may be appropriate.

○ **Name seven primary actions of cyclic antidepressant overdose:**

1. Inhibition of amine reuptake
2. Sodium channel blockade, which causes negative inotropy
3. Anticholinergic effects, primarily antimuscarinic
4. CNS depression
5. α-Adrenergic antagonism, which contributes further to hypotension
6. GABA antagonism
7. Q-T prolongation

○ **What is the appropriate treatment for QRS widening in tricyclic antidepressant (TCA) poisoning?**

$NaHCO_3$ is administered intravenously for patients with a QRS > 100 ms; 0.5–2.00 mEq/kg are initially administered and repeated until the blood pH is between 7.45 and 7.55. A continuous infusion of $NaHCO_3$, 3 amps in 1 L of D5W, may then be initiated and titrated in over 4–6 hours to maintain an appropriate pH. Potassium levels must be closely monitored as supplementation may be required to prevent hypokalemia. To arrhythmias not responsive to the above, consider lidocaine (1 mg/kg IV).

○ **What is the appropriate treatment for TCA-induced seizures?**

Benzodiazepines (clorazepam or diazepam) and barbiturates (phenobarbital) are the agents of choice. Phenytoin is not generally effective but may be tried for recurrent seizures or those unresponsive to treatment. Bicarbonate and alkalosis are the main stays of treatment.

○ **What is the treatment for TCA-induced hypotension?**

Isotonic saline and peptid alkalinization. If the patient is resistant to fluid resuscitation, a direct-acting α-adrenergic agonist, such as norepinephrine, should be started. Dopamine acts in part by releasing norepinephrine. This agent may already be depleted by the reuptake inhibition of the cyclic antidepressant and by stress.

○   **What period of observation is required prior to medically clearing a TCA overdose?**

6 hours.

○   **What level of lithium is generally considered toxic?**

2.0 mEq/L.

○   **Will charcoal bind lithium?**

No.

○   **What are the signs and symptoms of lithium toxicity?**

Neurological signs and symptoms include tremor, hyperreflexia, clonus, fasciculations, seizures, and coma. GI signs and symptoms consist of nausea, vomiting, and diarrhea. Cardiovascular effects include ST-T wave changes, bradycardia, conduction defects, and arrhythmias.

○   **What is the treatment for lithium toxicity?**

Supportive care, normal saline diuresis, hemodialysis for patients with clinical signs of severe poisoning, i.e., seizures and arrhythmias, renal failure, or decreasing urine output.

○   **What are the typical CNS findings in mild lithium toxicity?**

Rigidity, tremor, and hyperreflexia.

○   **What are the typical CNS findings in severe lithium toxicity?**

Seizures, coma, and myoclonic jerking.

○   **What are the indications for hemodialysis in lithium toxicity?**

Serum lithium level above 4.0 mEq/L, renal failure, and severe clinical symptoms (stupor, seizures etc.).

○   **True/False: Permanent neurologic sequelae (encephalopathy) can develop from lithium toxicity:**

True.

○   **A 30-year-old man presents to the emergency department 20 minutes after ingesting 30 tablets of amitriptyline. What is the preferred method of gastric emptying?**

Immediate gastric lavage using a large (34–36 French) orogastric tube. Ipecac should not be used due to the potential for a rapid deterioration in mental status and seizures.

○   **What is the initial treatment for hypotension in antidepressant overdose?**

Intravenous fluids—normal saline or Ringer lactate.

○   **What vasopressor should be used to treat hypotension not responsive to IV fluids in antidepressant overdose?**

Norepinephrine should be used because it is a direct-acting α-adrenergic agonist.

○ **The onset of toxicity of monoamine oxidase inhibitors (MAOI) can occur up to what period of time after ingestion?**

12 to 24 hours.

○ **What over-the-counter cold medications should not be used by people taking MAOIs?**

Decongestants, antihistamines, and products containing dextromethorphan.

○ **A 45-year-old patient presents with a diagnosis of depression, anxiety, and insomnia and is currently taking tramadol, flecainide, and tamoxifen. Can you prescribe an SSRI for her?**

No. SSRIs are cyp 450 2D6 inhibitors. The drugs she is on utilize the cyp 450 2D6 for their metabolism.

○ **Describe the signs, symptoms, and ECG findings associated with lithium toxicity:**

Tremor, weakness, and flattening of the T waves, respectively.

○ **What is the treatment of lithium overdose?**

Saline diuresis and hemodialysis.

○ **What is the difference between low-potency and high-potency neuroleptics and give examples of drugs in each category.**

Low-potency neuroleptics have greater sedative, postural hypotensive, and anticholinergic effects. High-potency neuroleptics have greater extrapyramidal effects.

Low potency: Chlorpromazine (Thorazine)

Medium potency: Perphenazine (Trilafon)

High potency: Haloperidol, droperidol (Inapsine), thiothixene (Navane), fluphenazine (Prolixin), trifluoperazine (Stelazine)

○ **You are considering chemical restraint. List your options:**

Benzodiazepines:

1. Lorazepam (Ativan), 1–2 mg IV, or 2–6 mg orally every 30 minutes
2. Midazolam (Versed), 2–4 mg IV every 30 minutes
3. Diazepam (Valium), 5 mg IV or orally every 30 minutes

Sedative hypnotics:

Haloperidol (Haldol), 1–5 mg IM/IV, titrate to clinical response

Droperidol (Inapsine), 1–2 mg IV every 30 minutes

Benzodiazepines may be given in combination with the sedative hypnotics above to both hasten and potentiate their effect. Titrate to effect and monitor appropriately.

○ **Is phenobarbital more quickly metabolized by children or by adults?**

Adults. Neonates are especially slow at metabolizing phenobarbital.

○ **A 32-year-old female patient is prescribed meperidine (Demerol) for an open fracture. The patient is chronically on fluoxetine (Prozac). What is a potential complication?**

The serotonin syndrome.

○ **What signs and symptoms are typical of the serotonin syndrome?**

Agitation, anxiety, altered mental status, ataxia, diaphoresis, incoordination, sinus tachycardia, hyperthermia, shivering, tremor, hyperreflexia, myoclonus, muscular rigidity, and diarrhea.

○ **What are potential pharmacological treatments for the serotonin syndrome?**

Serotonin antagonists, such as methysergide and cyproheptadine. Benzodiazepines and propranolol have also been successfully employed.

○ **A patient ingests a toxic quantity of an MAOI inhibitor and is in a hyperadrenergic state with a blood pressure of 240/160. What is the appropriate treatment?**

Short-acting antihypertensives, such as phentolamine and nitroprusside, should be employed because the patient may soon develop refractory hypotension.

○ **What are the major pharmacological effects of neuroleptics?**

Blockade of dopamine, α-adrenergic, muscarinic, and histamine receptors.

○ **What findings occur with neuroleptic malignant syndrome?**

Altered mental status, muscular rigidity, autonomic instability, hyperthermia, and rhabdomyolysis.

○ **What are the pharmacological effects of barbiturates and benzodiazepines?**

Both enhance chloride influx through the GABA receptor associated chloride channel. Benzodiazepines increase the frequency of channel opening, whereas barbiturates increase the duration of channel opening.

○ **Alkalization of the urine is beneficial in the management of what barbiturates?**

Long-acting barbiturates such as phenobarbital.

○ **What is the pharmacological basis of the anticonvulsant effect of phenytoin?**

Sodium channel blockade. Phenytoin causes an increasing efflux or a decreasing influx of sodium ions across cell membranes in the motor cortex during generation of a nerve impulse

○ **What are the signs and symptoms of phenytoin toxicity?**

Seizure, heart blocks, bradyarrhythmias, tachyarrhythmias, hypotension, and coma. All dangerous cardiovascular complications of phenytoin OD result from parenteral administration. High levels after PO doses do not cause such signs in a stable patient.

○ **What is the treatment for a phenytoin overdose?**

Systemic support, charcoal, atropine for bradyarrhythmias, and phenobarbital, 20 mg/kg IV, for seizures.

○ **What is the treatment for an opiate overdose?**

Naloxone, 0.4–2.0 mg in an adult and 0.01 mg/kg in a child. Naloxone duration of action is about 1 hour. Higher doses and continuous infusion may be required.

○ **What herbal remedies are associated with CNS stimulation?**

Guarance, ma huang, St. John wart, yohimbe, and ginseng.

○ **What four mechanisms induce tricyclic toxicity?**

1. Anticholinergic atropine-like effects secondary to competitive antagonism of acetylcholine
2. Reuptake blockage of norepinephrine
3. A quinidine-like action on the myocardium
4. An α-blocking action

○ **What is the most common neurologic complication of IV drug abuse?**

Nontraumatic mononeuritis (i.e., painless weakness 2–3 hours after injection).

● ● ● ANTIBIOTICS ● ● ●

○ **Name the four potential adverse effects that can happen with antibiotics:**

Allergic, toxic, idiosyncratic, and changes to the normal body flora.

○ **What is the most common overgrowth of bacteria as a result of antibiotic use?**

The superinfection of *clostridium difficile*, which is the causative agent of pseudomembranous colitis.

○ **Which laboratory test is the most helpful in determining the proper use of an antibiotic?**

The culture and sensitivity test. This will give you the mean inhibitory concentration for the bacteria, thus narrowing down your choices of antibiotics.

○ **What is the action of antibiotics such as penicillin, cephalosporin, and vancomycin?**

They all work by inhibiting cell wall synthesis of the bacteria.

○ **What is a potentially fatal reaction from penicillin?**

Hypersensitivity reaction.

○ **Name some other common adverse reactions with penicillin use:**

Urticaria, GI intolerance, and skin rashes (usually 72 hours or later).

○ **What are the four syndromes of penicillamine-induced lung toxicity?**

Chronic pneumonitis, hypersensitivity lung disease, bronchiolitis obliterans, and pulmonary-renal syndrome.

○ **Which generation cephalosporin can be used to penetrate the CNS?**

Third generation. These are typically used for treatment of infections such as meningitis.

○ **What is the cross reactivity of cephalosporin's in relation to penicillin?**

7%–18%, depending on the study.

○ **A 73-year-old female with a history of atrial fibrillation and on chronic warfarin therapy is diagnosed with a mild cellulitis of her forearm. You would like to prescribe her a first-generation cephalosporin as the first-line treatment. Is this a good choice for this patient?**

No. Cephalosporins can have an antivitamin K effect. Given that this patient is on chronic warfarin therapy, this may adversely affect her INR and bleeding rate. Your best bet is to choose another antibiotic.

○ **Name some adverse effects of using vancomycin:**

Ototoxicity—tinnitus, hightone deafness, hearing loss, and deafness.

○ **Which class of antibiotics acts by gaining entry into the cells and binds to intracellular proteins?**

Protein synthesis inhibitors, which include aminoglycosides, tetracyclines, macrolides, clindamycin, streptogramins, and chloramphenicol.

○ **Name three potential side effects of aminoglycosides:**

Ototoxicity, nephrotoxicity, and neuromuscular toxicity.

○ **When administering tetracycline, how is the medication to be taken to ensure proper absorption?**

They must be taken on an empty stomach to maximize absorption.

○ **A 15-year-old male adolescent has been diagnosed with acne. One of the possible treatment options is the use of tetracycline. Would this be a good choice for this type of patient?**

No. Tetracycline can cause staining of the teeth, retardation of bone growth, and photosensitivity and should be avoided in children as well as pregnant patients.

○ **Mnemonic for erythromycin for the drug of choice in these bacteria:**

Legionnaires **C**amp on **M**y **B**order (legionella, *Campylobacter, Mycoplasma, Bordetella*).

○ **What is the one bacteria that chloramphenicol is not sensitive in eradicating?**

Pseudomonas aeruginosa.

○ **What is gray baby syndrome?**

It is a fatal syndrome by which infants cannot conjugate chloramphenicol. The antibiotic absorbs into the cerebrospinal fluid. The infants will get abdominal distention, vomiting, cyanosis, hypothermia, decreased respiration, and vasomotor collapse.

○ **Which antibiotic has been listed as the most susceptible in contracting *Clostridium difficile* superinfections?**

Clindamycin.

○ **What is the effect of macrolide antibiotics (erythromycin, clarithromycin) on mucus hypersecretion?**

Some macrolide antibiotics have the ability to down/regulate mucus secretion by an unknown mechanism. This is thought to be due to an anti-inflammatory activity.

○ **Why are quinolones contraindicated in young adults and children?**

Quinolones are contraindicated because they can suppress the epiphyseal plate and cartilage formation in young adults. In all patients, quinolones can cause tendon rupture, most notably Achilles tendon ruptures.

○ **What are the possible side effects?**

Quinolones are contraindicated because they can suppress the epiphyseal plate and cartilage formation in young adults. In all patients, quinolones can cause tendon rupture, most notably Achilles tendon ruptures.

○ **How do quinolones work?**

They inhibit DNA gyrase synthesis, which is responsible for DNA replication of bacteria.

○ **Which bacteria do quinolones effectively kill?**

They are broad-spectrum killers (gram-negative mostly) and most effective in treating respiratory, bone and joint, urinary tract, and prostatitis. Some are effective in treating *Pseudomonas aeruginosa*.

○ **What is the mechanism of action of isoniazid?**

It is a simple inhibitor of mycolic acids, which are responsible for the formation of bacterial cell wall envelopes.

○ **What two side effects are causes of isoniazid?**

Hepatotoxicity and peripheral neuropathy. Both can be reversed by stopping the drug.

○ **What is the antidote for isoniazid-induced seizures?**

Pyridoxine.

○ **What is a serious side effect of rifampin?**

Hepatotoxicity. LFTs need to be monitored while patient is on either rifampin or isoniazid. Rifampin will also turn the urine and secretions orange while on the medication.

○ **What is the drug of choice for the treatment of leprosy?**

Dapsone.

○ **Fungal infections in general are more difficult to eradicate than bacterial infections. How do drugs like amphotericin B and nystatin function?**

They act by binding to ergosterol, which is the prinicipal sterol in fungus.

○ **How can nystatin be taken?**

It is limited to topical applications and oral liquids. Systemic nystatin is too toxic and therefore not used.

○ **What is the most serious and most common toxicity of amphotericin B?**

Nephrotoxicity.

○ **Why do patients with tinea infections that require griseofulvin need to take such a prolonged course of the medication?**

These infections must have new skin, hair, and nails that are new—keratin-containing griseofulvin. This usually takes several weeks to accomplish.

○ **What is the drug of choice for the treatment of trematodes (flukes)?**

Praziquantel.

○ **Name three drugs that can be used for the treatment of nematodes (roundworms):**

Albendazole, mebendazole, and pyrantel. Filarial infections must be treated with Ivermectin or diethylcarbamazine.

○ **What is the mechanism of action of albendazole and mebendazole?**

They inhibit tubulin polymerization in worms, which prevents replication.

○ **What is the treatment for lymphatic filariasis?**

Diethylcarbamazine.

○ **What are the three mechanisms of controlling viral illnesses?**

Vaccination, chemotherapy, and stimulation of the hosts natural resistance mechanisms.

○ **What is the function of reverse transcriptase inhibitors?**

All three types (nucleoside, nonnucleoside, and nucleotide) inhibit the formation of viral DNA from RNA by reverse transcriptase.

○ **Protease inhibitors are commonly used in the treatment and suppression of HIV. How do these medications work?**

They interfere with the production of viral proteins, thus preventing replication of new viral particles.

○ **What is the most effective treatment for HIV?**

The triple drug therapy (or cocktail) is the use of two reverse transcriptase inhibitors, and a protease inhibitor.

○ **What is the most effective prevention method for influenza?**

Vaccination.

○ **Which type of influenza does amantidine work effectively against?**

Influenza A.

○ **Which class of drugs is effective in reducing the length of both influenza A and B?**

Neuraminidase inhibitors. They are effective if the medication can be started within 30 hours of onset of symptoms of flu.

○ **Which antiviral is effective in the treatment of respiratory syncytial virus (RSV)?**

Ribavirin.

○ **How is ribavirin administered?**

By aerosol form.

○ **What is the treatment of choice for *trichomoniasis* and *giardiasis*?**

Metronidazole.

○ **Name some common side effects of metronidazole:**

Nausea, vomiting, and diarrhea. It will also cause your secretions to turn dark or red-brown in color. Some patients will get a metallic taste.

○ **Metronidazole, when mixed with alcohol, will cause a disulfiram like reaction to occur. What are some symptoms that you should look for in this scenario?**

Abdominal cramping, flushing, vomiting, and headache.

○ **What is the one drug that has shown resistance in treating plasmodium falciparum?**

Chloroquine.

○ **Which antiprotozoal drug must be avoided in patients with G6PD deficiency?**

Primaquine, which can cause hemolytic anemia.

○ **Chloroquine is a commonly prescribed drug for the treatment of malaria. What are two ophthalmologic side effects of the drug that need to be monitored?**

Corneal deposits containing melanin can develop. This can lead to blindness.

○ **What is the main goal of most anticancer drugs?**

They are either cytotoxic drugs, which will block cell replication, or they are drugs, which act on hormonal-sensitive tumors.

○ **Patients undergoing chemotherapy are at risk for bleeding and infections. Why?**

The chemotherapeutic agents' most serious side effect is bone marrow toxicity. This will cause a drop in the production of all blood products including white cells and platelets.

○ **What are the main gastrointestinal side effects of chemotherapy?**

Nausea and vomiting, which is thought to be a centrally acting effect.

○ **Some chemotherapeutic agents can have cardiotoxicity. Name some possible cardiac effects from these drugs:**

Patients can develop arrhythmias, decreased ventricular function (cardiomyopathy), and focal necrosis of tissue.

○ **Why does hair loss occur so frequently in chemotherapy?**

Most chemotherapeutic agents block the telophase stage of hair production, thus causing a stoppage of hair growth. This will cause hair death. Stopping the chemo will reverse this side effect.

Common chemotherapeutic agents and their serious side effects:

Drug	Side effect
Cisplatin	Renal tubular damage
Cyclophosphamide	Hemorrhagic cystitis
Doxorubicin/daunorubicin	Cardiotoxicity
Bleomycin	Pulmonary fibrosis
Vincristine	Central nervous system toxicity
Methotrexate	Renal tubular damage

○ **A 66-year-old female patient is currently under treatment for malignant myeloma. Her calcium is measured at 19 mg/dL and she is showing signs of hypercalcemia on examination. What treatment can be given to help lower the calcium level?**

Bisphosphonates, creating the volume status of the patient to be euvolemic are the two initial goals. An additional therapy for life-threatening hypercalcemia is plicamycin.

○ **How do drugs such as Tamoxifen and toremifene act on breast cancer cells?**

They are competitive antagonists of estrogen receptors.

○ **An acute chest pain syndrome can occur with which chemotherapeutic agents?**

Methotrexate and bleomycin.

○ **What are four distinct presentations of bleomycin lung toxicity?**

Chronic pulmonary fibrosis, hypersensitivity lung reaction, acute pneumonitis, and acute chest pain syndrome.

○ **What are the risk factors for methotrexate (MTX) pulmonary toxicity?**

Primary biliary cirrhosis, frequency of administration, adrenalectomy, tapering of corticosteroid therapy, and use in multidrug regimens.

○ **What drug will produce hilar and mediastinal adenopathy as a toxic reaction?**

Methotrexate.

● ● ● ENDOCRINE SYSTEM ● ● ●

○ **What is the main glucocorticoid and mineralocorticoid produced by the adrenal gland?**

Glucocorticoid—hydrocortisone (cortisol)
Mineralocorticoid—aldosterone

○ **What is the function of glucocorticoids?**

They promote the catabolism of proteins and gluconeogenesis.

○ **Why is there an increased risk of infection for those patients on steroids?**

Glucocorticoids inhibit inflammatory and immunologic responses, which make them more susceptible to infection.

○ **What is a potential long-term complication for chronic glucocorticoid use?**

Osteoporosis.

○ **Where does the primary source of estradiol originate?**

From the ovary.

○ **What are the most common side effects of estrogen use?**

Nausea and vomiting.

○ **Which antiestrogen is used to stimulate ovarian function for the purpose of treating infertility?**

Clomiphene.

○ **What are the most common side effects when using progestins?**

Weight gain, edema, and depression. More serious problems are with the hematologic system. Increased clotting can occur; thrombophlebitis and pulmonary embolus are serious adverse effects of progestins.

○ **Progestin alone used in contraceptives can cause what main side effect?**

Irregular uterine bleeding.

○ **The main androgen in the body is testosterone. What are some of the effects that androgens cause in the body?**

Virilization of women, including deepening of voice, acne, growth of facial hair, and excessive muscle development.

○ **What is the treatment of choice for hypothyroidism?**

Levothyroxine.

○ **Name two medications that inhibit thyroid synthesis:**

Propylthiouracil and methimazole.

○ **What is the most common side effect of insulin?**

Hypoglycemia.

○ **What is the treatment for the crystallization of tissue from repetitive use of insulin at the same site of skin?**

Injections of glucagon to the site will reverse the problem.

○ **What is the mechanism of sulfonylureas in the treatment of diabetes?**

They act to stimulate the β cells of the pancreas.

○ **A 65-year-old male patient has a history of diabetes for which he takes metformin. He is having an MI and will be in need of a cardiac catheterization. Is there anything special that this patient needs before the cath?**

Yes. The metformin needs to be stopped prior to the cath as the dye in combination with the metformin can impair renal function.

○ **Describe which histamine receptors act on different systems of the body:**

H_1 receptors act on intestinal and smooth muscle whereas the H_2 receptors control gastric secretions.

○ **What are H_1 antagonists used to treat?**

They are commonly used to treat allergic rhinitis, motion sickness, and in some cases to help induce sleep.

• • • RESPIRATORY SYSTEM • • •

○ **What is the main delivery system for β-agonists for respiratory diseases?**

Inhalation by either aerosol nebulizer or metered dose inhaler.

○ **What is the inhaled drug of choice for the treatment of COPD?**

Ipratropium.

○ **Is cromolyn useful in the treatment of acute asthma attacks?**

No.

○ **True/False: β-adrenergic antagonists in massive overdose may cause severe bronchospasm in normal individuals:**

False.

○ **What conditions or commonly used medications result in an increase in serum theophylline concentration?**

Cimetidine, macrolides, quinolones, verapamil, fever, congestive heart failure, and liver failure.

○ **What drugs, activities, and cooking habits are associated with an increased clearance of theophylline (decreasing the theophylline level)?**

Phenytoin, phenobarbital, cigarette smoking, and charcoal barbecuing.

○   **What is the appropriate initial treatment of theophylline-induced seizures?**

Benzodiazepines and barbiturates. Theophylline-induced seizures warrant hemodialysis or charcoal hemoperfusion.

○   **What is the treatment of theophylline-induced hypotension?**

Fluid administration and β-blockers. Theophylline-induced cardiovascular instability is secondary to β-agonist effects. Therefore, β-blockers can be beneficial in the treatment of arrhythmias and hypotension.

● ● ● GASTROINTESTINAL SYSTEM ● ● ●

○   **Of all the H_2-blockers used for gastrointestinal complaints, which one has the most potential side effects and why?**

Cimetidine because it binds to cytochrome P-450.

○   **What instructions do you need to give patients that you prescribe sucralfate and why?**

They must take on an empty stomach because the drug binds to protein.

○   **What are the two major types of drugs used to treat constipation?**

There are bulk-forming agents, which absorb water and soften the stool, and the second is the cathartics and stimulants, which increase water and electrolytes in the stool to increase bowel motility.

Two other types are saline salts to draw water into the colon, and docusate, which absorbs into stool to soften.

○   **Which drugs are utilized in the treatment of Crohn disease?**

Sulfasalazine, which is metabolized into 5-ASA and sulfapyridine.

● ● ● MUSCULOSKELETAL SYSTEM ● ● ●

○   **What is the main mechanism of non-steroidal anti-inflammatory (NSAIDs)?**

They act by inhibiting prostaglandin synthesis.

○   **What are the most common side effects associated with NSAIDs?**

GI upset, bleeding, oliguria, fluid retention, renal insufficiency, decreased sodium excretion, and renal failure. They can also prolong bleeding times.

○   **What is the only non-reversible COX inhibitor?**

Aspirin.

○   **Why are children not to be given aspirin?**

Aspirin can cause Reyes syndrome to occur.

○ **What are some of the characteristics associated with Reyes syndrome?**

CNS damage, liver injury, and hypoglycemia.

○ **What is the incidence of aspirin-induced bronchospasm in patients with nasal polyps?**

Up to 75%.

○ **True/False: In aspirin-induced bronchospasm, there can be cross-reactivity with nonsteroidal anti-inflammatory drugs:**

True.

○ **What is the major side effect associated with the inhalation of *N*-acetylcysteine?**

Cough and bronchospasm, most likely due to irritation from the low pH (2.2) of the aerosol solution.

○ **Which acid–base disturbance is typical for salicylate poisoning?**

Mixed respiratory alkalosis, secondary to central respiratory center stimulation, and metabolic acidosis, secondary to uncoupling of oxidative phosphorylation.

○ **What order are the kinetics of elimination for an ASA overdose?**

Zero-order elimination with hepatic enzymatic clearance saturated and renal clearance becoming important.

○ **What is the "magic number" for the dose of a nonenteric coated ASA that must be exceeded to cause toxicity (mg/kg)?**

150 mg/kg.

○ **What dose of ASA will cause mild to moderate toxicity?**

200–300 mg/kg. Greater than 500 mg/kg is potentially lethal.

○ **Is hemodialysis used to treat salicylate toxicity?**

Yes. For severely poisoned patients, i.e., coma, ARDS, cardiac toxicity, serum levels > 100 mg/dL, and for patients who are unresponsive to maximal therapy.

○ **What is the treatment for a prolonged prothrombin time in salicylate poisoning?**

Parenteral vitamin K administration. Salicylates inhibit vitamin K epoxide reductase in poisoning, resulting in an ability for the inactive vitamin K epoxide to be regenerated into the active vitamin K.

○ **Can a patient present with salicylate poisoning and a therapeutic level?**

Yes. Patients with chronic salicylate poisoning have a large Vd (volume of distribution) and thus may present with mental status changes and a therapeutic level.

○ **What is the X-ray finding in a patient with salicylate toxicity?**

Noncardiogenic pulmonary edema.

○   **Describe the effects of salicylate poisoning on the central nervous system:**

Lethargy, confusion, seizures, and respiratory arrest.

○   **Salicylate levels should ideally be checked how long after an ingestion?**

6 hours.

○   **What is the minimum toxic dose of salicylates?**

150 mg/kg.

○   **What salicylate level, measured 6 hours after ingestion, is associated with toxicity?**

45 mg/dL.

○   **What acetaminophen level, measured 4 hours after ingestion, is associated with toxicity?**

150 μg/mL.

○   **What are the signs of salicylate poisoning?**

Hyperventilation, hyperthermia, mental status change, nausea, vomiting, abdominal pain, dehydration, diaphoresis, ketonuria, metabolic acidosis, and respiratory alkalosis.

○   **A child presents with lethargy, seizures, and hypoglycemia. He has had viral syndrome symptoms for several days. Mom states she has only been giving him aspirin. What two disorders should be considered:**

Reye syndrome and salicylate intoxication.

○   **When does acetaminophen become toxic?**

When there is no glutathione to detoxify its toxic intermediate.

○   **Would you like to have four Aces?**

Of course! So check ACEtaminophen levels 4 hours after ingestion.

○   **Which type of acid–base disturbance initially occurs with a salicylate overdose?**

Respiratory alkalosis. Approximately 12 hours later, an anion gap metabolic acidosis or mixed acid–base picture may occur.

○   **Is hyperglycemia or is hypoglycemia expected with a salicylate overdose?**

Expect either hyperglycemia or hypoglycemia.

○   **What are the common signs and symptoms of chronic salicylism?**

Fever, tachypnea, CNS alterations, acid–base abnormalities, electrolyte abnormalities, chronic pain, ketonuria, and noncardiogenic pulmonary edema.

○ **A patient presents with an acute salicylate ingestion. What symptoms are expected with a mild, moderate, and severe overdose?**

Mild: Lethargy, vomiting, hyperventilation, and hyperthermia

Moderate: Severe hyperventilation and compensated metabolic acidosis

Severe: Coma, seizures, and uncompensated metabolic acidosis

○ **What is the treatment for a salicylate overdose?**

Decontaminate, lavage and charcoal, replace fluids, supplement with potassium, alkalize the urine with bicarbonate, cool for hyperthermia, administer glucose for hypoglycemia, place on oxygen and PEEP for pulmonary edema, prescribe multiple dose–activated charcoal, and initiate dialysis.

○ **What are the four stages of acetaminophen (APAP) poisoning?**

Stage I: 30 minutes to 24 hours, nausea and vomiting

Stage II: 24–48 hours, abdominal pain and elevated LFTs

Stage III: 72–96 hours, LFTs peak, nausea, and vomiting

Stage IV: 4 days to 2 weeks, resolution or fulminant hepatic failure

○ **Which measure of hepatic function is a better prognostic indicator in APAP overdose: liver enzyme levels or bilirubin level and prothrombin time?**

Bilirubin level and prothrombin time.

○ **An acutely intoxicated, nonalcoholic, otherwise healthy patient ingests APAP. Is this patient more or less likely to develop hepatotoxicity?**

Less likely. An acute ingestion of alcohol will tie up the P-450 system thereby inhibiting the formation of NAPQI. A chronic alcoholic has an induced P-450 system and will suffer greater APAP hepatic toxicity through increased NAPQI formation.

○ **What is the minimum dose of APAP that can cause hepatotoxicity in the child? In the adult?**

Child: 140 mg/kg. Adult: 140mg/kg (or about 7.5 g).

○ **What is the antidote for APAP poisoning?**

Mucomist (NAC) 140 mg/kg followed by 17 doses of 70 mg/kg every 4 hours.

○ **According to the Rumack-Matthew nomogram, at what 4-hour APAP level should treatment be initiated?**

150 mg/mL.

○ **What is the treatment goal in the management of osteoporosis?**

First is the prevention of further bone loss, and second is the treatment of the osteoporosis already present.

○ **What is the mechanism of bisphosphonates?**

They inhibit osteoclast activity to prevent further bone destruction.

• • • TOXICOLOGY AND OVERDOSE • • •

○ **What is the most important treatment of all poisoned and toxic patients?**

Supportive care.

○ **What is the difference between methadone and heroin?**

Methadone causes analgesia, but does not cause euphoria. Habituation occurs with both drugs. The withdrawal symptoms of methadone are less severe, but they last longer.

○ **What is the treatment for cocaine toxicity?**

Acidify the urine and administer neuroleptics and phentolamine
Sedate with benzodiazepine
Treat unresponsive hypertension with nitroprusside or phentolamine

○ **Name some over-the-counter and "street" drugs that may produce delirium or acute psychosis:**

Salicylates, antihistamines, anticholinergics, alcohols, phencyclidine, LSD, mescaline, cocaine, and amphetamines.

○ **Hallucinogens affect what neurotransmitter?**

Serotonin.

○ **What is the treatment for a "bad trip" on LSD?**

Constantly remind patients that their perceptions are only distortions due to the drug. This is called "talking down." Chlorpromazine can be used IM for severe or uncontrollable anxiety.

○ **PCP most commonly affects what brain system?**

The vestibulocerebellar system. This has a positive analgesic effect. However, the side effects, including dizziness, muscular incoordination, nystagmus, delirium, anxiety, irritability, and catalepsy, weigh heavily against any positive effect.

○ **How is a patient with PCP overdose treated?**

Acidify the urine with cranberry juice or NH4Cl, give a benzodiazepine, and restrain the patient.

○ **Which types of nystagmus are expected with a PCP overdose?**

Vertical, horizontal, and rotary. Vertical nystagmus is not common with other conditions/ingestions. The most common findings of a PCP overdose are hypertension, tachycardia, and nystagmus.

○ **How can the pesticide PCP enter the body?**

Through inhalation, skin, and ingestion

○ **What is the clinical presentation of PCP intoxication?**

Irritation of skin, eyes, and upper respiratory tract, headache, vomiting, weakness, sweating, hyperthermia, tachycardia, tachypnea, convulsions, coma, pulmonary edema, cardiovascular collapse, and death.

○ **Describe the features of the three stages of PCP intoxication:**

Stage I: agitation or violence, normal vital signs

Stage II: tachycardia, hypertension, no response to pain

Stage III: unresponsive, depressed respirations, seizures, death

○ **Should the urine be acidified in the treatment of PCP intoxication?**

Although acidification of the urine is theoretically advantageous, clinical experience has not shown this to be efficacious. Let's call that a "no."

○ **What is a dystonic reaction?**

A very common side effect of neuroleptics seen in the emergency department. It involves muscle spasms of the tongue, face, neck, and back. Severe laryngospasm and extraocular muscle spasms may also occur. Patients may bite their tongues, leading to an inability to open the mouth, to tongue edema, or to hemorrhage.

○ **How do you treat dystonic reactions?**

Diphenhydramine (Benadryl), 25–50 mg IM or IV, or benztropine (Cogentin), 1–2 mg IV or PO. Remember that dystonias can recur acutely.

○ **A patient has ingested a phenothiazine and arrives hypotensive. What intervention(s) may be considered?**

IV crystalloid boluses usually suffice. Severe cases best managed with norepinephrine (Levophed) or metaraminol (Aramine). These pressors stimulate α-adrenergic receptors preferentially. β-Agonists, such as isoproterenol (Isuprel), are contraindicated because of risks of β-receptor–stimulated vasodilation.

○ **What are some common side effects of phenothiazine use?**

Malaise, hyperthermia, tachycardia, anticholinergic effects, and quinidine-like membrane stabilization. The most dangerous side effect is neuroleptic malignant syndrome.

○ **How should stable ventricular tachyarrhythmias associated with phenothiazine overdose be treated?**

Lidocaine and phenytoin.

○ **What factors and substances decrease theophylline metabolism and increase theophylline levels?**

Factors: Age greater than 50 years, prematurity, liver and renal disease, pulmonary edema, CHF, pneumonia, obesity, and viral illness in children

Substances: Drugs that increase theophylline levels include cimetidine, erythromycin, allopurinol, troleandomycin, BCPs, and quinolone antibiotics

In smokers, the theophylline half-life is decreased, which causes the levels of serum theophylline to decrease. Phenobarbital, phenytoin, rifampin, carbamazepine, marijuana smoking, exposure to environmental pollutants, and the consumption of charcoal-broiled foods can also decrease serum theophylline levels.

○ **Can theophylline be dialyzed?**

Yes.

○ **Why should the use of atropine be considered in a pediatric patient prior to intubation?**

Many pediatric patients develop bradycardia associated with intubation, which can be prevented by pretreatment with atropine (0.01 mg/kg).

○ **What is a "Mickey Finn"?**

A mixture of alcohol and chloral hydrate.

○ **At what rate is alcohol metabolized in an acutely intoxicated person?**

About 20 mg/dL/h.

○ **What is the pharmacological treatment for alcohol withdrawal?**

Benzodiazepines or barbiturates.

○ **What is a normal osmolar gap?**

<10 mOsm.

○ **What is the toxic metabolic end product in methanol poisoning?**

Formic acid.

○ **What cofactor is required to convert formic acid to carbon dioxide and water?**

Folate. Leucovorin, folinic acid, the active form of folate, is preferentially administered at 1 mg/kg. Folate may be substituted at the same dose if leucovorin is not available.

○ **Is sodium bicarbonate ($NaHCO_3$) beneficial in the management of methanol poisoning?**

Yes. In animal models, maintenance of a normal pH through bicarbonate administration decreased toxicity, including visual impairment.

○ **What methanol level mandates dialysis?**

50 mg/dL. Other indications include visual impairment, severe metabolic acidosis, and ingestion of greater than 30 cc.

○ **What cofactors are administered to a patient with ethylene glycol poisoning?**

Thiamine and pyridoxine. These cofactors will aid in transforming glyoxylic acid to nontoxic metabolites. Both are administered intravenously in 100 mg increments.

○ **Name the three clinical phases of ethylene glycol poisoning:**

Stage I: Neurological symptomatology (i.e., inebriation)
Stage II: Metabolic acidosis and cardiovascular instability
Stage III: Renal failure

○ **When should dialysis be initiated for an ethylene glycol poisoning case?**

When the serum level is >25 mg/dL, or when renal insufficiency or severe metabolic acidosis occurs.

○ **What is the toxic dose of naloxone?**

None. Narcan is a safe drug and may be given in large quantities. The usual adult dosage is 2 mg IV; the usual pediatric dose is 0.01 mg/kg. Narcan may precipitate acute withdrawal and may therefore be titrated to effect.

○ **What syndrome is associated with Jimson Weed?**

Anticholinergic poisoning.

○ **What are absolute indications for hemodialysis or hemoperfusion in theophylline toxicity?**

Seizures or arrhythmias that are unresponsive to conventional therapy—a theophylline level >100 μg/mg in an acute overdose or 50 μg/mg in a chronic overdose

○ **What are the four stages of iron poisoning?**

Stage I (0–6 hours): Abdominal pain, nausea, vomiting, and diarrhea secondary to the corrosive effects of iron. In more severe cases, hematemesis, hypotension and altered mental status.

Stage II (6–24 hours): Quiescent period during which iron is absorbed (in severe poisoning, a latent period may be absent).

Stage III: (12–24 hours): GI hemorrhage, shock, metabolic acidosis, heart failure, CV collapse, coma, seizures, coagulopathy, hepatic, and renal failure.

Stage IV: (4–6 weeks postingestion): Gastric outlet or small bowel obstruction secondary to scarring.

○ **What dose of iron is expected to produce clinical toxicity?**

20 mg/kg of elemental iron. For example, a toddler ingests 10 tablets of 324 mg ferrous sulfate, i.e., 20% elemental iron; this equals 648 mg of elemental iron. The dose would be toxic to a 20 kg child at 32.4 mg/kg.

○ **What 4-hour iron level is generally considered toxic?**

300–350 μg/dL.

○ **What are the indications for deferoxamine therapy?**

All symptomatic patients exhibiting more than merely transient symptomatology.

Patients with lethargy, significant abdominal pain, hypotension, mental status changes, hypovolemia, or metabolic acidosis.

Patients with a positive KUB.

Any symptomatic patient with a level greater than 300 mg/dL.

○ **What oral chelator reduces iron absorption in animal model studies?**

Magnesium hydroxide or milk of magnesia.

○ **What historical disclosure warrants an evaluation after a hydrocarbon ingestion?**

Coughing. Any patient who coughs after ingesting a hydrocarbon has the potential for developing chemical pneumonitis.

○ **At what point can a patient who has ingested a hydrocarbon be safely discharged?**

After 6 hours, asymptomatic patients, with a normal chest X-ray and pulse oxygen, may be discharged to home.

○ **Chronic solvent abusers develop what metabolic complication?**

Renal tubular acidosis.

○ **Methylene chloride is metabolized to which toxin?**

Carbon monoxide.

○ **A 2-year-old child is asymptomatic after ingestion of a button battery. A KUB reveals the foreign body in his stomach. What is the disposition for this patient?**

Discharge to home. If the battery is lodged in the esophagus, an endoscopy must be performed immediately. Otherwise, reassure the patient's parents and instruct them to check their son's stools.

○ **What is the potent ingredient in Sarin?**

An organophosphate.

○ **What enzyme is inhibited by organophosphates?**

Acetylcholinesterase.

○ **How do organophosphates enter the body?**

They can be inhaled, ingested, or absorbed through the skin.

○ **What are the signs and symptoms of organophosphate poisoning?**

1–2 hours after poisoning patients may have GI upset, bronchospasm, miosis, bradycardia, excessive salivation and sweating, tremor, respiratory muscle paralysis, muscle fasciculations, agitation, seizures, coma and death. *Remember:* SLUDGE (**S**alivation, **L**acrimation, **U**rinary incontinence, **D**iarrhea, **G**astric upset, and **E**mesis).

○ **What antihypertensive agent may induce cyanide poisoning?**

Nitroprusside. One molecule of sodium nitroprusside contains five molecules of cyanide. To prevent toxicity with long duration infusions, sodium thiosulfate should be infused with sodium nitroprusside at a ratio of 10:1, thiosulfate to nitroprusside. Beware of thiocyanate toxicity!

○ **What is corn picker's pupil?**

Mydriasis from contact of the eye with Jimson weed. Jimson weed contains atropine, scopolamine, and hyoscyamine. It is a common plant and is available through health food stores.

○ **What is the most common cause of chronic heavy metal poisoning?**

Lead.

○ **Organophosphates are found in what kinds of compounds?**

Pesticides, flame retardants, and plasticizers.

○ **What is the rate-limiting step in the metabolism of ethanol?**

The conversion of ethanol to acetaldehyde by alcohol dehydrogenase.

○ **In a nondrinker, what blood ethanol level will cause confusion or stupor?**

180–300 mg/dL. The minimum blood alcohol level that can cause coma in a nondrinker is 300 mg/dL.

○ **In chronic alcohol users, alcohol withdrawal seizures occur approximately how many hours after cessation of heavy alcohol consumption?**

6–48 hours from the time of the last drink.

○ **Delirium tremens occurs how long after the cessation of alcohol consumption?**

On average, 3–5 days.

○ **Is there a role for phenytoin in the prevention or treatment of pure alcohol withdrawal seizures?**

No. Careful titration of benzodiazepines or phenobarbital should be used if necessary.

○ **True/False: Status epilepticus is commonly seen in alcohol withdrawal seizures:**

False. Status epilepticus is rare in alcohol withdrawal seizures and should suggest the need to find other causative pathology.

○ **What is the classic triad of Wernicke encephalopathy?**

Global confusion, oculomotor disturbances, and ataxia.

○ **What constellation of findings should prompt consideration of ethylene glycol toxicity?**

Ethanol-like intoxication (with no odor), large anion gap acidosis, increased osmolal gap, altered mental status leading to coma, and calcium oxalate crystals in the urine.

○ **In life-threatening theophylline overdose, what is definitive management?**

Charcoal hemoperfusion.

○ **True/False: Lithium has a narrow therapeutic toxic range:**

True. Therapeutic lithium levels are between 0.5 amd 1.5 mEq/L and must be monitored closely.

○ **How is lithium eliminated after metabolism?**

By renal excretion.

○ **Name five herbal remedies associated with bleeding:**

Ginger, garlic, ginkgo, ginseng, and feverfew.

○ **If a patient has a sulfa or ASA allergy, can they be prescribed a COX II inhibitor?**

No.

○ **Which opiate combination is associated with arrhythmias, pulmonary edema, and hepatic failure?**

Propoxyphene N 100 plus APAP.

○ **Ethylene glycol is the alcohol that is present with hypocalcemia in one-third of the cases. Where does the calcium go?**

Oxalic acid is one of the metabolites of ethylene glycol. Calcium precipitates with oxalate and forms calcium oxalate crystals. The positive birefringent calcium oxalate dihydrate crystals are pathognomonic of this ingestion.

○ **Methanol intoxication causes early death as a result of:**

Respiratory arrest. The pathophysiology is unknown.

○ **Activated charcoal is not an effective treatment for which poisonous substances?**

Alcohols, ions, acids, and bases.

○ **Describe the clinical characteristics of carboxyhemoglobin concentrations, specifically for ranges of 10% to 70%:**

10%: Frontal headache
20%: Headache and dyspnea
30%: Nausea, dizziness, visual disturbance, fatigue, and impaired judgment
40%: Syncope and confusion
50%: Coma and seizures
60%: Respiratory failure and hypotension
70%: May be lethal

○ **What is the appropriate treatment for cyanide poisoning?**

Amyl nitrite and sodium nitrite IV, followed by sodium thiosulfate IV.

○ **What is the most common cause of chronic heavy metal poisoning?**

Lead. Arsenic is the most common cause of acute heavy metal poisoning.

○ **Cyanide binds to metals and disrupts the function of metal-containing enzymes. Which is the most important of these enzymes?**

Cytochrome A (also known as cytochrome oxidase) is necessary for aerobic metabolism.

○ **Why administer nitrites for cyanide poisoning?**

Nitrites form methemoglobin and methemoglobin, which strongly bind to cyanide.

○ **Why prescribe sodium thiosulfate for cyanide poisoning?**

Rhodanese, an intrinsic enzyme, transfers cyanide from its attachment to methemoglobin to sulfur, thereby forming thiocyanate. Thiocyanate is excreted. Sodium thiosulfate acts as a sulfur donor for this process.

○ **What is the antidote for ethylene glycol?**

Ethanol and dialysis.

○ **What is the antidote for gold?**

British anti-Lewisite (BAL).

○ **What are the potential complications of excess sodium bicarbonate?**

Cerebral acidosis, hypokalemia, hyperosmolality, and an increased binding of hemoglobin to oxygen.

○ **What are common entities in the differential diagnosis of pinpoint pupils?**

Narcotic overdose, clonidine overdose, and sedative hypnotic overdose, including alcohol, cerebellar pontine angle infarct, and subarachnoid hemorrhage.

○ **What mnemonic may assist in recalling the signs of life-threatening cholinergic poisoning?**

DUELS:

Diaphoresis

Urination

Eye changes (miosis)

Lacrimation

Salivation

○ **Name six common drugs that can cause hyperthermia:**

SANDS-PCP:

1. **S**alicylates

2. **A**nticholinergics

3. **N**euroleptics

4. **D**initrophenols

5. **S**ympathomimetics

6. **P**hencyclidine (**PCP**)

○ **What drugs cause an acetone odor on the breath?**

Ethanol, isopropanol, and salicylates. Ketosis is often accompanied by the same odor.

Substances or drugs that have an induced odor on breath:

Type of odor on breath	Drugs or substances that induce the abnormality
Almonds	Cyanide, laetrile, and apricot pits (latter two contain amygdalin)
Garlic	DMSO, organophosphates, phosphorus, arsenic, arsine gas, and thallium
Peanut	Vacor (RH-787)
Pear	Chloral hydrate and paraldehyde
Rotten eggs	Hydrogen sulfide, mercaptans, and sewer gas

○ **What is the mnemonic for remembering drugs that are radiopaque?**

BAT CHIPS:

Barium
Antihistamines
Tricyclic antidepressants
Chloral hydrate, calcium, cocaine
Heavy metals
Iodine
Phenothiazine, potassium
Slow-release (enteric-coated)

○ **What three toxicologic emergencies require immediate dialysis?**

Ethylene glycol, methyl alcohol, and Amanita phalloides.

○ **What is the antidote for isoniazid?**

Pyridoxine.

○ **What drugs are commonly excreted by using alkaline diuresis?**

Long-acting barbiturates, INH, tricyclic antidepressants, salicylates, and less commonly, lithium.

○ **What are the signs and symptoms of a cyanide overdose?**

Dryness and burning in the throat, air hunger, and hyperventilation. If the individual is not removed from the toxic environment, loss of consciousness, seizures, bradycardia, and apnea will occur followed by asystole.

○ **What drugs can cause methemoglobinemia?**

Nitrites, local anesthetics, silver nitrate, amyl nitrite and nitrites, benzocaine, commercial marking crayons, aniline dyes, sulfonamides, and phenacetin.

○ **For which type of overdoses is atropine used?**

Organophosphate and carbamate.

○ **For which type of an overdose may the drug pralidoxime (2-PAM) be used?**

Organophosphate.

○ **Chronic bromism is treated with what drug?**

Sodium chloride.

○ **Isoniazid and *Gyromitra* mushroom poisoning is best treated with what drug?**

Pyridoxine.

○ **Name some side effects of alkalization of the urine:**

Hypernatremia and hyperosmolality.

○   **What is the antidote for phosphorus poisoning?**

Copper sulfate, 1% solution. Remove phosphorus within 30 minutes of exposure. Phosphorus may be identified by the formation of an insoluble black precipitate when swabbing with copper sulfate.

○   **What local anesthetics may cause anaphylaxis?**

The ester derivatives containing para-aminobenzoic acid (PABA) are known to stimulate IgE antibody formation and thereby cause anaphylaxis. Such anesthetics include procaine and tetracaine.

○   **What is the best diluent for treating the ingestion of solid lye?**

Milk.

○   **What is the most commonly abused volatile substance?**

Toluene.

○   **A patient presents with hypokalemia of 2.0, hyperchloremia, and acidosis. What is the most likely toxicologic cause?**

Chronic toluene abuse.

○   **A patient has been abusing nitrous oxide for a long time. What symptoms might be expected?**

Paresthesias and motor weakness may be present in chronic abusers. Such symptoms are often mistaken for symptoms of multiple sclerosis.

○   **A patient presents with belladonna alkaloid poisoning resulting in anticholinergic effects. Explain the dangers of treating this patient with physostigmine:**

Physostigmine acts to increase acetylcholine levels. In doing so, it can precipitate a cholinergic crisis resulting in heart block and asystole. As a result, it is recommended to reserve physostigmine for life-threatening anticholinergic complications.

○   **What is the ferric chloride test and what toxic ingestion does it detect?**

Add a few drops of 10% ferric chloride solution to a few drops of urine. A purple color indicates presence of salicylic acid. Ketones or phenothiazine can lead to falsely positive results.

○   **What is the treatment for chloral hydrate overdose?**

Hemodialysis and/or charcoal hemoperfusion will clear the active metabolite, trichloroethanol.

○   **What are the common effects of barbiturate overdose?**

Hypothermia, hyperventilation, vasodilation with hypotension, and negative inotropic effect on the myocardium. Clear vesicles and bullae may also be seen.

○   **What is the pediatric dose of naloxone?**

0.01–0.8 mg/kg; may need to repeat.

○   **What is the antidote for magnesium sulfate overdose?**

Calcium gluconate infusion.

○   **What are the effects of using ketamine in a pediatric patient?**

The child's eyes will be wide open with a glassy stare. He or she will have nystagmus, hyperemic flush, and hypersalivation. There will also be a slight rise in the heart rate. A very rare complication of ketamine use is laryngospasm. Hallucinations are a common side effect in children older than 10 years; as a consequence, ketamine should be restricted to use only in patients younger than 10 years.

Note: Ketamine may also cause sympathetic stimulation, which increases intracranial pressure and may cause random movements of the head and extremities. Thus, it is not a good sedative for children going to CT scan.

○   **You are having a hard time remembering which anesthetics are amides and which anesthetics are esters. What is a fairly easy way of telling these two classifications apart?**

With the exception of the suffix -caine, the anesthetics only in the amide classification include the letter I.

Amides esters
Lidocaine (Xylocaine)
Bupivacaine (Marcaine)
Mepivacaine (Carbocaine)
Procaine (Novocain)
Cocaine
Tetracaine (Pontocaine)
Benzocaine

○   **Activated charcoal is not indicated for which types of overdose?**

Alcohol ingestion, electrolytes, heavy metals, lithium, hydrocarbons, and caustic ingestions.

○   **How should barbiturate poisoning be treated?**

Support, charcoal, alkalinization of the urine, charcoal hemoperfusion, or hemodialysis.

○   **A heroin addict presents with pulmonary edema. What is the best treatment?**

Naloxone, O_2, and ventilatory support (not diuretics).

○   **What alcohol poisoning is suggested by a plasma bicarbonate level of zero?**

Methanol. It also produces a large osmolar gap and a large anion gap. Methanol poisoning is treated with IV ethanol and hemodialysis.

○   **Positive birefringent calcium oxalate crystals in the urine are pathognomonic for poisoning with what substance?**

Ethylene glycol. The lethal dose of ethylene glycol is 100 mL.

○   **What are the signs and symptoms of ethylene glycol poisoning?**

Hallucinations, nystagmus, ataxia, papilledema, and a large anion gap.

○ **How should ethylene glycol poisoning be treated?**

This should be treated with gastric lavage, sodium bicarbonate, thiamine and pyridoxine, IV ethanol, and hemodialysis.

○ **A patient presents with ataxia, altered mental status, and sixth nerve palsy. What is your diagnosis?**

Wernicke encephalopathy.

○ **Alkalinization of urine will increase the excretion of which drugs?**

Cyclic antidepressants, salicylates, and long-acting barbiturates.

○ **What laboratory test can aid in the evaluation of a possible toxic iron ingestion?**

Total iron-binding capacity measured 3–5 hours after ingestion. If serum iron level is significantly less than the total iron-binding capacity, a toxic iron ingestion is less likely.

○ **What is the antidote for a toxic ingestion of iron?**

Deferoxamine chelates only free iron. It should be given if the iron level is greater than 350 μg/dL.

○ **Which type of hydrocarbons are most toxic?**

Substances with low viscosities (measured in Saybolt Seconds Universal (SSU)) are more toxic than compounds with high viscosities. Gasoline, kerosene, and paint thinner (all aliphatic hydrocarbons with SSUs < 60) are all more toxic than motor oil, tar, and petroleum jelly, which all have SSUs > 100.

Of the compounds with SSUs < 60, the most toxic are those that are not aliphatic, including benzene, toluene, xylene, and tetrachloroethylene.

○ **Where is the most reliable site for detecting central cyanosis?**

The tongue.

○ **What are two frequently observed organisms causing septic arthritis in drug addicts?**

Serratia and *Pseudomonas*. These are rare causes in nonaddicts.

○ **An alcoholic patient presents with complaints of abdominal pain and blurred vision. The patient is very photophobic, and blood gases reveal a metabolic acidosis. Diagnosis?**

Methanol poisoning. Patients may describe seeing something resembling a snowstorm.

○ **What is the lethal dose of methanol?**

30 mL. Formate levels in methanol poisoning are greatest in vitreous humor.

○ **What is clonidine mechanism of action?**

Clonidine is a centrally acting α-agonist. It leads to decreased sympathetic outflow and lowers catecholamine levels.

○   **What is a common complication of pancuronium?**

Tachycardia from its vagolytic action.

○   **Of the following anesthetics, which has the shortest duration of action—lidocaine, procaine, bupivacaine, or mepivacaine?**

Procaine.

○   **Hepatic failure is commonly associated with what anticonvulsant?**

Valproic acid.

○   **What are the end products of methanol, ethylene glycol, and isopropyl alcohol metabolism?**

Methanol: Formate

Ethylene glycol: Oxalate and formate

Isopropyl alcohol: Acetone

○   **Which type of alcohol ingestion is associated with hypocalcemia?**

Ethylene glycol.

○   **Which type of alcohol ingestion is associated with hemorrhagic pancreatitis?**

Methanol.

○   **Name some hydrocarbons that are considered to be the most toxic and have SSUs under 60:**

Aromatic hydrocarbons, halogenated hydrocarbons, mineral seal oil, kerosene, naphtha, turpentine, gasoline, and lighter fluid. Those considered less toxic (with SSUs over 100) include grease, diesel oil, mineral oil, petroleum jelly, paraffin wax, and tar.

○   **What drug is absolutely contraindicated when treating hydrocarbon poisoning?**

Epinephrine, as it sensitizes the myocardium and potentially leads to arrest.

○   **What drug is contraindicated in a glue-sniffing patient?**

Epinephrine. Like solvent abusers, these patients may be scared to death.

○   **What is a delayed complication of acid ingestion?**

Pyloric stricture.

○   **What is the difference between carbamates and organophosphates?**

Carbamates produce similar symptoms as organophosphates; however, the bonds in carbamate toxicity are reversible.

○ **A patient presents with miotic pupils, muscle fasciculations, diaphoresis, and diffuse oral and bronchial secretions. The patient has a garlic odor on his breath. What is your diagnosis?**

Organophosphate poisoning.

○ **What ECG changes may be associated with organophosphate poisoning?**

Prolongation of the QT interval, and ST and T wave abnormalities.

○ **What is the key laboratory finding in the diagnosis of organophosphate poisoning?**

Decreased RBC cholinesterase activity. The serum cholinesterase level (pseudocholinesterase) is more sensitive but less specific. RBC cholinesterase is regenerated slowly and can take months to approach normal levels.

○ **What is the treatment for organophosphate poisoning?**

Decontaminate, charcoal, atropine, and pralidoxime PRN.

○ **What signs and symptoms are expected after radiation exposures of 100 REM, 300 REM, 400 REM, and 2000 REM, less than 2 hours after exposure?**

100 REM: Nausea and vomiting
300 REM: Erythema
400 REM: Diarrhea
2000 REM: Seizures

○ **Psilocybin mushroom is associated with what?**

Hallucinations.

○ **How is pancuronium reversed?**

Atropine and neostigmine.

○ **Of patients who die from CA overdose, what percent are awake and alert at the time of first prehospital contact?**

25%.

○ **What are the contraindications to TAC?**

Mucus membranes, burns, and large abrasions. TAC used on the tongue and mucus membranes has led to status epilepticus and patient death.

○ **What is the most reliable test for determining the severity of radiation poisoning 48 hours after exposure?**

Absolute lymphocyte counts. Presence or absence of GI symptoms following near lethal doses is a good indicator of mortality.

Lead poisoning (clinical features):

Learning disability

Encephalopathy

Anemia

Developmental

Poisoning (contraindications for charcoal use):

Cyanide

Hydrocarbon

Acid/alkali

Relative small compounds

Charged (iron, heavy metals)

Organophosphate

Alcohol

Lithium

○ **Match the poison with the antidote:**

1. Acetaminophen	**a.** Deferoxamine
2. Anticholinergics	**b.** Digoxin antibody
3. Arsenic	**c.** Dimercaptosuccinic acid or penicillamine
4. Carbon monoxide	**d.** Acetylcysteine (Mucomyst)
5. Digoxin	**e.** Oxygen
6. Iron	**f.** Atropine
7. Lead	**g.** Physostigmine
8. Mercury	**h.** Calcium EDTA or penicillamine
9. Methanol or ethylene glycol	**i.** Naloxone (Narcan)
10. Narcotics	**j.** Ethanol
11. Organophosphates	**k.** Penicillamine

Answers: (1) d, (2) g, (3) k, (4) e, (5) b, (6) a, (7) h, (8) c, (9) j, (10) i, and (11) f.

○ **What percentage of poisons have specific antidotes?**

5%.

○ **What agent usually causes anaphylactic reactions?**

Contrast media. Other causative agents include NSAIDs, thiamine, and codeine. Conversely, parenteral penicillin and hymenoptera stings are the most common causes of anaphylactic reactions. Anaphylactic reactions are IgE-mediated reactions in previously sensitized people, while anaphylactoid reactions are due to direct release of mediators, including histamine and leukotriene.

○ **Describe the action and side effects of diazoxide:**

Action begins within 1–2 minutes and lasts up to 12 hours. Side effects may include nausea, vomiting, fluid retention, and hyperglycemia. Diazoxide is a direct arterial vasodilator. It is contraindicated in patients with aortic dissection or angina.

● ● ● **REFERENCES** ● ● ●

Brunton Laurence L, L. J. *Goodman and Gilman's the Pharmacological Basis of Therapeutics.* 11th ed. New York, NY: McGraw-Hill; 2006.

Fauci AS, Braunwald E, Kasper DL, et al., eds. *Harrison's Principles of Internal Medicine,* 17th ed. New York: McGraw-Hill; 2008.

McPhee Stephen J, PM. *Current Medical Diagnosis and Treatment 2009.* New York, NY: McGraw-Hill; 2009.

Stringer J. *Basic Concepts in Pharmacology—A Students Survival Guide.* 3rd ed. New York, NY: McGraw-Hill; 2005.

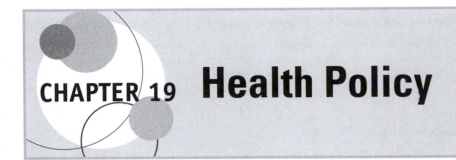

CHAPTER 19   Health Policy

Michael Dryer, PA-C, DrPH

○ **How do Health Maintenance Organizations (HMOs) differ from traditional indemnity health plans?**

In an HMO, the plan takes responsibility for the financing and delivery of health care services to a defined group of beneficiaries. The payment is usually prospective with a fixed payment for each person served regardless of the actual services provided (capitation). Indemnity insurance is based upon the fee-for-service model where the plans responsibility is limited to financial reimbursement and payment is made after services are rendered.

○ **In what sector of the U.S. health care system is the most money spent each year?**

Hospital care represents the largest component of health care spending representing about one-third of the costs of health care in the United States. Prescription drugs are the fastest growing expense consuming 11% of the nation's health care dollar.

○ **What is the largest source of funding for health care services in the United States?**

Private health insurance is the largest source financing 37% of all health care expenditures. Medicare and Medicaid rank second and third at 18% and 17%, respectively.

○ **What is the definition of physician group practice?**

The American Medical Association (AMA) defines group practice as three or more physicians organized to provide medical care, consultation, diagnosis, and/or treatment through the joint use of equipment and personnel with the practice income distributed utilizing a predetermined methodology.

○ **Which component of Medicare is mandatory for all enrollees?**

Part A is provided to all Medicare enrollees. It covers hospital care, home health care, hospice care, and limited care in skilled nursing facilities. Medicare Parts B, C, and D are all optional.

○ **What are the key elements of financial success for a primary care provider working with patients enrolled in a managed care plan?**

Avoid unnecessary hospitalizations; keep patients out of the emergency department for services that can be rendered in the office and limit referral to specialists. These are all high cost services that can impact withhold and bonus payments from managed care plans.

O   **What are the differences between community-rated health insurance plans and experience-rated plans?**

In community-rated health plans, the premium is based upon utilization in a defined geographic area without regard to age, gender, occupation or health status. In essence, healthy people subsidize the costs for the unhealthy, which leads to adverse selection. In experience-rated health plans, the premium is based upon demographic characteristics, occupation, and/or the actual experience of the group.

O   **Who is eligible for coverage under the Medicare Program?**

U.S. citizens or permanent residents older than 65 years who have paid into Social Security system for 10 or more years and those eligible for benefits from the Railroad Retirement Board are eligible for Medicare coverage. In 1974, individuals who were disabled were added to the eligibility list and in 1978 individuals with end stage renal disease were included.

O   **What services are covered under Medicare Part B?**

Medicare Part B Supplemental Medical Insurance covers Physician/Physician Assistant services, outpatient care, and durable medical equipment (DME).

O   **Who funds Medicaid Programs?**

While individual states administer their own Medicaid programs, the federal government pays between 50% and 76% of the costs with larger contributions going to states with lower per capita incomes.

O   **How good are the health outcomes for Medicaid recipients?**

There is general agreement that health outcomes for Medicaid recipients lag behind those for the privately insured. This gap is due in large part to the lack of access to care. Comparisons between Medicaid coverage and the uninsured are not quite as definitive. Studies have shown the Medicaid recipients fare somewhat better than the uninsured for some conditions; however, in many instances the health outcomes are as poor as those without insurance.

O   **What is the impact of not having health insurance?**

It is estimated that in 2008, 47 million Americans did not have health insurance. People who lack health insurance delay treatment for care and have worse health outcomes than people who are insured. The uninsured also have a higher overall mortality rate. In 2004, the Institute of Medicine estimated that 18,000 deaths in the United States could be attributed to the lack of health insurance.

O   **How does gender impact health care?**

According to the Agency for Healthcare Research and Quality (AHRQ), there are significant disparities between the care received by men and women in the United States. In a 2004 study, AHRQ found that women received better care than men for 18% of measures, worse care for 22%, and comparable care for 59%. The study also showed that women tend to receive better preventive care for cancer and cardiovascular disease than men, while men tend to receive better treatment for end stage renal disease and heart disease.

O   **How much does the United States spend on health care each year?**

Total U.S. health care expenditures reached $2.2 trillion in 2007; this translates to $7,421 per person or 16.2% of the nation's Gross Domestic Product. This represents nearly half of the $4.7 trillion that the World Health Organization estimates was spent worldwide on health care.

○   **What is the difference between a medical error and an adverse event?**

According to the Institute of Medicine, an error is the failure of a planned action to be completed as intended or the use of a wrong plan to complete an aim. An adverse event is an injury caused by medical management rather than the underlying condition of the patient.

○   **What are the key elements that define primary care?**

In 1992, Barbara Starfield identified four elements that help delineate the breadth and depth of primary care. First, is that primary care is the point of first contact for a patient. It is the entry point into the health care system. The second element is coordination of care. In primary care, the practitioner must coordinate and integrate the services provided by other members of the health care system. This is closely aligned with the gatekeeper function of the primary care provider where they are expected to control referrals for specialist and diagnostic services. The third element is comprehensiveness. Primary care addresses the routine medical needs of a population. It is centered on the patient rather than a disease or body system. The fourth element is longitudinality, which refers to the management of the health care needs of a patient over an extended period of time. This is in contrast to episodic care provided by emergency departments and urgent care centers.

○   **Is there a shortage of physicians in the United States?**

There are approximately 283 physicians per 100,000 population in the United States. The Department of Health and Human Services projects that number will increase to 313 per 100,000 population by 2020. While this increase suggests an improvement in physician supply, it does not reflect the impact of growing demand for medical services. The increase in demand is related to the aging of the population, the feminization of the physician workforce and the expansion of services to the 47 million Americans currently without health insurance. Current forecasts suggest that there will be a physician shortage for the foreseeable future with the greatest shortfall occurring in primary care.

○   **Are hospital emergency departments required to treat all patients even if they do not have health insurance?**

The Emergency Medical Treatment and Labor Act of 1986 (EMTLA), also known as the Antidumping Act, requires that a hospital emergency department provide an appropriate medical screening examination within the capability of the hospital, to determine whether or not an emergency medical condition or active labor exists. They must also provide necessary stabilizing treatment and admission if necessary regardless of the patient's ability to pay. Failure to meet comply with this federal statue can lead to penalties of up to $50,000 per incident.

○   **Who is eligible for hospice care?**

Hospice services are considered to be palliative care with an emphasis on pain management and psychosocial and spiritual support. To be eligible for hospice services, patients must be terminally ill with a life expectancy of 6 months or less.

○   **What is the difference between a copay and a deductible?**

Copays and deductibles are both cost-sharing mechanisms designed to reduce unnecessary utilization of health care services. A copayment is a set dollar amount or a percentage of a bill for services that is paid by the enrollee in conjunction with the benefits paid by a health plan. A deductible is an amount of money that must be paid out of pocket before insurance benefits are paid by a health plan.

○   **What proportion of physicians in the United States are International Medical Graduates?**

As of 2005, approximately one in four physicians in the United States was an International Medical Graduate (IMG). Their numbers have grown in response to a need to fill geographic and specialty gaps. International Medical Graduates have also helped hospitals fill vacant residency slots, particularly in those hospitals with a large proportion of indigent patients.

○ **Why does the United States rank poorly in life expectancy and infant mortality compared to other developed nations?**

According to the Central Intelligence Agency Fact Book, the United States ranks 50th among nations for life expectancy and 180th for infant mortality out of the 224 nations studied. The main reason for this poor performance is the disparity in access to care most evident in the fact that there are 47 million Americans without health insurance.

○ **What is the ratio of specialist physicians to primary care physicians?**

The ratio of specialist physicians to primary care physicians is 60:40. This proportion is fairly unique to the United States. In most other countries, there are far more primary care physicians than specialists. Medical students gravitate to the specialty areas due to the prestige and higher levels of compensation associated with specialty practice.

○ **What is the largest component of the health care workforce?**

The largest component of the health care workforce is registered nurses. There are 2.4 million registered nurses and 531,000 licensed practical nurses in the United States.

○ **What are diagnosis related groups (DRGs)?**

Diagnosis related groups is a prospective payment system established by the federal government in 1983 to control hospital costs. The system assigns a numeric value to an acute care inpatient hospital episode of care. The patient's diagnosis determines how much a hospital is paid, not the number of inpatient days or the procedures performed in the hospital. This provides financial incentives for hospitals to discharge patients as early as possible.

○ **How does Medicare's "incident to" provision impact physician assistants?**

Physician assistants providing outpatient services may bill under Medicare's "incident to" provisions, if Medicare billing guidelines are met. This allows for payment at 100% of the physician's Medicare fee schedule instead of the standard 85% normally paid for PA services.

○ **What are the defining features of public health care as compared to personal health care?**

Personal health care focuses on the health care needs of an individual. The distinguishing feature of public health care is its central focus on the health of a population. The population-based approach uses a defined population as the organizing principle for determining interventions for the prevention and treatment of disease. The population can be any type or size of community; from an entire nation to a panel of patients in a managed care plan.

○ **Must physician assistants accept Medicare assignment?**

When a provider accepts Medicare assignment, they agree to be paid by Medicare, to charge only the amount Medicare approves for their service, and to only charge the patient or their insurance plan the Medicare deductible or coinsurance amount. If they provide a Medicare covered service physician assistants must accept assignment.

○ **What is Medigap insurance?**

On average, Medicare covers less than half of a beneficiary's total annual health care costs. To minimize their out of pocket expenses, Medicare beneficiaries can purchase a supplemental policy from an insurance company. This additional policy is known as Medigap insurance.

○ **Can providers waive Medicare copayments and deductibles?**

Routine waiver of Medicare deductibles and copayments by providers is unlawful because it may result in false claims, violations of the anti-kickback statute, and excessive utilization of services paid for by Medicare. Providers may forgive the copayment if a patient demonstrates a financial hardship. This hardship exception, however, cannot be used routinely; it should be used only occasionally to address the special financial needs of a particular patient. Except in such special cases, the provider must make a good faith effort to collect deductibles and copayments. Penalties for violating this regulation can include imprisonment, criminal fines, civil damages, and forfeitures.

• • • REFERENCES • • •

Shi L, Singh D. *Delivering Health Care in America; A Systems Approach*. 4th ed. Sudbury, MA: Jones and Bartlett; 2008.

Williams SJ, Torrens PR. *Introduction to Health Services*. 7th ed. Clifton Park, NY: Delmar; 2008.

Sultz HA, Young KM. 2009. *Health Care USA; Understanding Its Organization and Delivery*. Sudbury, MA: Jones and Bartlett; 2009.

Bodenheimer TS, Grumbach K. 2009. *Understanding Health Policy; A Clinical Approach*. 5th ed. New York, NY: McGraw-Hill; 2009.

Women's Healthcare in the United States; Selected Findings From the 2004 National Healthcare Quality and Disparities Reports, Agency for Health care Research and Quality.

Historical health care expenditure data. Centers for Medicare & Medicaid Services. http://www.cms.hhs.gov/NationalHealthExpend Data/02_NationalHealthAccountsHistorical.asp#TopOfPage

To Err is Human; Building a Safer Health Care System. Institute of Medicine, National Academy Press; 2000.

Starfield B. *Primary Care: Concept, Evaluation, and Policy*. New York, NY: Oxford University Press, 1992.

Lee P, Estes C. *The Nation's Health*. Sudbury MA: Jones and Bartlett; 2003.

U.S. Census Bureau; Facts for Features. http://www.census.gov/PressRelease/www/releases/archives/facts_for_features_special_editions/004491.html

American Academy of Physician Assistant, Third party reimbursement. Issue brief. http://www.aapa.org/images/stories/Advocacy-issue-briefs/3rdParty_transitional_6-09.pdf.

Williams SJ, Torrens PR. *Introduction to Health Services*. 7th ed. Clifton Park, NY: Delmar; 2008.

Medicare.gov

Department of Health and Human Services, Office of Inspector General, Special Fraud Alert: Routine Waiver of Copayments or Deductibles Under Medicare Part B, May 1991.